Newborn Respiratory Care

Newborn Respiratory Care

Edited by

MARVIN D. LOUGH, R.R.T.

*Technical Director of Pediatric Respiratory Therapy
and Pulmonary Function,
Rainbow Babies & Childrens Hospital;
Clinical Instructor, School of Respiratory Therapy,
Cuyahoga Community College, Cleveland, Ohio*

THOMAS J. WILLIAMS, B.S., R.R.T.

*Clinical Specialist, Bourns Medical Systems, Inc.,
Riverside, California*

JOHN E. RAWSON, M.D.

*Clinical Associate Professor, Department of Pediatrics,
University of Mississippi;
Chief of Newborn Section, Heines General Hospital, Jackson, Mississippi;
Attending Neonatologist, University of Mississippi Hospitals*

YEAR BOOK MEDICAL PUBLISHERS, INC.
CHICAGO • LONDON

Library of Congress Cataloging in Publication Data

Main entry under title:
Newborn respiratory care.

Includes index.
1. Respiratory insufficiency in children. 2. Infants
(Newborn) – Diseases. 3. Inhalation therapy for children.
4. Neonatal intensive care. I. Lough, Marvin D.
II. Williams, Thomas J. III. Rawson, John E.
[DNLM: 1. Respiratory tract diseases – In infancy and
childhood. 2. Infant, Newborn, Diseases – Therapy.
3. Respiratory tract diseases – Therapy. WS280 L887n]
ISBN O-8151-5635-9

*This book is dedicated
to our families, who greatly
supported our efforts:*

KATHY, BRAD, GREG and TODD LOUGH

NANCY and TOM WILLIAMS

MARY, KATHERINE and WIN RAWSON

Contributors

BERNARD BLUMENTHAL, M.D., Assistant Professor of Radiology, University of Mississippi Medical Center, Jackson, Mississippi

STEPHEN J. BOROS, M.D., Assistant Professor, Department of Pediatrics, University of Minnesota; Director of Newborn Medicine, St. Paul Children's Hospital, St. Paul, Minnesota

JANE H. DAVIS, A.S.S.S., A.C.S.W., Department of Social Work Services, Kennedy Memorial Hospital for Children, Boston, Massachusetts

DONNA deMONTERICE, R.N., M.N., Nurse Clinician, Neonatology; Assistant Clinical Professor of Pediatric Nursing, Case Western Reserve University and Rainbow Babies & Childrens Hospital, Cleveland, Ohio

MICHAEL GALGOCZY, M.S., C.R.T.T., Pediatric Respiratory Therapy, Rainbow Babies & Childrens Hospital, Cleveland, Ohio

ROSANNE GUGINO-TOUFEXIS, R.N., M.S., Regional Education Coordinator, Cleveland Regional Perinatal Network, Cleveland, Ohio

MARVIN D. LOUGH, R.R.T., Technical Director of Pediatric Respiratory Therapy and Pulmonary Function, Rainbow Babies & Childrens Hospital; Clinical Instructor, School of Respiratory Therapy, Cuyahoga Community College, Cleveland, Ohio

GERARD W. OSTHEIMER, M.D., Assistant Professor of Anaesthesia, Harvard Medical School, Anesthesiologist, Boston Hospital for Women, Boston, Massachusetts

BRUCE R. PARKS, JR., PH.D., Assistant Professor of Pediatrics; Instructor in Pharmacology, University of Mississippi Medical Center, Jackson, Mississippi

JOHN E. RAWSON, M.D., Clinical Associate Professor, Department of Pediatrics, University of Mississippi; Chief of Newborn Section, Heines General Hospital, Jackson, Mississippi; Attending Neonatologist, University of Mississippi Hospitals

BRADFORD RICHMOND, M.S., C.R.T.T., Pediatric Respiratory Therapy, Rainbow Babies & Childrens Hospital, Cleveland, Ohio

BARBARA SCHUCHARDT, R.R.T., Pediatric Respiratory Therapy, Rainbow Babies & Childrens Hospital, Cleveland, Ohio

THOMAS J. WILLIAMS, B.S., R.R.T., Clinical Specialist, Bourns Medical Systems, Inc., Riverside, California

Preface

THIS BOOK was conceived as part of an effort to assist students and postgraduate health personnel, including respiratory therapists, nurses and physicians interested in the care of ill newborn infants. The text represents a compilation of the experience of many dedicated individuals with a primary concern for the health care of the newborn infant. In the past decade, the field of neonatology has grown tremendously and texts have been published that deal with the over-all care of the newborn infant. We will not attempt to duplicate the already-existing texts but instead place greater emphasis on newborn respiratory care at the clinical level. Attempts have been made to provide a learning venture from the time of conception through the newborn period. The information provided on the development of the cardiorespiratory system as related to health and disease has been brought together in a concise and useful manner. Methodology and techniques for newborn respiratory care have been provided from the time of delivery through the intensive care period. Since continuous positive airway pressure and mechanical ventilation play such an important role in newborn respiratory care, we have devoted separate chapters to each. The section dealing with disease is oriented to a description of those problems requiring respiratory care. Radiologic findings and effects of drugs are detailed as they relate to infants. The nursing chapter provides comprehensive coverage of those nursing procedures that are related to pulmonary care. The chapter on care of the parents details the psychologic problems associated with having an ill infant.

The information provided in this text is based on the broad experience of many health care professions. It is clear that the perinatal mortality rate over the past 25 years has declined but its associated problems are far from solved. It is our hope that the knowledge and experience detailed in this text will help to improve the morbidity so that the surviving infants can lead productive lives.

We wish to acknowledge the invaluable assistance of Barbara Schiffhauer, who typed the manuscript, and Angel Martinez for his help with the illustrations.

We especially wish to thank all members of our families for their patience and understanding.

MARVIN D. LOUGH
THOMAS J. WILLIAMS
JOHN E. RAWSON

Introduction

"Everything ought to be done to ensure that an infant be born at term, well-developed, and in a healthy condition. But in spite of every care, infants are born prematurely . . . ." — PIERRE BUDIN, *The Nursling*, 1907

OUR CHILDREN are our future. The care of children has always been a major activity of mankind. The modern era in special care for premature infants began in Paris, in 1892, when Dr. Pierre Budin became interested in the congenitally feeble and weakling infant. He opened his consultation service for nurslings at the Charity Hospital in that year and published his book *The Nursling* in 1907. Martin Cooney, one of Doctor Budin's students, recognized the public's interest in prematurely born infants and established exhibits to which he charged admission. One of his first exhibits was at the Chicago Exposition in 1914.

The shift of childbirth from the home, with lay-trained assistants, to the hospital, with well-trained health specialists, has made birth a medical rather than a family-centered event. Before the antibiotic era of the 1940s, hospitals enforced stringent controls on the patient, health care personnel and visitors to the maternity area in hopes of preventing the spread of infection. This resulted in the "hands off" concept, the practice of isolating the infant from its parents and the total exclusion of visitors, for sterility's sake alone. The safeguards provided by a hospital environment were soon accepted, and the popularity of hospital births soared.

The establishment of neonatal intensive care units, in the late 1960s, has been one of the most significant contributions toward reduction of perinatal mortality. One of the most common problems in the neonatal intensive care unit today, and the major cause of mortality, occurring in 0.5–1.0% of all deliveries, is hyaline membrane disease. This disease is characterized by increased work of respiration and cyanosis. Most of the early research was empirical and designed to decrease cyanosis and improve ventilation. Not all of these efforts have been without risk. The use of oxygen had a beneficial effect but was later shown to contribute to retrolental fibroplasia and blindness. When this association was recognized, it led to a severe curtailment in the use of oxygen. The result was a reduction in the incidence of retrolental fibroplasia and blindness but an increase in the number of premature infants who were neurologically damaged. Although the use of oxygen has been the most publicized problem associated with serious complications in the search for ways of improving the outcome of premature infants, many of the new techniques have introduced new complications or diseases.

Mechanical ventilation of newborns was first introduced as a resuscitative technique in the delivery room for infants who failed to quickly establish normal respiration. The earlier devices were crude and suitable only for short-term use. In the 1960s, infants were placed on scaled-down negative-pressure ventilators or adult positive-pressure ventilators modified for the newborn. In the 1970s, newborn ventilation gradually became an acceptable medical practice outside the research institution. This was possibly because of the development of reliable neonatal ventilators and the availability of equipment for microsample blood gas analysis. The technologic advances in mechanical ventilation, patient monitoring and laboratory support equipment have provided the tools for respiratory care of newborn infants.

The requirements for an effective neonatal intensive care unit are so stringent in terms of clinical equipment, laboratory equipment, space and trained personnel that only a select few hospitals can meet the financial obligation. To deal with this problem, a national policy on regionalization of perinatal care has been developed by the American Medical Association, the American College of Obstetrics and Gynecology, the American Academy of Pediatrics and the American Academy of Family Physicians. These sponsoring organizations recommended that the nation be divided into regions with 12,000–14,000 deliveries per year. Hospitals in each region are to be divided into 3 classes; in each area there would be one institution that would accept the responsibility for coordinating perinatal health care activities. This would include providing specialized facilities for high-risk obstetric and newborn patients, organizing referral and transporting systems in other regions and coordinating both public and professional education for perinatal care in their region.

The federal government has recognized this concept as policy and has classified hospitals in the following manner: Level 1 (primary care) hospitals will provide service primarily for uncomplicated maternal and neonatal patients. These units exist primarily because of geographic or cultural situations that limit access to units with greater care and capabilities. Level 2 (secondary care) facilities are those hospitals that have larger maternity and newborn services. In addition to providing a full range of maternal and newborn services for perinatal patients who have no complications, they will also provide services for some more complicated obstetric and neonatal problems that fall within their capabilities. These capabilities will depend on the resources available. Level 3 (tertiary care) facilities, in addition to the resources and capabilities of a Level 2 unit, are able to provide a full range of services for all serious maternal illnesses and newborn intensive care. Established arrangements should be provided for early access of high-risk pregnant women and prompt referral among levels of care as appropriate.

The initial efforts of implementing this plan have required local adaptation to special needs in each location. The requirement of maintaining 1500 deliveries per year to be classified as a Level 2 center has posed problems in many states with low populations. Each state now has a health service area council and/or state health planning council with the authority to issue a "certificate of need" for all new services. The guidelines set forth by these councils are serving as the basis for decisions on the need for new perinatal services.

Perinatal health care is rapidly changing with the advent of new technologies, new approaches to patients, new funding mechanisms and the organization of new services. The successful delivery of high-quality care to perinatal patients requires not only excellence from physicians, therapists, nurses and other health professionals as individuals but also a mechanism or system of organization that permits them to function as a cohesive and well-coordinated team. This book focuses primarily on the respiratory complications of the newborn infant and discusses medical, technical and social issues related to the care delivered by this invaluable team.

JOHN E. RAWSON

Contents

1 / Development of the Cardiorespiratory System

BRADFORD RICHMOND, M.S., C.R.T.T.

AND

MICHAEL GALGOCZY, M.S., C.R.T.T.

AN UNDERSTANDING of the developmental aspects of the cardiovascular and respiratory systems is crucial to the proper management of postpartum complications that occur in infants involving these organ systems. The selection of supportive modes of therapy, as well as the type of equipment used, may be dependent on the gestational age of the fetus. This point is especially important when considering cardiorespiratory support. The lungs require a greater amount of time to develop sufficiently to support life than does the cardiovascular system. Knowledge of the embryologic origins of the heart is essential in order to understand the various abnormalities that are associated with this organ system. Knowledge of fetal circulation and the transition of circulation that occurs pre- to postpartum is important to facilitate treatment of an infant in distress. Comprehension of newborn developmental aspects of the unborn infant may be fully appreciated only after clinical exposure to a newborn suffering from a respiratory and/or cardiac problem.

INTRODUCTORY CONCEPTS

Like all multicellular species, humans have a limited life span and thus require some mechanism to perpetuate and produce successive generations of their species. This mechanism is called reproduction, which is effected by a complicated process that requires the presence of two sexes, male and female, each of which contributes specialized sex cells called gametes. The organs that produce the gametes are known as the gonads, or primary sex organs. Gonads of the male are the testes, which produce gametes called spermatozoa or sperm. The female gonads are the ovaries, which produce ova or eggs.

1

The gametes are produced by their respective gonads through a series of mitotic (mitosis) and meiotic (meiosis) events that occur in gametogenesis or the formation and maturation of germ cells. In the male this process is referred to as spermatogenesis, and in females it is called oogenesis. Mitosis is the process of cell division in which each chromosome, that is, the hereditary material composed of strands of deoxyribonucleic acid (DNA) responsible for an individual's genetic make-up, is duplicated and passed on to daughter cells. Thus, mitosis is extremely important in higher forms of life. It ensures that each daughter cell will be genetically alike to its parent cell and, therefore, compatible with every other cell in the individual's body. Mitosis occurs primarily in the somite or body cells. Meiosis is the specialized form of cell division that seems to occur only in the germ cells (i.e., gametes), resulting in the formation of daughter cells that contain a haploid number of chromosomes. The haploid number of chromosomes is one-half the normal complement of chromosomes that normally are present in an organism. In humans, the haploid number is 23 as opposed to the diploid number of chromosomes, 46, that results from mitosis of the somatic cells.

In addition to the primary sex organs, each sex usually is characterized by the presence of accessory sex organs or secondary sex characteristics. These are required to transmit the gametes that have been generated by the gonads. In the male, the accessory sex organs include the penis, which enables the sperm cells to be deposited in the female genital tract. The accessory sex organs in the female include the vagina, which is a special receptacle for the sperm cells, and the uterus, for reception and incubation of the zygote, which will be discussed below.

Development of an organism begins with fertilization. A sperm unites with an oocyte (egg) to form a zygote (from the Greek *zygōtos*, meaning "yoked"), which requires approximately 24 hours. Fertilization (stage 1 of development) of the ovum occurs in the ampulla portion of the oviduct. An ovum contains a half set of 23 chromosomes with a nutrient supply (the yolk), which is required for the initial developmental activity. The fertilizing sperm donates the other 23 chromosomes for a complete set of genes. In general, only one sperm cell penetrates the ovum. Figure 1–1 illustrates the penetration of the oocyte by the sperm and the procession of events that lead to the formation of the zygote once penetration has occurred. The sex of the embryo is determined at the time of fertilization by the kind of sperm that fertilizes the oocyte. Human cells contain 46 chromosomes; 22 pairs of these chromosomes are somatic, whereas the twenty-third pair

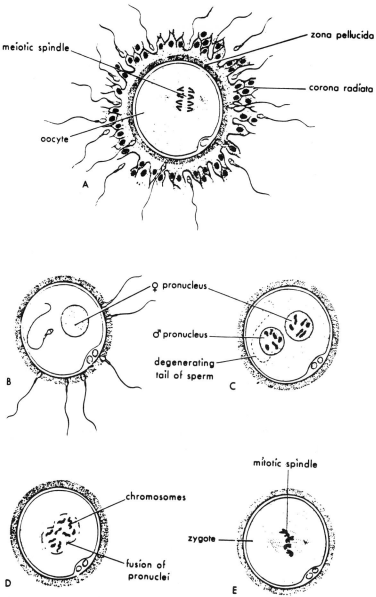

Fig. 1–1. — Fertilization, the process of sperm and egg uniting to establish a full complement of chromosomes (46) forming a zygote (not all chromosomes are shown). **A,** secondary oocyte about to be fertilized; **B,** sperm entered oocyte; **C,** male pronucleus forms containing chromosomes of sperm; **D,** pronuclei of male and female fuse; **E,** zygote with full chromosome complement is formed. (From Moore, K. L.: *The Developing Human* [2d ed.; Philadelphia: W. B. Saunders Company, 1977]. Reprinted by permission.)

are the sex chromosomes. Male sperm cells contain two types of sex chromosomes: an X and a Y chromosome. Fertilization of the ovum, which contains only an X chromosome, by an X-bearing sperm results in an XX zygote, which develops into a female. Fertilization by a Y sperm produces an XY zygote, which develops into a male. Within 3–5 days, the zygote moves down the oviduct and attaches to the wall of the uterus.

Fertilization initiates development of the organism by stimulating the zygote to undergo a series of rapid mitotic cell divisions called cleavage. Initial cleavage of the zygote begins within a few hours after fertilization occurs. It is preceded by a burst of biochemical activity; that is, the activation of various enzyme systems, DNA synthesis and protein biosynthesis. This biochemical activity prepares the cell for further stages of cleavage that result in the formation of a multicellular organism. About 30 hours after fertilization, the zygote divides into two daughter cells called blastomeres, which are duplicate and equal in size (stage 2 of development). After formation of the blastomere, further divisions follow rapidly, producing 4-cell, 8-cell and 16-cell stages. Each progressive stage of cleavage forms progressively smaller blastomeres. The 16-cell stage of the blastomere is called a morula and develops after about 3 days postfertilization. As the morula forms, it begins to enter the uterus. Figure 1–2 illustrates the successive stages following the initial cleavage to the development of the morula.

In approximately 4 days (stage 3), fluid from the uterine cavity flows into the morula and occupies the intercellular spaces. As the fluid volume increases in the morula, it causes a separation of the cells, which now range in number from 50 to 200, into two distinct parts. The first group of cells is centrally located in the morula and is called the inner cell mass (or embryoblast), which gives rise to the embryo, the amnion and the yolk sac. The other cell mass forms the outer layer of the morula, called the trophoblast, which will develop into part of the placenta and the chorion. At this point, the yolk from the original ovum is the main nutrient source for the cells. After a brief time lapse, the fluid-filled spaces fuse to form a single, large space known as the blastocyst cavity. This phase converts the morula into a blastocyst. The inner cell mass projects into the blastocyst cavity and the trophoblast forms the wall of the blastocyst. The blastocyst lies free in the uterine secretions for approximately 2 days, then the zona pellucida (the noncellular, secreted layer surrounding the ovum) degenerates and disappears, heralding the start of the implantation stage (Fig. 1–3).

In order for further development of the embryo to occur, implantation of the blastocyst in the uterine wall is essential. During the fifth

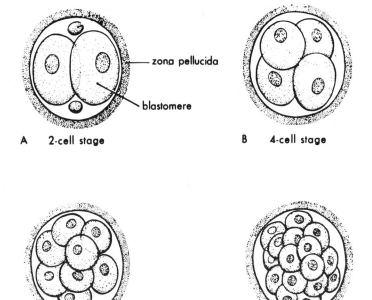

A 2-cell stage B 4-cell stage

C 8-cell stage D morula

Fig. 1–2.—Illustrations of cleavage of the zygote to morula stage. (From Moore, K. L.: *The Developing Human* [2d ed.; Philadelphia: W. B. Saunders Company, 1977]. Reprinted by permission.)

Fig. 1–3.—Formation of blastocyst through further cleavage and formation of a cavity. (From Moore, K. L.: *The Developing Human* [2d ed.; Philadelphia: W. B. Saunders Company, 1977]. Reprinted by permission.)

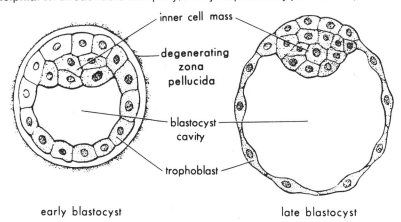

early blastocyst late blastocyst

and sixth days (stage 4 of development), the blastocyst attaches to the endometrial epithelium, which is shortly thereafter invaded, along with the endometrial stroma, by trophoblastic cells through finger-like processes. By the end of the first week, the blastocyst is superficially implanted in the endometrium. On implantation, the chorionic membrane, amniotic membrane and placenta develop. The trophoblast begins to proliferate. The blastocyst usually implants in the upper part of the uterus (intrauterine site). However, ectopic or extrauterine implantation (i.e., outside the uterus) does occur, with ectopic tubal pregnancy (fallopian tube) being the most common.

The blastula stage of development is succeeded by the gastrulation stage (Fig. 1–4), which results from the changes in position and displacements of the various presumptive regions of the blastula. It is in this stage that rearrangement of cells establishes the three primary germ layers, which are formed by the end of the third week of development, bringing the presumptive organs of the embryo into the positions in which they will undergo further development. The first germ layer formed is the endoderm. By the end of stage 6 (about 16 days), the ectoderm (the second germ layer) and the mesoderm (the third germ layer) are developed, which results in the formation of the trilaminar embryo giving rise to all tissues and organs of the embryo. Organs develop (a process referred to as organogenesis) from the different cell layers, and the main derivatives from the germ layers include the following: ectodermal organs are the central (brain and spinal cord) and peripheral nervous systems, the sensory epithelia of the eyes, ears and nose, the epidermis and its appendages; mesodermal organs are connective tissue, cartilage, bone, striated and smooth muscle, the urinary tract, the heart, blood and lymph vessels with their cells and reproductive organs; endodermally derived organs are the gastrointestinal tract, mouth and pharynx region, lungs, liver and pancreas.

The gastrula stage is followed by one in which the neural plate and the axial embryonic structures are elaborated. This stage is called neurulation (neurula), which begins at about 20 days (stage 9), when the mesoderm begins to divide into paired cuboidal bodies called somites (or body), and is known as the somite period. By the end of this stage of development, the general pattern of the embryo is well established.

Intrauterine life consists of two phases. Up to the first trimester, that is, the first 3 months of pregnancy, the embryonic or embryo phase exists. From conception until the end of the first trimester, organogenesis occurs. Further development, in both refinement and size of

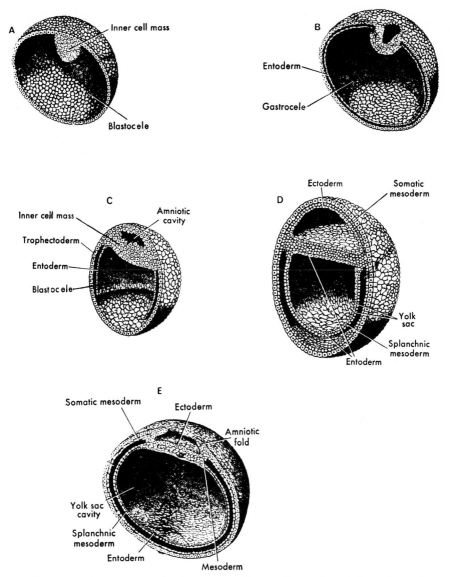

Fig. 1–4. — Gastrulation in the mammalian embryo. **A** and **B,** embryonic knob forms from the inner cell mass; **C,** later it will form the embryonic shield; **D,** delamination of the inner cell mass forms the amniotic cavity; **E,** yolk sac formation occurs. (Modified from Huettner, A. F.: *Fundamentals of Comparative Embryology of the Vertebrates* [Toronto: The Macmillan Company, 1949].)

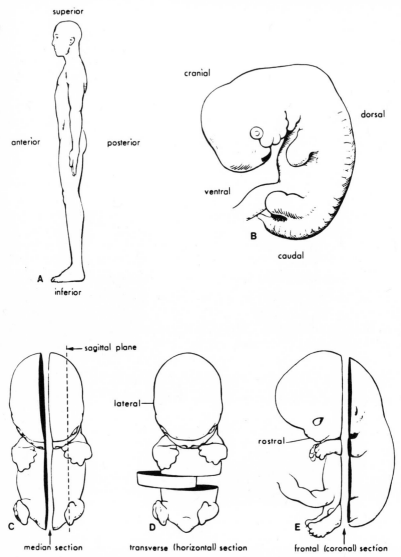

Fig. 1–5.—Anatomic positions of the body. **A,** lateral view of an adult human; **B,** lateral view of embryo at 5 weeks; **C** and **D,** ventral view of embryo at 6 weeks; **E,** lateral view of embryo at 7 weeks. (From Moore, K. L.: *The Developing Human* [2d ed.; Philadelphia: W. B. Saunders Company, 1977]. Reprinted by permission.)

organs plus general growth, takes place in the fetal phase, which is the beginning of the fourth month until delivery occurs.

Before proceeding with the developmental aspects of the respiratory and cardiovascular systems, it would be helpful to present some terms that are used frequently in descriptive anatomy and embryology. The anatomic position (i.e., the body is erect, with the arms by the sides and the palms directed forward) is used to describe the adult (Fig. 1–5). The terms anterior or ventral and posterior or dorsal are used to describe the front and back of the body; in embryos, ventral and dorsal are used. Superior and inferior are used to indicate the relative levels of different structures. In embryos, cranial (cephalic) and caudal (tail end) commonly are used to describe relationships of the head and tail ends, respectively. Rostral is used to indicate the relationships of structures to the nose.

The median plane is a vertical plane passing through the center of the body that divides the body into right and left halves. A sagittal plane is any plane passing through the body parallel to the median plane. A frontal plane is a vertical plane that intersects the median plane at right angles, whereas a transverse or horizontal plane is any plane that is at right angles to both the median and frontal planes. Sections through the embryo play an important role in descriptive embryology. A median section is one cut through the median plane; sagittal sections are longitudinal sections parallel to the median plane but

TABLE 1–1.—SUMMARY OF EARLY EMBRYOLOGIC GROWTH

STAGE* OF DEVELOPMENT	APPROXIMATE TIME OF OCCURRENCE	DEVELOPMENTAL EVENT
1	First day	Passage of sperm through the corona radiata and penetration of the zona pellucida
2	About 30 hours after fertilization to about 4 days	Blastomere formation with resulting morula development
3	About 4 days	Trophoblast and blastocyst formation
4	5–6 days	Blastocyst attachment to the endometrial epithelium
5	7–12 days	Invasion of the endometrium Endoderm formation
6	15–21 days	Ectoderm, endoderm and mesoderm formation

*Stage is the term used to denote the period or level of development of an organism.

not through it. Transverse or cross sections are through the transverse plane, and oblique sections are slanted or inclined.

In summary, development of the embryo begins with the union of the sperm and egg, which results in the formation of a zygote. Within a day or so, cleavage of the zygote begins, which results in the formation of the morula and passage of the fertilized egg into the uterus. Once in the uterus, the blastocyst begins the series of steps that lead to the implantation of the developing egg into the endometrial epithelium of the uterine wall. Following the blastula stage, the embryo enters the gastrula phase of development. It is in this stage where development of the three primary germ layers occurs. These germinal layers — endoderm, mesoderm and ectoderm — give rise to all tissues and organs of the embryo. Gastrulation is succeeded by the neurula stage, in which the general pattern of the embryo has been determined. Table 1–1 presents a brief summary of events in the early development of the embryo.

DEVELOPMENT OF THE RESPIRATORY TRACT

In humans, completion of the embryonic respiratory system occurs late in fetal life and, as a result, the lung is considered a nonfunctional organ until near term. Thus, in utero, the respiratory system develops independently of the functional demands of the growing embryo and fetus. Physiologic lung activity prior to birth is limited to some respiratory movements, growth and secretion of various substances during specific times in development. The system, therefore, must be so developed that the lung is capable of immediate function at birth. At birth, the fetus is expelled from its aquatic surroundings and the partially collapsed, fluid-filled lung must be able to adapt immediately to air-breathing, thus facilitating oxygen and carbon dioxide diffusion, which provides for continuation of life for the neonate. The transition to an air-breathing organism is extremely hazardous to the fetus. The chief cause of perinatal death in the period from about 26 weeks after fertilization to about 4 weeks after birth is failure of the respiratory system to function adequately.

The Upper Respiratory Tract

In the 4th week of gestation, the buccopharyngeal (oropharyngeal) membrane disintegrates, allowing communication between the primitive oral cavity of the ectoderm and the endoderm of the foregut. The primitive nasal cavities (nasal sacs) originate in the 4th week as two ectodermal thickenings (Fig. 1–6). Mesenchymal cells, which will become the nasal septum and primary palate, separate the ectodermal

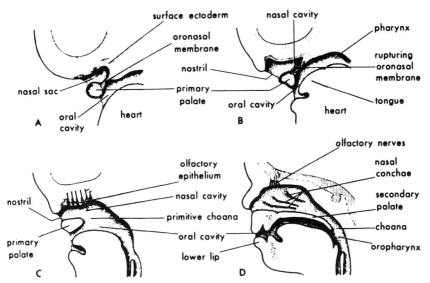

Fig. 1–6. – Development of the nose. **A,** buccopharyngeal membrane separating nasal sac and oral cavity; **B** and **C,** buccopharyngeal membrane disintegrates, forming communication between oral and nasal cavities; **D,** nasal development at 12 weeks. (From Moore, K. L.: *The Developing Human* [2d ed.; Philadelphia: W. B. Saunders Company, 1977]. Reprinted by permission.)

thickenings. Mesenchymal cells are derived from the layer of intraembryonic mesoderm and form a loose embryonic connective tissue called mesenchyme, which functions as a supporting tissue of the embryo. An oronasal membrane separates the growing nasal sacs from the oropharynx. The disintegration of this membrane occurs during the 7th week, allowing nasal choana to form. Connection of the nasal cavities to the anterior oropharynx then is complete. At this time, lateral sheets of tissue begin to form the secondary palate while the nasal septum develops from the primary palate. The secondary palate is completed at 10–12 weeks of gestation. Posterior nasal septal tissue extends to complete the posterior choana, thereby forming the nasopharynx. Occasionally, plugging by remaining epithelial tissue of the choana results in the formation of a membranous sheet that occludes the nasal passage. This condition, known as choanal atresia, can result in death of the obligate nose-breathing neonate if medical intervention is not prompt. The tongue grows along the floor of the oral cavity during the 4th to 7th week.

Endodermal foregut produces the pharynx at 4 weeks. The laryngotracheal groove along the floor of the pharynx will give rise to the res-

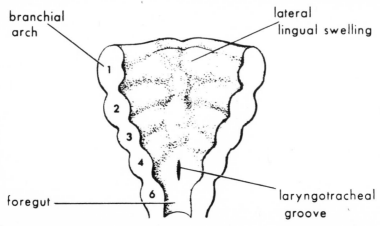

Fig. 1–7.—The laryngotracheal groove. Precursor of the respiratory tract. (Modified from Moore, K. L.: *The Developing Human* [2d ed.; Philadelphia: W. B. Saunders Company, 1977].)

Fig. 1–8.—Formation of the laryngeal orifice by arytenoid swellings. **A,** laryngeal orifice occluded by epithelial tissue at 6 weeks; **B,** epithelial tissue disintegrates, forming patent laryngeal orifice.

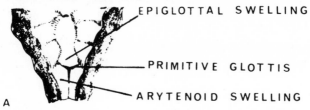

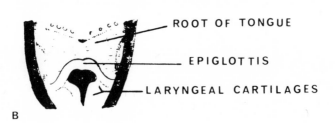

piratory tract (Fig. 1–7). The cranial portion of the tube forming the primordial respiratory tract will become the larynx. At approximately the 6th week, epiglottal tissue has formed, with arytenoid swellings developing toward the tongue. These swellings will form the laryngeal orifice (Fig. 1–8). Until the 10th week of gestation, the orifice is occluded by epithelial tissue. At 10 weeks, the epithelium disintegrates. Vocal cords, yellowish elastic connective tissue, appear as folds during the 8th week. The cords are necessary for normal breathing, cough, Valsalva maneuvering and intonation by acting as a sphincter.

The Lower Respiratory Tract

Lung development may be divided into three general phases or stages. First is the glandular phase (about 5–15 weeks), including tracheobronchial development, in which the air-conducting system is established (Fig. 1–9). Respiration is not possible during this period because the conducting airways are blind-ending tubules. In the 16th week, the canalicular phase begins and continues to about the 25th

Fig. 1–9.—The three stages of lung development. **I,** glandular phase, formation of conducting airways; **II,** canalicular phase, lung circulatory system forms; **III,** alveolar phase, respiratory portion of lung develops.

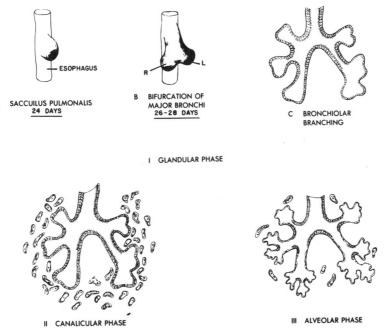

A   SACCULUS PULMONALIS
    24 DAYS

B   BIFURCATION OF
    MAJOR BRONCHI
    26-28 DAYS

C   BRONCHIOLAR
    BRANCHING

I   GLANDULAR PHASE

II   CANALICULAR PHASE

III   ALVEOLAR PHASE

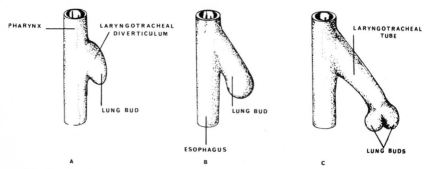

Fig. 1–10.—Lung bud (laryngotracheal diverticulum). **A,** the beginning of the respiratory tract; **B** and **C,** elongation of the lung bud, with development of buds of the major bronchi.

week. During this period, the circulatory system of the lung develops, and by the end of 24 weeks each terminal bronchiole has given rise to two or more respiratory bronchioles. Respiration is possible near the end of this phase because primitive alveoli or terminal sacs have developed. Also, these regions now are highly vascularized. The vast amount of alveoli formed in the fetus begins at approximately the 24th week and continues to about 8 years of age. This phase constitutes the alveolar period of lung development.

An anlage (the primordial forerunner of an organ), the laryngotracheal groove, appears at approximately 24 days of embryonic development. This anlage is an endodermal outgrowth from the pharynx and, together with mesenchyme from the foregut, appears as a sac ventral to the pharynx. This sac is the primordia of the larynx, trachea and buds of the main bronchi. This outgrowth is called the sacculus pulmonalis (lung bud), and from the onset its growth is continuous and unceasing (Fig. 1–10).

Fig. 1–11.—Normal separation of the trachea and esophagus. Transverse sections showing the formation of the tracheoesophageal septum and the subsequent separation of the foregut into the laryngotracheal tube and the esophagus.

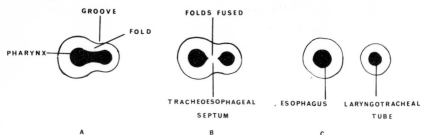

Figure 1–11 illustrates the development of the tracheoesophageal septum and the subsequent separation of the foregut into the laryngotracheal tube and the esophagus. The tracheoesophageal septum results from the laryngotracheal diverticulum (see Fig. 1–10). Longitudinal grooves appear on the lateral portions of this diverticulum, forming internal tracheoesophageal folds. Starting at the caudal end of this diverticulum, the folds grow toward each other and eventually fuse to form the tracheoesophageal septum. This septum divides the foregut into the laryngotracheal tube and esophagus. The laryngotracheal tube opens into the pharynx, giving rise to the larynx, trachea, bronchi and lungs, and into the esophagus.

The Trachea

The lung bud elongates in the caudal direction while beginning to form the trachea. Almost from the onset of elongation, the buds of the major bronchi are present on the most caudal end of the trachea (see

Fig. 1–12.—**A,** mesenchyme surrounding the trachea; **B,** formation of cartilage and connective tissue from the mesenchyme; **C,** smooth muscle and glands further develop from the mesenchyme.

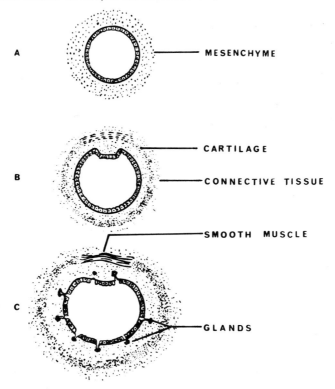

Fig. 1 – 10). During this elongation, the endodermal outgrowth forms the epithelial lining of the trachea and its glands. Early in the development of the trachea, the epithelial lining consists of columnar cells that later undergo transformation into pseudostratified columnar epithelial cells. By 10 weeks of gestation, ciliary development has begun in these cells.

Mesenchyme that surrounds the trachea forms the cartilage, connective tissue, muscle and vascular system (Fig. 1 – 12). Tracheal cartilage can be seen at approximately the 7th week of gestation. However, during the 4th week of gestation, the process of cell aggregation to form these structures occurs. From the 10th to the 20th week, most of the glands of the trachea are formed, and by 16 weeks the goblet cells are well developed. Continual elongation of the trachea permits movement of the bronchial buds into the region of the developing thorax, where further bronchial development and refinement will occur.

The Bronchi

At approximately 26 – 28 days, the two main bronchi are the first of the conductive airways to form. The bronchi are derived from the buds at the caudal end of the trachea (see Fig. 1 – 10). The left main bronchus develops at a slightly greater angle than the right main bronchus. This difference in angles is needed to accommodate the heart on the left side of the thorax. Mesenchyme surrounds the bronchi while the bronchioles are forming, and the bulk of the lung tissue is formed from these mesenchymal cells. The bronchioles migrate in the mesenchyme in wave-like movements. Tissue culture studies have demonstrated that the endodermal epithelium forming the bronchi will not form the tubules in the absence of mesenchyme.

In examining bronchiolar development it is noted that the lung is a self-developing entity. A predetermined pattern governs the formation of a specific differentiation in the branching pattern of the bronchial tree. This specific branching pattern cannot be demonstrated among individuals. What can be said is that a relatively constant number of branchings occur in each individual. Various numbering systems are used to identify the number of generations of bronchi, and two of the schemes are presented in Figure 1 – 13.

From the two main bronchi, through dichotomous branching, the second generation of bronchioles develop. This second generation, in turn, gives rise to another generation. Continuation of this pattern can be seen for an average of 19 generations per lung segment (range 8 – 32). Variations in bronchial branching patterns occur not only from

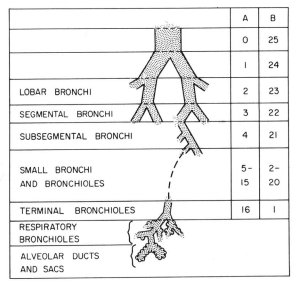

		A	B
		0	25
		I	24
LOBAR BRONCHI		2	23
SEGMENTAL BRONCHI		3	22
SUBSEGMENTAL BRONCHI		4	2I
SMALL BRONCHI AND BRONCHIOLES		5- 15	2- 20
TERMINAL BRONCHIOLES		I6	I
RESPIRATORY BRONCHIOLES			
ALVEOLAR DUCTS AND SACS			

Fig. 1–13.—Numbering systems for successive generations of bronchi. **A,** counting begins at upper airways; **B,** counting starts at final conducting airway. (From Lough, M. D., Doershuk, C. F., and Stern, R. C. [eds.]: *Pediatric Respiratory Therapy* [Chicago: Year Book Medical Publishers, Inc., 1974].)

lung to lung but can be observed in lobe-to-lobe and segment-to-segment relationships. No further development of new nonrespiratory bronchioles occurs after this point. However, elongation and widening of the existing airways is found in proportion to the crown-rump length of the body. By 24 weeks, approximately 17 orders of branches have formed, and after birth 5–8 additional orders of conductive airways (respiratory bronchioles, alveolar ducts and sacs) will develop up to about 8 years of age. Once the total of approximately 25 orders of airways is established, development of this particular portion of the respiratory tract will cease.

Histologically, the epithelium lining the conducting airways of the embryonic bronchioles is predominantly nonciliated columnar cells, which increase significantly as gestation progresses from the 12th to the 17th week. In addition to their increase in number, these cells are transforming from their original columnar appearance into cuboid-shaped or low columnar epithelial type cells. By 20 weeks, all bronchiolar epithelial cells assume a cuboid shape and are becoming closer in proximity. Development of cilia on these cuboid-shaped cells begins at approximately 12 weeks; by 13 weeks, the segmental bronchi contain ciliated cells; by 20 weeks, the terminal bronchioles are lined by cuboid-shaped cells, and, at birth, cilia are present in the terminal bronchioles.

CARTILAGE, SMOOTH MUSCLE, CONNECTIVE TISSUE AND LYMPHATICS OF THE BRONCHI. — In the bronchi, the mesenchymal cells that surround the bronchial tubes differentiate into the lymphatics, connective tissue and cartilage. Cartilaginous plates or rings are found at the 10th week of gestation. Initially, they are in a fibril form and are present in all airways that will contain cartilage. As development continues until the 24th week, these primordial fibrils differentiate into the circular (ring) cartilage surrounding the airway. Cartilage is found in the first 8 generations of airways; the bronchi contain cartilaginous rings but the bronchioles do not. The proximal airways contain cartilage by birth; however, maturity of the cartilage of the most distal airways continues beyond birth.

From the 7th week, smooth muscle cells, derived from the splanchnic mesenchyme, appear on the bronchi and bronchioles. By 12 weeks of gestation, the smooth muscle aids in the support of the posterior wall of the larger proximal bronchi.

During this same period, fibroelastic tissue also begins to appear as thin fibrils in the mesenchyme that surrounds the developing airways. Mature collagen and fibrous tissue bundles can be seen at the 12th week. This collagenous tissue, found surrounding the airways, in the septa and in the blood vessels, is considered the major connective tissue of the respiratory tract. Elastic tissue does not develop to any extent in the fetus or infant, as compared to the adult. The elastic tissue that does develop in the fetus is primarily at the opening of the developing alveolar sacs and is present at approximately 26 weeks.

The lymphatic tissue of the fetus develops in the form of channels at 20 weeks and arises from the mesenchyme. Three distinct cellular forms of lymphocytes can be demonstrated. At 30 weeks, small lymphocytic aggregates, which may be the origin of the macrophages in the adult lung, are prominent in the connective tissues. A second aggregation of lymphocytes is found associated with the terminal bronchioles and alveoli and juxtaposed to the septa. Last, lymph node tissue is diffuse in lung tissue. These lymphatics generally do not follow the airways but travel through the interstitial tissue in random form.

Glands

Endodermal epithelium forms the lumen of the bronchioles. The lumina of these bronchioles give rise to the mucous glands that form in the folds or lateral wall of the epithelial tissue at the 12th week.

These glands appear as clusters of mucous cells that migrate to the basement membrane. While these cell clusters are migrating, tubules are developing and thus provide a duct between the basement membrane and the lumen.

Mucous glands are found only in the upper third of the bronchi, and additional glands continue to differentiate until approximately the twenty-sixth week. After this time, further differentiation is limited to the individual mucous glands already present and to development of additional glands. However, serous glands begin to appear during this time. The density of the mucous glands begins to decrease after birth to approximately one-third the number found in the fetus. In the adult lung there is a further decrease in number, resulting in a much lower density of mucous glands. In addition, the composition of the mucus secreted by the infant's mucous glands is different from that of the adult. This difference in composition of mucoid secretions is of short

Fig. 1–14.— Mucus-secreting components of the human respiratory tract. Beginning at the airway lumen, goblet cells of the epithelium are found interspersed among the ciliated cells. They comprise no more than 1 of 5 surface epithelial cells and discharge mucus in a thin layer. Submucosal glands are coiled, compound tubular glands with portions containing largely mucous cells and other portions containing serous (granular) cells. Submucosal gland secretions are discharged via a duct that is ciliated near the surface. The cartilage is found deep in the wall of the trachea and bronchi. (From Lough, M. D., Doershuk, C. F., and Stern, R. C. [eds.]: *Pediatric Respiratory Therapy* [Chicago: Year Book Medical Publishers, Inc., 1974].)

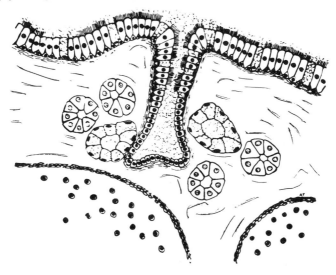

duration, and within several months the composition of the infant's lung is identical to that of the adult lung.

Goblet cells appear by the 13th week. By 16 weeks, they are fully developed and appear only in the proximal intrasegmental bronchi. By 32 weeks, they are found in the same areas and in the same plane as that of the mucous glands (Fig. 1–14).

RESPIRATORY PORTION OF THE LUNG

The Alveoli

During the late canalicular period (about 24 weeks), numerous terminal sacs develop, and capillaries begin to bulge into the sacs. These respiratory structures (the respiratory bronchioles, alveolar ducts, sacs and alveoli) are lined with a flattened continuous sheet of epithelial cells of endodermal origin and differentiate into two different cell types. The first are type I alveolar epithelial cells that have a small perinuclear body with long cytoplasmic extensions spreading out thinly over the alveolar walls. Type II alveolar cells are larger, rounder and contain "lamellar inclusion" called osmiophilic bodies and lack the cytoplasmic extensions. A continuous adepithelial membrane, approximately 30 millimicrons thick, separates the respiratory epithelium from the mesenchyme.

The extremely thin epithelial lining of the alveoli is composed of type I cells. The respiratory bronchioles and alveolar ducts are composed of both type I and type II cells. The alveoli form by mono- and dichotomous branching of the alveolar ducts. At birth, approximately 2.4 million alveoli are present, and thick intra-alveolar septa are found. Respiratory bronchiolar sacs terminate in clusters of thin-walled sacs that are separated by loose connective tissue and represent the future

Fig. 1–15.—Respiratory section of lung demonstrating the terminal bronchiole *(TB)* giving rise to 3 orders of respiratory bronchioles *(RB),* the alveolar ducts *(AD),* alveolar sacs and alveoli in early alveolar stage. (From Lough, M. D., Doershuk, C. F., and Stern, R. C. [eds.]: *Pediatric Respiratory Therapy* [Chicago: Year Book Medical Publishers, Inc., 1974].)

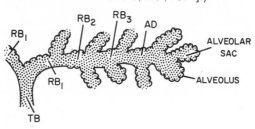

alveolar ducts. Until the event of air-breathing, these primitive alveoli are shallow bulges that protrude from the walls of the terminal sacs and respiratory bronchioles (Fig. 1–15) and are the primordia for future alveolar development. Alveoli increase tenfold from birth to age 8 years. After 8 years of age, increase in alveolar size results in a larger air-surface interface. Also, the mean number of generations of conductive airways is increased in the respiratory portion to a total of about 25 generations. Thus, transformation of the lungs from gland-like surfaces into highly vascular, alveolus-containing organs occurs during the late fetal period; characteristic mature alveoli do not form for some time after birth.

Surfactant

As discussed above, the alveoli are lined by two main types of cells. The type I alveolar epithelial cells appear to have a role in the structural support of the alveoli, have a rapid turnover rate, are oxygen sensitive and involved early in oxygen toxicity, and have low energy requirements. The large type II alveolar cells are fewer in number and contain inclusion bodies thought to be involved in the synthesis and secretion of surfactant. Type II cell energy requirements probably are high; these cells require glucose, lipids, fatty acids and amino acids, all necessary ingredients for biosynthetic activity. Surfactant mechanically aids in lowering the surface tension of alveoli during expiration. Therefore, alveoli remain open, resulting in less effort required to ventilate in the next inspiratory phase. A deficiency or absence of surfactant promotes alveolar instability and collapse on expiration. A deficiency in surfactant is found in the idiopathic respiratory distress syndrome (IRDS) of premature infants.

The fetal lung is metabolically active during its anatomical development and secretes at least two important substances: lung fluid (which is discussed below) and surfactant. This surface-active substance first appears in the lung at 22–24 weeks of gestation. Surfactant is a complex substance containing principally phospholipids plus small amounts of protein and possibly carbohydrate. Surfactant derives its activity primarily from certain phospholipids, the most active being dipalmitoyl lecithin.

There are at least two pathways for the biosynthesis of the surface-active lecithins. The first pathway for lecithin synthesis appears at about 22–24 weeks, with the substrate primarily being palmitoyl-myistol lecithin, and is catalyzed by the methyltransferase system. Although this system increases activity with gestational age, it is easily inhibited by hypoxia, hypothermia and acidosis. Lecithin synthesized by the methyltransferase system, however, is not the major pathway for surfactant production in the lung. The second and more important pathway for lecithin synthesis is the phosphocholine transferase system, which normally develops at about 35 weeks of gestation. After birth, it provides the major pathway for surfactant lecithin synthesis. Surfactant from this pathway is predominantly dipalmitoyl lecithin and denotes maturation of the lung. Fetal maturation can be determined by examining surfactant collected from amniocentesis, which is discussed below.

Hormonal influence, in addition to an intact nervous system and pituitary gland, may be important in the development of the inclusion bodies within type II cells as well as development of the functional lung. Although it has not been conclusively proved, there is a possible role for glucocorticosteroids in the activation of surfactant production in the stressed fetus. Clinically, the incidence of RDS seen by Dlubolucky *et al.* (1976) has decreased 75% with the administration of hydrocortisone to high-risk mothers threatening premature delivery. This effect of lowering the incidence of RDS was seen only when the injection was given at least 24 hours prior to delivery.

Biochemical Aspects of the Developing Lung

Before the outgrowth of the lung bud there is a rapid build-up of glycogen in that area and also a marked increase in ribonucleoprotein is observed. These compounds are contained in the cytoplasm of the epithelial cells. High concentrations of glycogen and ribonucleoprotein are indicative of cell division. Glycogen is found in high concentrations in the most distal ends of the pulmonary tree, demonstrating that lung development proceeds in a proximal to a distal direction. As the lung reaches its later stages of development, the glycogen level rises. Due to its exocrine gland shape in early development, the lung is considered by some to be a storage depot of glycogen for liver metabolism. Villee (1954) found that when fetal lung tissue was placed in culture, the synthesis of glycogen was continuous. Glycogen stores in the lung may also be important at birth to meet the high energy demands required to initiate respiration.

The presence of ribonucleoprotein indicates that growth is occurring. This substance is found in high concentrations throughout the connective tissue of the fetal lung. The enzyme alkaline phosphatase also indicates a rapid rate of growth and is present in high concentrations in the most distal lung buds or developing bronchioles. This enzyme is highly concentrated in the embryo but decreases to a low concentration shortly after bronchiolar development.

Fluid of the Fetal Lung

Although the fetal lung does not carry on its primary function of gas exchange, it is metabolically active. Lung fluid is actively secreted into the developing lumen of the conducting airways, which not only fills the lungs but enters the amniotic fluid. The lung fluid may enter the amniotic fluid via fetal respiratory movements. However, the glottis probably acts as a sphincter that releases lung fluid, as it accumulates in excess, into the amniotic fluid; ligation of the trachea of the fetal animal causes distention of the lungs, which verifies that secretion does indeed occur. The volume of lung fluid approximately equals the functional residual capacity of the lung after birth. Constituent concentrations of the lung fluid have similarities to fetal plasma and/or lymph fluid (for example, sodium and potassium levels). Lung fluid is more acidic, hyperchloremic and lower in bicarbonate than plasma or lymph. The nature of the lung fluid has not yet been determined but there are some constituents of the fluid, such as surfactant, where the origins are well established.

Vasculature of the Lung

Pulmonary artery development begins in the 4th week. The truncus arteriosus, ventral portions of the sixth (pulmonary) aortic arches and vessels from the lung combine to form the pulmonary arteries. Only the terminal air sac capillaries are supplied by these vessels.

Muscle mass in fetal pulmonary arteries increases with gestational age. The muscle mass of these vessels is much greater than that found in the aorta. After birth, the muscle atrophies to a large degree in the first week. The degree of atrophy varies with the cardiovascular status and continues until the lesser amount of muscle mass found in the adult is achieved.

Adult branching patterns of the pulmonary arteries are present at birth. These branches elongate into the mesenchyme connecting with the capillary plexus (from another aortic arch) that developed during the 16th week. This capillary network pushes the adepithelial layer away from the epithelial cells of the lung. As the capillary vessels make contact with the epithelium, cytoplasmic extensions are released to meet the capillaries. These structures form the blood-air barrier and by 24 weeks the capillary development surrounding the terminal air sac is nearly complete.

Pulmonary veins also originate during the 4th week. They appear as an anlage of the developing atrium of the left heart. Initially, only one pulmonary vein develops and later it divides to form a right and left vein, both of which undergo further division to produce four pulmo-

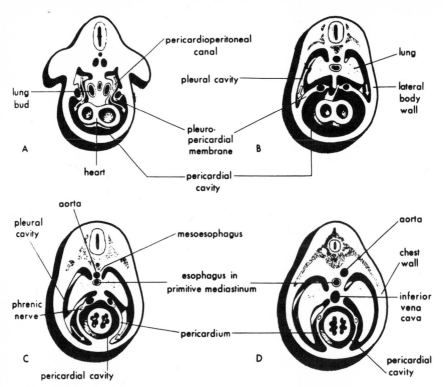

Fig. 1–16.—Drawings of transverse sections through an embryo illustrating successive stages in the separation of the pleural cavities from the pericardial cavity. Also shown are the growth and development of the lungs and the expansion of the pleural cavities. **A,** the communications between the pericardial cavity and the pericardioperitoneal canals are indicated by the arrows in a 5-week embryo; **B,** at 6 weeks, the arrows show the development of the pleural cavities as extensions of the pericardioperitoneal canals and the expansion of the pleural cavities into the body wall; **C,** at 7 weeks, the pleuropericardial membranes are fused in the midline and the pleural cavities have expanded ventrally around the heart; **D** illustrates the continued expansion of the lungs and pleural cavities and the formation of the chest wall in an 8-week embryo. (From Moore, K. L.: *The Developing Human* [2d ed.; Philadelphia: W. B. Saunders Company, 1977]. Reprinted by permission.)

nary veins. As the fetal heart develops, the four pulmonary veins become incorporated into the left atrium. The pulmonary veins also migrate into the surrounding mesenchyme and connect with the venous side of the capillary plexus.

The bronchial arteries develop in the 8th week of gestation. The lymph nodes, nerves, bronchi, the vasa vasorum of the major pulmonary arteries and visceral pleura are supplied by the bronchial arteries. Blood from these arteries empties into the pulmonary venous side via the bronchial veins. This blood volume contributes to the normal anatomic shunt of the lung.

Pleural Cavities and the Diaphragm

During the 2d week, the embryonic mesoderm splits into layers, which results in the formation of two intraembryonic coeloms (body cavities), which are completed in the 3d week. Further development results in the formation of pericardial and peritoneal coeloms that are connected. Two canals, the pleural canals, comprise the pericardial coelom. Mesothelium lining these canals becomes the parietal pleura and secretes a slimy substance. At approximately the 6th week, lung buds begin to migrate into the pleural canals and at the same time the heart migrates upward and midline between them. Pleuropericardial membranes begin developing in the 4th week. These membranes begin to fold, thereby causing the separation of the lung tissue into their respective pleural canals. This folding action also isolates the

Fig. 1–17. — Diagram illustrating the diaphragm of a newborn infant. (Modified from Moore, K. L.: *The Developing Human* [2d ed.; Philadelphia: W. B. Saunders Company, 1977].)

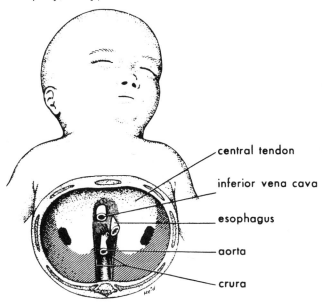

central tendon

inferior vena cava

esophagus

aorta

crura

heart from the pleural canals and thus creates the mediastinum. A second membrane, the pleuroperitoneal membrane, also arises during the 4th gestational week. The formation of this membrane results in the separation of the pleural canals from the peritoneal coelom, resulting in two pleural cavities, each containing a developing lung (Fig. 1–16). By 8 weeks, the mediastinum and the peritoneal cavity have been completed.

Diaphragmatic development begins in approximately the 3d week.

TABLE 1–2.—SUMMARY OF RESPIRATORY
TRACT DEVELOPMENT

APPROXIMATE TIME OF OCCURRENCE	DEVELOPMENTAL EVENT
24 days	Laryngotracheal groove develops
26–28 days	Bronchial buds form
2 weeks	Intraembryonic coeloms form
3 weeks	Diaphragm development begins
4 weeks	Primitive nasal cavities
	Tongue development
	Pharynx formation begins
	Pulmonary artery development
	Pulmonary vein development
	Phrenic nerves originate
5 weeks	Glandular phase begins
6 weeks	Arytenoid swellings (lead to formation of larynx)
	Lung bud migration into pleural canals
7 weeks	Oropharynx
	Tracheal cartilage development begins
	Smooth muscle cells of bronchi develop
8 weeks	Bronchial arteries develop
10 weeks	Secondary palate
	Vocal cords
	Ciliary development
	Cartilaginous rings of trachea
11 weeks	Lymphatic tissue appears
12 weeks	Mucous glands appear
13 weeks	Goblet cells appear
15 weeks	Glandular phase ends
16 weeks	Canalicular phase begins
22 weeks	Methyltransferase system for lecithin synthesis
	Lecithin appears
24 weeks	Alveolar phase begins
	Respiratory bronchioles
	Alveoli develop
26–28 weeks	Alveolar-capillary surface area of respiratory system developed sufficiently to support extrauterine life
35 weeks	Phosphocholine transferase system for lecithin synthesis

During the 7th week, convergence of the transverse septum, the diaphragmatic cervical myotomes, the condensed mesentery of the esophagus and the pleuroperitoneal folds, in addition to other lesser tissue masses, combine to form the diaphragm (Fig. 1–17). Three permanent hiatuses (the caval, esophageal and aortic) and two temporary hiatuses (the pleuroperitoneals) are found in the diaphragm. The phrenic nerves originate in the 4th week, and their migration into the connecting tissue between the pericardium and pleural canals leads to diaphragmatic innervation. A summary of the major developmental aspects of the respiratory system appears in Table 1–2.

Congenital malformations of the lower respiratory tract, as in all other organ systems in humans, have a number of defects that are associated with it and are the direct result of deviations from normal in the

TABLE 1–3.—CONGENITAL MALFORMATIONS OF THE LOWER RESPIRATORY TRACT

CONGENITAL MALFORMATION	EMBRYOLOGIC ORIGIN	REMARKS
Tracheoesophageal fistula (four different varieties)	Results from incomplete division of the foregut into respiratory and digestive portions during the fourth and fifth weeks	Occurs in about 1 of 2500 births, predominantly in males
Tracheal stenosis Tracheal atresia	Probably results from unequal partitioning of the foregut into the esophagus and trachea	Rare malformations
Laryngeal web	A membranous web forms around the vocal cords, causing airway obstruction. Results from the incomplete recanalization of the larynx during the tenth week	Rare
Congenital bronchial cysts	Cysts may develop when abnormal saccular enlargements occur in the terminal bronchioles	Occurrence is rare
Agenesis of the lung (absence of the lung)	Results from failure of the lung bud(s) to develop	Unilateral more frequent than bilateral; however, both are rare
Hypoplasia of the lung	Lungs unable to develop normally because they are compressed by abnormally positioned abdominal viscera	Rare; seen in infants with posterolateral diaphragmatic hernia

developing fetus. Tracheoesophageal fistula (TE fistula) is the most common congenital defect of the respiratory tract and commonly is associated with esophageal atresia; TE fistula alone is not common. It occurs once in about 2500 births and there exist four different varieties, the most common being the blind ending of the upper portion of the esophagus (esophageal atresia) and the lower portion joining the trachea near its bifurcation. Other congenital defects of the lower respiratory tract are summarized in Table 1–3.

FETAL MONITORING – AMNIOCENTESIS

Amniotic Fluid

Amniotic fluid is thought to be an ultrafiltrate of maternal plasma that accumulates during early gestation. Composition of the fluid, early in the 1st trimester, is similar to that of interstitial fluid, which substantiates the ultrafiltrate assumption. Amniotic fluid may also be contributed from the amnion, umbilical cord, vessel transudates, fetal skin, lung, gastrointestinal tract and kidneys. At various times during the development of the fetus, the origin of amniotic fluid changes. Although the range of volume of amniotic fluid present at any given gestational age varies with the individual fetus, certain mean amounts of fluid can be found during different times in development. By the end of the first trimester, approximately 30 ml of fluid is present and the volume increases until it peaks at approximately 34 weeks of gestation. At midgestation, about 350 ml is present, the volume increasing to about 700 ml at term. During the time that the fluid volume is increasing, a change in its composition occurs and a decrease in osmolarity, electrolytes and bilirubin is seen. Increases in urea, uric acid, lipids, phospholipids and estriol are noted as gestation continues. With further progression, a larger proportion of fluid is contributed from the fetal lung and the kidneys, which are excreting a hypotonic urine.

Amniotic fluid itself has a rapid turnover time in the fetus. Approximately every 3 hours the fluid is replaced. This occurs primarily in two ways: maternal circulation absorbs the fluid or the fetus swallows it and then absorbs it into the fetal circulation.

Amniocentesis

Amniocentesis is the removal of amniotic fluid by needle aspiration. When the needle is introduced, care must be taken to avoid puncturing the fetus, umbilical cord or placenta. This procedure is not without complications; amniocentesis can induce abortion and can cause fetal death, maternal peritonitis, feto-maternal hemorrhage and Rh sensitization. It is used diagnostically to determine fetal sex and fetal maturation and to detect biochemical defects and genetic abnormalities.

Genetic defects may include translocation of chromosomes, X-linked (sex-linked) disorders, autosomal dominant disorders, inherited biochemical disorders and immune deficiencies that may be considered genetic. Cells from amniotic fluid can be examined for overt chromosomal abnormalities, such as trisomies or chromosomal translocations. Culturing of cells obtained from the amniotic fluid can elucidate certain immunologic and biochemical defects with appropriate testing. Many of the biochemical abnormalities tested for have a low incidence of expression in the population. Most of the testing procedures used are not easily performed nor are they easily available due to the cost and technology involved. In both karyotyping (chromosome detection) and culturing procedures, the problem of contamination from maternal cells exists.

Cell types may be differentiated to determine from which organ of the fetus each was derived for use in performing the appropriate biochemical analysis. Enzyme concentrations in the amniotic fluid may give clues to the status of the fetus. One such determination is the examination of diamine oxidase (DAO) levels. This test allows estimates as to the outcome of fetuses with Rh-isoimmunization. A relatively normal DAO level in fluid from fetuses with Rh disease denotes a favorable outcome (i.e., survival) and abnormally low levels of DAO correlate with poor fetal outcome and an increased incidence of disseminated intravascular coagulation. Diamine oxidase estimations are used as an adjunct to the amniotic bilirubin levels in this disease. Bilirubin concentration can be determined by spectrophotometric analysis of the amniotic fluid to help determine the severity of Rh disease present.

Other biochemical tests can be performed to detect specific organ maturation defects; an example is in the determination of alpha-fetoprotein (α-fetoprotein). This protein is produced by the fetal liver, and during 20–34 weeks of gestation there is a rapid drop of α-fetoprotein levels in amniotic fluid. Defects of the central nervous system have been correlated with very high levels of this protein at 15–22 weeks of gestation. The defects that have been associated with high protein levels are those that result in an open central nervous system, such as spina bifida and anencephaly. Neural tube defects have also been diagnosed in the fetus by use of an antibody precipitation reaction with B trace vitamins. If a precipitation reaction occurs, a cerebrospinal fluid leak must be present; therefore, a neural tube defect will also be present. The neural tube is derived from the folding of the embryonic ectoderm and is developed by the end of the third week.

Genetic counseling is performed when the determination of risk or a proved hereditary disorder or chromosomal aberration in the fetus is made. The counselor provides professional advice and explanations as to the future problems that may arise from the defect. Alternatives to deal with the fetal problem at birth or the option of abortion are discussed. Before terminating the pregnancy by aborting the fetus, certain minimal criteria should be met in addition to that of the personal considerations of the counselor and family. Other criteria that are needed include a diagnostic amniocentesis, a family history to ascertain prior hereditary problems and disorders, plus placental and family karyotypes.

By far the most common and important use of amniocentesis is the determination of fetal maturation. Many constituents of amniotic fluid are utilized for this purpose, including cells and proteins. The benefits are definitely greater than most risks associated with performing amniocentesis when a fetus with immature lungs is suspected.

Of all the tests performed for fetal maturity, the most important are those used for the determination of fetal lung maturation. IRDS is the major cause of mortality in the neonate. Prevention or early diagnosis of a fetus, by amniocentesis, with immature lungs has decreased the mortality from the disease.

Amniotic fluid levels for amylase activity that are greater than 200 IU have been used to correlate with mature fetuses of gestational age greater than 36 weeks. However, overlap in the 200–250 IU range included some immature infants. Activity of this enzyme, a component of saliva and urine, rises gradually until 36 weeks, at which time an abrupt increase in activity can be noted. Amylase activity of greater than 200 IU correlated fairly well with a weight of 2.5 kg, with some exceptions (DeCastro *et al.*, 1973).

Gauthier *et al.* (1972) demonstrated that creatinine levels of amniotic fluid have a 94% accuracy in correlating gestational age and a 92% accuracy for fetal weight. A creatinine level of 1.6 mg/100 ml was correlated with gestational age of 36 weeks and a fetal weight of 2.5 kg. Creatinine levels are indicative of fetal kidney maturation. Cytologic studies were also performed on amniotic fluid, using Nile blue dye, which stains cells that are thought to be derived from the sebaceous glands orange. A level of these cells of 50% or greater correlated with a 93% accuracy for a gestational age of 38–40 weeks. Fat cells or "ghosts," however, do not stain orange; therefore, false results may be obtained (Myers *et al.*, 1975).

Presently, the most valuable test of fetal maturity is the lecithin/ sphingomyelin (L/S) ratio. Good correlations have been found between an L/S ratio of greater than 2 and gestational age of 35–36 weeks. Amniotic fluid lecithin is derived primarily from the fetal lung and exhibits an abrupt rise at 35–36 weeks. Prior to this point, sphingomyelin is predominant or equal to lecithin in concentration. Criticism of this method is that desaturated lecithin, that is, the lecithin associated with surfactant, is not examined; therefore, the surfactant lecithin is assumed to be present in a total lecithin determination (Ogawa et al., 1976). The L/S ratio also correlates fairly well with the presence of pulmonary surfactant. Prenatally, the L/S ratio can be assayed in amniotic fluid obtained by amniocentesis. Postnatally, determination of the L/S ratio from a specimen of the neonate's gastric aspirate will yield a reliable prediction of the surfactant level present and the possibility of developing RDS.

King et al. (1975) demonstrated that apoproteins of surfactant may be detected by antibodies to them. The apoproteins are absent at 29 weeks of gestation but demonstrate a marked rise in concentration that peaks at 37 weeks and then remains constant. This test may provide yet another means of determining fetal lung maturity.

Amniocentesis is an important tool in determining fetal maturity and status. Its use must be dependent on the benefit-to-risk ratio to both the fetus and the mother. Measurement of fetal lung maturity seems to be most applicable in determining fetal maturity as well as the ability of the respiratory system to meet the demands of independent life.

Other methods for the determination of fetal maturity and fetal distress are available. Amnioscopy provides for direct visualization of membranes, amniotic fluid and placenta and can also be used to collect blood samples or take biopsies of skin tissue. Probably the optimal time for this procedure is at 18 weeks, because the amniotic sac is large enough to allow easy passage of the amnioscope and also the fetus can be maneuvered for inspection. Blood taken from the fetal scalp is used for determining the fetal pH; a fetal scalp pH of less than 7.2 is a strong indication of fetal distress. The Doppler principle may be used to monitor fetal heart rate. Ultrasonography is also used to determine placental and fetal size, abnormal presentation of the fetus, multiple births; also, the chorionic sac may be visualized during the embryonic period. Serial ultrasound determinations are used to demonstrate patterns of fetal growth.

RESPIRATION—FETUS TO NEONATE

Fetal respiration has been demonstrated in various animals at relatively early gestational age. By the ultrasound method, breathing movements in fetal lambs have been found to occur 50–90% of the time at rates of 70–90 breaths per minute (Fox, 1976). Prior to this observation, fetal respirations have been noted to start and then abruptly stop. This phenomenon is attributed to possible neural control overriding the respiratory movement. Data for the origin, central control or frequency of fetal respiration are not yet conclusive. Boyce *et al.* (1976) have measured fetal chest movements and, by using ultrasound techniques, have found them to be 1–3 cm/sec in humans. It was also observed, in human fetuses studied, that fetal respiratory movements are initiated as early as 32 weeks of gestation. Fox (1976) proposes that fetal respiration may require sufficient maturation for lung expansion to occur. Presently, the point in gestation at which fetal respirations begin is questionable.

Fetal lungs are filled with fluid because they have not yet had any contact with air. As the fetus traverses the birth canal, a portion of this fluid is squeezed out of the upper airways due to uterine contractions that result in intrathoracic pressures of 70 cm H_2O being generated. In addition, gravity may allow leakage of some fluid out of the mouth. Initially, not all the fluid is removed from the lung but is later removed by swallowing, tracheal regurgitation, coughing and sneezing. In the more distal airways and alveoli, fluid is cleared by the pulmonary lymphatics; lymphatic clearance is facilitated by grunting or crying, which increases the intrathoracic pressure and forces fluid of low oncotic pressures into the lymphatic tissues. Deficient clearance of excess fluid from the airways and alveoli during the birth descent and the first few breaths after birth may lead to transient respiratory distress in the neonate.

When the first breath occurs, numerous factors work in opposition to the lung opening. Atelectasis in areas from which fluid has been removed leaves a region of high tissue resistance to gas flow. Up to this point, the lung has not been stretched to any degree as occurs in air-breathing man; therefore, in general, the tissue resistance that exists does so without decreased compliance. The viscosity of the lung fluid is another factor resisting the opening of the lung. Finally, initial surface tension of the alveoli together with the air-liquid interface that must be established for a functional air-breathing lung requires high pressures at the first breath. Surfactant that is present in the fetal lung lowers surface tension in the alveoli at birth after the first breath and helps to promote alveolar stability. Negative intrathoracic pressures required for the first breath have been reported from 20 to 70 cm H_2O or higher. Figure 1–18 demonstrates the pressure-volume relationships of the first and subsequent breaths. These large pressures are applied transiently for only 0.5–1 second. After the first few breaths, the neonate has established both its tidal volume and functional residual capacity. By the third or fourth extrauterine breath, only 20 cm H_2O are needed to achieve an adequate inspiration.

Why the first breath occurs has been attributed to many factors. As the uterine contractions generate the high pressures on the thorax, elastic recoil of the thorax immediately allows a small volume of air to enter the lungs. The initial breath has been ascribed to tactile and thermal stimuli. Keatinge and Nadel (1965) demonstrated a rapid respiratory response to immediate cooling in adults. These investigators suggest that cooling from fluid evaporation on fetal skin serves this purpose in initiating the first breath. As the birth process proceeds, and when the umbilical cord is clamped, hypoxia and hypercapnia result. Peripheral chemoreceptors in the neonate have been demonstrated to be functional. Hypoxia has been shown to be a respiratory

Fig. 1–18. — Pressure-volume relationships during the first (—), second (---) and third (xxx) breaths.

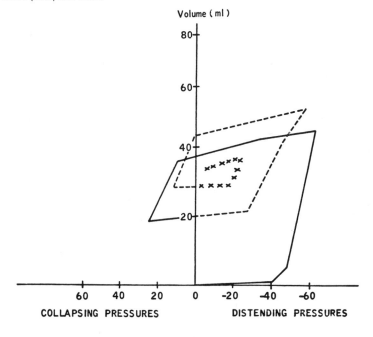

stimulant in the newborn lamb (Purves, 1966a). This response was attenuated with carotid sinus nerve ligation; hypoxia resulted in a rise in minute ventilation with intact carotid sinus nerves. Hypercapnia has also been demonstrated to increase minute volume with intact carotid sinus nerves (Purves, 1966b). Although hypoxia and hypercapnia may not play a major role in the initiation of the first breath, they are definitely the primary cause of subsequent breaths. The Hering-Breuer inspiratory inhibiting reflex in term human infants has been demonstrated; however, it is not as pronounced in the term infant as it is in the premature infant (Kirkpatrick et al., 1976). Bodegard (1976) has demonstrated two types of responses by newborns to inhalation of 4% carbon dioxide. The type A infants were shown to be capable of increasing their rate and depth of respiration on inhalation of 4% carbon dioxide. The type B infants were those of less than 37 weeks of gestation and could increase their rate of breathing only with carbon dioxide inhalations. Bodegard believes that the gamma fibers in the striated muscles are absent in the preterm infants. The "rate only" compensation of these infants (type B) is suggested to be due to the Hering-Breuer deflation reflex, a low grade of neuromuscular development and decreased chest wall stability. He also describes a mixed-type infant exhibiting type A (stable) and type B (unstable) responses. Respiratory centers of the medulla function in newborns, as in adults, for normal rhythmicity of respiration.

Complete aeration of the lung does not occur with the first breath. Tidal volumes on inspiration are larger than expired tidal volumes. This discrepancy facilitates the build-up of the functional residual capacity. Newborns usually cry after the first breath; crying helps to redistribute gas to unventilated areas of the lung and increases intrathoracic pressure to maximize gas distribution. Lung compliance increases whereas airway resistance decreases over the first week to 10 days. Chiswick and Milner (1976) have shown that crying vital capacities in neonates increased significantly from the 1st day post partum to the 10th day. Vital capacity as related to chest circumference was shown to have a rapid increase in the 24–48-hour period, leveling off at 10 days.

The fluid remaining in the lung after the first breath is absorbed by the pulmonary blood flow and lymphatic flow. Pulmonary blood flow increases five- to tenfold after the first breath. This results from a decrease in pulmonary artery resistance (described in the circulation section). Boston et al. (1965) demonstrated a fourfold increase in lymph flow at birth, with a decrease in protein content. Lung weight to body weight ratios were shown to decrease rapidly in the first 2 hours after birth, with a decrease in the rate of weight loss after 5 hours; these findings suggest a loss of fluid. The hypotonicity of the amniotic fluid facilitates its removal via blood and lymph channels. Boston *et al*. also conclude that the high capillary fluid permeability found in the fetus also facilitates fluid clearance.

Breathing Patterns

Apnea may be observed in newborn infants. Apnea is characterized as the cessation of respirations for a time interval greater than 30 seconds and with associated changes in body function, such as bradycardia or acidosis. At birth, two basic types of apnea are observed and both are related to the degree of asphyxia that has occurred at birth. Primary apnea is seen following a rapid increase in the rate and depth of respiration. Cessation of breathing occurs immediately after birth, its duration lasting approximately 1 minute. Gasping follows for several minutes, after which secondary apnea, the complete cessation of breathing, occurs. Primary apnea responds to a variety of stimuli, such as pain, cold or bag-breathing with oxygen. Gasping will occur following these intervening measures, which can lead to the establishment of normal respiration or to secondary apnea. Secondary apnea does not respond to any of the above stimuli and requires prompt resuscitative measures. In general, the longer the duration of the apnea the longer the duration of resuscitation required. In addition to the two basic apneas discussed above, another form of apnea is seen in approximately 30% of all premature infants. This form of apnea lasts for more than 30 seconds, with a decrease in oxygen saturation accompanying it. The frequency of occurrence is much higher in premature infants than in term infants. Apneic periods have been associated with a variety of respiratory disorders: upper airway occlusion from formula, milk or secretions; neurologic disorders; acid-base disturbances; and electrolyte disorders, among other problems. The chemical or physiologic basis for these apneic spells is not clear but it has been suggested that they are due to immature respiratory control mechanisms. Oxygen does not prevent this type of apnea and may even prolong the apneic period. Regular respiration may be reinstituted through tactile stimulation. Continuous positive airway pressure (CPAP) has proved useful in preventing the apneic episodes in some instances.

Periodic breathing is seen in the first few weeks of life. It is believed to be due to respiratory center immaturity and has no pathologic significance. Periodic breathing expresses itself as brief apneic periods in a series of breaths usually lasting 10–20 seconds with no concomitant alterations in other body functions. Respiratory rates immediately after the apneic episode are elevated slightly and are believed to be a physiologic hyperventilation pattern. Periodic breathing is more frequent during sleep. Fenner and associates (1973) have shown a lower Pa_{CO_2} at the onset of the cessation of breathing than at the initiation of respiration again. With the addition of 3.15% carbon dioxide, almost all periodic breathing was abolished. Also, the administration of high concentrations of oxygen, which was believed to cause mild cerebral acidosis from cerebral vasoconstriction, converted periodic breathing to regular respirations of 30–40 breaths per minute. This supports the explanation of immaturity of the respiratory center causing the episodes of periodic breathing.

CIRCULATION – FETAL AND TRANSITIONAL

The Placenta

Prior to birth, the embryonic or fetal membranes, which include the chorion, the amnion, the yolk sac, the allantois and the placenta, perform the following functions: protection, nutrition, respiration and excretion. At birth, they are expelled from the uterus as the afterbirth.

Development of the placenta begins as soon as the implantation of the zygote in the uterine wall occurs. Within 3 weeks, lacunar spaces and villi have developed, allowing placental-fetal circulation. Spiral arterioles that open at the intervillous space may be seen at 6 weeks. After 12 weeks, no further new arteriolar development occurs. Dilation of the existing arterioles, however, does continue until birth. Developing vessels from the fetus enter the placenta at the chorionic plate, diverging to allow a large surface area for exchange between the maternal and fetal blood. Figure 1–19 illustrates the structure of the placenta.

In fetal placental circulation, the deoxygenated blood of the fetus leaves and passes in the umbilical arteries to the placenta. As the umbilical cord attaches to the placenta, the umbilical arteries divide into a number of radially disposed vessels that branch in the chorionic plate before entering the villi. The blood vessels form an extensive arterio-capillary-venous system within the villus, bringing the fetal blood in very close proximity to the maternal blood. The oxygenated fetal blood passes into veins that follow the placental arteries back to the site of attachment of the cord and then converge to form the umbilical vein. This large vessel carries the oxygenated blood to the fetus. In the umbilical circulation, the rate of blood flow is relatively high and is regulated by blood pressure and vascular resistance.

In maternal placental circulation, the blood enters the intervillous space through the spiral arteries (see Fig. 1–19). The flow from these

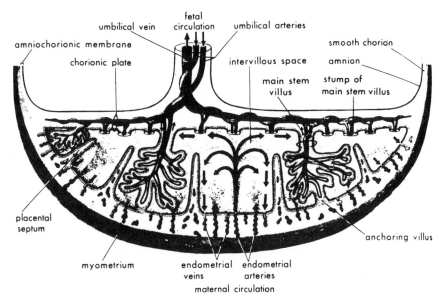

umbilical vein

fetal circulation

umbilical arteries

amniochorionic membrane

chorionic plate

smooth chorion

intervillous space

amnion

main stem villus

stump of main stem villus

placental septum

anchoring villus

myometrium

endometrial veins

endometrial arteries

maternal circulation

Fig. 1–19.—Placental blood flow. Fetal blood enters the placenta through arteries, circulating in the intervillous spaces and returning to the fetus via the vein. (From Moore, K. L.: *The Developing Human* [2d ed.; Philadelphia: W. B. Saunders Company, 1977]. Reprinted by permission.)

vessels is pulsatile and is propelled in jet-like streams by the maternal blood pressure. This blood, on entry, is at a significantly higher pressure than that of the intervillous space and spurts toward the chorionic plate of the intervillous space. As the pressure dissipates, the blood flows over and around the surface of the villi, allowing the exchange of metabolic and gaseous products with the fetal blood. The maternal blood eventually reaches the decidual plate of the intervillous space, where it then enters the endometrial veins.

Briefly, under normal circumstances, the maternal and fetal blood do not come into any gross physical contact. A series of fetal capillary networks enter the intervillous space, in which a lower-pressure, slower-flow maternal blood exchanges nutrients and metabolic products with fetal blood. Fetal blood is carried to the placenta via the umbilical arteries and returns to the fetus via the umbilical veins. The rate of blood flow is regulated through the interaction of blood pressure and vascular resistance.

The placenta has three main functions: (1) metabolism, (2) transfer and (3) endocrine secretion; all of these activities are essential for maintaining pregnancy and promoting normal embryonic development.

Oxygen and carbon dioxide movement across the placenta occurs by simple diffusion. Interruption of oxygen transport for even a few minutes can endanger fetal survival. Diffusion of these gases is affected by both maternal and fetal blood pressure and the rate of blood flow. Higher oxygen tensions of the maternal side result in oxygen diffusion to fetal blood. Not only does the fetal blood have a lower oxygen tension than maternal blood but it also has a higher affinity for oxygen due to its unique hemoglobin. Fetal blood has a higher hemoglobin content than maternal blood (4–8 gm/100 ml more Hb). This feature of fetal blood allows it to carry more oxygen at lower saturations than maternal blood. Carbon dioxide diffuses from fetal to maternal blood. Regulation of acid-base in the fetus is dependent on the carbon dioxide diffusion process, and the kidneys of the fetus play no role in acid-base or electrolyte regulation. In addition to the function of gas exchange via simple diffusion, the placenta, through various transport mechanisms, which include facilitated diffusion, active transport, pinocytosis and several others, supplies nutrients and allows electrolytes to pass freely to the fetus. Also, the placenta synthesizes various enzymes and hormones, one of which helps maintain the pregnant state of the mother.

Fetal Circulation

Development of the fetal heart and circulation results in the first system to function in the embryo, with blood beginning to circulate by the end of the third week. This early development is required because the rapidly growing embryo needs an efficient method of acquiring nutrients and disposing waste products. This rapid development is correlated with a significant decrease of nutritive yolk that once was found in the oocyte and yolk sac. The heart originates as two tubular structures that fuse to form the right and left sides of the heart. This development is first indicated at 18 or 19 days and two tubes fuse by 22 days (Fig. 1–20). At first, the heart is tubular in shape, but while developing, it assumes the adult appearance. After 8 weeks, with the exception of the interatrial foramen ovale and atrioventricular valves, the atrial and ventricular septa are formed. Also, rudimentary trunks of major vessels are developed. From the point that the fetal heart becomes functional, its size-to-surface-area ratio is significantly larger than the ratio found in the adult. At birth, this ratio is slightly higher than in the fetus. In the fetus, the right heart size is much larger in relation to the left heart. In the fetus, the right side of the heart is primar-

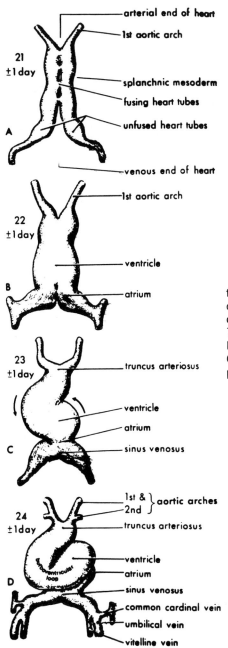

Fig. 1–20.—Development of the fetal heart schematically demonstrated. Refer to text for description. (From Moore, K. L.: *The Developing Human* [2d ed.; Philadelphia: W. B. Saunders Company, 1977]. Reprinted by permission.)

ily responsible for blood flow through the systemic circulation. Therefore, unlike the adult, the right heart is pumping blood against greater resistance than the left heart. After birth, with air-filled lungs, resistance to blood flow from the right heart is less than that from the left heart, which is pumping blood into the systemic circulation.

Early in the development of the heart, its pacemaker and conducting system regulate its function. However, by 8 weeks, chemoreceptors, baroreceptors and extrinsic nervous tissue are present. The point in time at which these tissues become important in fetal circulatory regulation is not clear. Term infants demonstrate a well-developed chemoreceptor and baroreceptor reflex system for circulation.

Fetal circulation differs markedly from adult circulation in that the lungs are poorly perfused while they are nonfunctional. Therefore, placental function alters the circulation to provide oxygen and appropriate nutrients to the fetus. From the placenta, oxygenated blood is carried through the umbilical vein to the fetus. As the vein enters the fetal abdomen, blood flow is directed into one of two vessels. Both the ductus venosus and branches of the portal vein receive approximately equal portions of blood. Portal vein flow passes through the liver to the hepatic veins and then to the inferior vena cava, where flow from the ductus venosus is met. Blood from the inferior vena cava also has two routes. The majority of the oxygenated blood enters the left atrium via the foramen ovale from the right atrium. This blood flow occurs due to higher right-sided pressures in the fetus, which open the foramen ovale. In addition, structural aspects of the inferior vena cava favor this route. The remainder of the blood from the inferior vena cava flows to the right ventricle, where it is met by blood from the superior vena cava that is also entering the right ventricle. The blood from the right ventricle enters the pulmonary arteries; however, only about 10% of the blood enters the pulmonary vessels, the remaining 90% or so of the blood from the right ventricle entering the ductus arteriosus. The ductus arteriosus is a vessel that connects the pulmonary arteries to the descending aorta. Since the pulmonary arteries are constricted, presumably due to the low Pa_{O_2} of the blood perfusing them, the larger diameter and low resistance of the ductus arteriosus allow most of the blood flow from the right ventricle to bypass the lungs. A schematic diagram of the fetal circulation is presented in Figure 1–21.

Blood flow that is directed to the brain contains the most highly oxygen-saturated blood due to the positioning of the ductus arteriosus. Approximately 60% of the blood flow from the descending aorta returns to the placenta for reoxygenation. Iliac arteries and umbilical

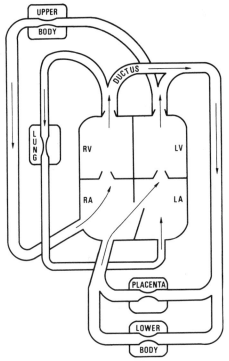

Fig. 1–21.—Fetal circulation. Right ventricle *(RV)*; left ventricle *(LV)*; left atrium *(LA)*; right atrium *(RA)*; the foramen ovale between RA and LA; ductus arteriosus shunts blood from high-resistance lung vessels. (From Lough, M. D., Doershuk, C. F., and Stern, R. C. [eds.]: *Pediatric Respiratory Therapy* Chicago: Year Book Medical Publishers, Inc., 1974].)

arteries carry the blood to lower the resistance of the placental circulation. The blood remaining in the descending aorta supplies the abdomen and lower extremities and returns via the inferior vena cava.

At birth, the umbilical vessels are clamped, causing contractions for a short time, which results in narrowing and elongation of the vessels and finally closure. At birth, a transitory change occurs as the first breath is taken (Fig. 1–22). An increase in arterial oxygen reaching the pulmonary arteries results in their dilation. A decreased resistance in the pulmonary circulation concomitant with closure of the foramen ovale results in the rerouting of almost all the blood flow through the right heart into the pulmonary circuit and closure of the ductus venosus. Only the delayed closure of the ductus arteriosus prevents all the blood flow from entering the pulmonary vessels. Closure of the ductus

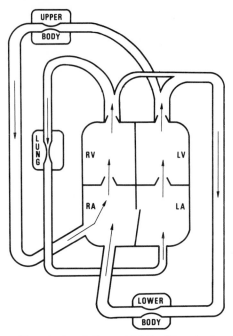

Fig. 1–22.—Transitional circulation at birth. The ductus arteriosus begins to close. The foramen ovale closes from rising left atrial pressure. (From Lough, M. D., Doershuk, C. F., and Stern, R. C. [eds.]: *Pediatric Respiratory Therapy* [Chicago: Year Book Medical Publishers, Inc., 1974].)

arteriosus results from the increasing Pa_{O_2} that occurs with each breath; also, closure appears to be mediated by bradykinin, which is a vasoactive substance released from the lungs during their initial infla-tion. The action of bradykinin appears to be dependent on the high oxygen content of the aortic blood that normally results from ventila-tion of the lungs at birth. If the neonate should become hypoxic short-ly after birth, the ductus arteriosus could reopen, establishing the "fe-tal" type of circulation that results in the re-establishment of the right-to-left shunt. Normally, within 15 hours, the right-to-left shunt from the ductus is closed, and permanent closure of the ductus arteriosus occurs after 72 hours. The status of the adult type of circulatory pattern is achieved when the ductus arteriosus right-to-left shunt is closed (Fig. 1–23).

Systemic resistance rises with the clamping of the umbilical cord, which results in higher left heart pressures, thereby closing the fora-

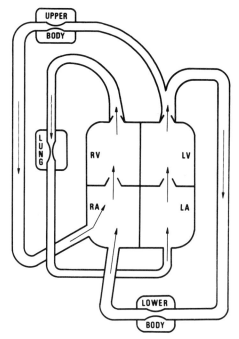

Fig. 1–23. — Adult circulation after the ductus arteriosus closes functional-ly. The foramen ovale functionally closes immediately after the first breath, with a drop in pulmonary resistance. (From Lough, M. D., Doershuk, C. F., and Stern, R. C. [eds.]: *Pediatric Respiratory Therapy* [Chicago: Year Book Medical Publishers, Inc., 1974].)

men ovale. Left atrial pressures rise above right atrial pressures due to rising systemic resistance whereas the pulmonary resistance falls. This type of closure is functional. Anatomic closure of the foramen ovale does not occur until 3 months or more after birth. In many adults, anatomical closure of the foramen ovale does not exist — only functional closure. Activity of the chemoreceptors and baroreceptors is well established at birth. With the above changes, the adult circulation pattern exists.

The critical period of cardiovascular development occurs from about the 20th day through the 50th. Since there are a number of critical events that occur in the development of the heart and great vessels, any deviation from the normal pattern at any one time may produce several cardiac defects. Due to the fact that partitioning of the heart is very complex, defects of the cardiac septa occur frequently,

TABLE 1–4.–CONGENITAL MALFORMATIONS OF THE CIRCULATORY SYSTEM

CONGENITAL MALFORMATION	EMBRYOLOGIC ORIGIN	REMARKS
Dextrocardia	Bending of the heart tube to the left instead of the right, resulting in transposition in which the heart and its vessels are reversed left to right as in a mirror image	Most frequent positional abnormality of the heart but still is relatively uncommon
Atrial septal defects (ASD)		Among the most common congenital heart defects
(1) Patent foramen ovale	Usually results from abnormal resorption of the foramen ovale valve (septum primum) during formation of the foramen secundum, resulting in abnormal location; short septum primum does not cover foramen ovale; large foramen ovale that cannot be covered or a combination of large foramen and excessive reabsorption of the septum primum	One of the most common congenital cardiac defects
(2) Endocardial cushion defect	Incomplete fusion of the endocardial cushions and septum primum, producing a large hole in the center of the heart	Relatively common occurrence; occurs in about 20% of persons with Down's syndrome
(3) Ventricular septal defect (VSD), numerous types	Incomplete closure of the interventricular foramen and failure of the membranous septum to develop	Ranks first in frequency of cardiac defects; isolated VSDs are detected at a rate of 10–12/10,000 between birth and 5 years

Complete transposition of the great vessels	Not clear	
Tetralogy of Fallot—, classic defect consisting of (1) pulmonary stenosis, (2) VSD, (3) dextroposition of aorta and (4) hypertrophy of the right ventricle	Thought to result from under-development of the pulmonary infundibulum	
Pulmonary stenosis (results in a variable degree of right ventricular hypertrophy)	Pulmonary valve cusps are fused together to form a dome with a narrow central opening	
Pulmonary atresia	Division of the truncus arteriosus is unequal, resulting in absence of a lumen in the pulmonary trunk or no orifice at the level of the pulmonary valve	
Aortic stenosis	The edges of the valve are fused, forming a dome with a narrow lumen	
Aortic atresia	Fusion of the valves, producing aortic obstruction or total valve obstruction	
Coarctation of the aorta	Cause not clearly understood; due to observations of the occurrence of this defect in, other syndromes (e.g., Turner's), genetic or environmental factors are attributed	Relatively common malformation
Patent ductus arteriosus (PDA)	Failure of the distal portion of the aortic arch (6th) to involute after birth and form the ligamentum arteriosum	Common; 2–3 times greater incidence in females than in males; most common cardiac malformation associated with maternal rubella

particularly ventricular septal defects. Other congenital malformations are the direct result of abnormal transformation of the aortic arches into the adult arterial pattern. A summary of some of the common congenital malformations of the circulatory system and the embryologic events that result in these defects is presented in Table 1–4.

REFERENCES

Cited References

Bodegard, G.: Control of respiration in newborn babies. IV, Acta Paediatr. Scand. 65:257, 1976.

Boston, R. W., Humphrey, P. W., Reynolds, E. D. R., and Strang, L. B.: Lymph-flow and clearance of liquid from the lungs, Lancet 2:473, 1965.

Boyce, E. S., Dawes, G. S., Gough, J. D., and Poore, E. R.: Doppler ultrasound method for detecting human fetal breathing in utero, Br. Med. J. 2:17, 1976.

Chiswick, M. L., and Milner, R. D. G.: Crying vital capacity, Arch. Dis. Child. 51:22, 1976.

DeCastro, A. F., Usategui-Gomez, M., and Spellacy, W. N.: Amniotic fluid amylase, Am. J. Obstet. Gynecol. 116:931, 1973.

Dlubolucky, S., Babic, J., and Taylor, I.: Reduction of incidence and mortality of respiratory distress syndrome by administration of hydrocortisone to mother, Arch. Dis. Child. 51:420, 1976.

Evans, H. E., Gloss, L., and Mandl, I.: α_1-Antitrypsin concentration in amniotic fluid, Biol. Neonate 27:232, 1975.

Fenner, A., Schalk, V., Hoenicke, H., Weidenburg, A. W., and Roehling, I. F.: Periodic breathing in premature and neonatal babies: Incidence, breathing pattern, respiratory gas tensions, response to changes in composition of ambient air, Pediatr. Res. 7:174, 1973.

Fox, H. E.: Fetal breathing movements and ultrasound, Am. J. Dis. Child. 130:127, 1976.

Gauthier, C., Jr., Desjardins, P., and McLean, F.: Fetal maturity: Amniotic fluid analysis correlated with neonatal assessment, Am. J. Obstet. Gynecol. 112:344, 1972.

Keatinge, W. R., and Nadel, J. A.: Immediate respiratory response to sudden cooling of the skin, J. Appl. Physiol. 20:65, 1965.

King, R. J., Ruch, J., Gikus, E., Platzker, C. F., and Creasy, R. K.: Appearance of apoproteins of pulmonary surfactant in human amniotic fluid, J. Appl. Physiol. 39:735, 1975.

Kirkpatrick, S. M. L., Olinsky, A., Bryan, M. H., and Bryan, A. C.: Effect of premature delivery on the maturation of the Hering-Breuer inspiratory inhibitory reflex in human infants, J. Pediatr. 88:1010, 1976.

Macri, J. N., Weiss, R. R., Joshi, M. S., and Evans, M. I.: Antenatal diagnosis of neural-tube defects using cerebral-fluid proteins, Lancet 1:14, 1974.

Myers, J. L., Harrell, M. J., and Hill, F. L.: Fetal maturity: Biochemical analysis of amniotic fluid, Am. J. Obstet. Gynecol. 121:961, 1975.

Ogawa, T., Okamato, T., Fukuda, M., Hiratami, T., and Ogawa J.: Estimation of surfactant lecithin in amniotic fluid and prediction of respiratory distress syndrome, Biol. Neonate 28:18, 1976.

Purves, M. J.: Respiratory and circulatory effects of breathing 100% oxygen in the newborn lamb before and after denervation of the carotid chemoreceptors, J. Physiol. 185:42, 1966a.

Purves, M. J.: The respiratory response of the newborn lamb to inhaled CO_2 with and without accompanying hypoxia, J. Physiol. 185:78, 1966b.

Rome, R. M., and Glover, J. L.: The benefits and risks of amniocentesis for the assessment of fetal lung maturity, Br. J. Obstet. Gynaecol. 82:662, 1975.

Rossi, F., Pescetto, G., and Reale, E.: Enzymatic activities in human ontogenesis: First synoptic tables in histochemical research, J. Histochem. Cytochem. 5:221, 1957.

Villee, C. A.: The intermediary metabolism of human fetal tissues, Cold Spring Harbor Symp. Quant. Biol. 19:185, 1954.

Ward, H., Whyley, G. A., and Miller, M. D.: The value of amniotic fluid diamine oxidase estimations in the management of severe rhesus isoimmunization, Acta Obstet. Gynecol. Scand. 55:63, 1976.

General References

Aladjem, S., and Brown, A. K.: *Clinical Perinatology* (St. Louis: The C. V. Mosby Company, 1974).

Barnes, A. C.: *Intra-Uterine Development* (Philadelphia: Lea & Febiger, 1968).

Burrow, G. N., and Ferris, T. F.: 1975. *Medical Complications During Pregnancy* (Philadelphia: W. B. Saunders Company, 1975).

Charnock, E. L., and Doershuk, C. F.: Development aspects of the human lung, Pediatr. Clin. North Am. 20:275, 1973.

Cheek, D. B.: *Fetal and Postnatal Cellular Growth* (New York: John Wiley & Sons, 1975).

Crelin, E. S.: Development of the lower respiratory system, Clin. Symp. 27(4):3, 1975.

DeHaan, R. L., and Ursprung, H.: *Organogenesis* (New York: Holt, Rinehart, and Winston, 1965).

Hamilton, W. J., Boyd, J. D., and Bossman, H. W.: *Human Embryology* (3d ed.; Baltimore: The Williams & Wilkins Company, 1962).

Huettner, A. F.: *Fundamentals of Comparative Embryology of the Vertebrates* (Toronto: The Macmillan Company, 1949).

Klaus, M. H., and Fanaroff, A. A.: *Care of the High-Risk Neonate* (Philadelphia: W. B. Saunders Company, 1973).

Lough, M. D., Doershuk, C. F., and Stern, R. C.: *Pediatric Respiratory Therapy* (Chicago: Year Book Medical Publishers, Inc., 1974).

McKay, D. G., Adams, E. C., Hertiz, A. T., and Danzier, S.: Histochemical horizons in human embryos, 15 mm embryo, Streeter Horizon XIII, Anat. Rec. 122:125, 1955.

McKay, D. G., Adams, E. C., Hertiz, A. T., and Danzier, S.: Histochemical horizons in human embryos, II, 6 and 7 mm embryos, Streeter Horizon XIV, Anat. Rec. 126:433, 1956.

Moore, K. L.: *The Developing Human* (2d ed.; Philadelphia: W. B. Saunders Company, 1977).

Patten, B. M.: *Human Embryology* (2d ed.; Philadelphia: Blakiston Co., Inc., 1953).

Potter, E. L., and Craig, J. M.: *Pathology of the Fetus and the Infant* (3d ed.; Chicago: Year Book Medical Publishers, Inc., 1975).

Walsh, S. Z., Meyer, W. W., and Lind, J.: *The Human Fetal and Neonatal Circulation* (Springfield, Ill.: Charles C Thomas, Publisher, 1974).

Selected Readings

Boyden, E. A., and Tompsett, D. H.: The changing patterns in the developing lungs of infants, Acta Anat. 61:164, 1965.

Buchner, V., and Reid, L.: Development of the mucus secreting elements in the human lung, Thorax 16:219, 1961.

Buchner, V., and Reid, L.: Development of the intrasegmental bronchial tree: The pattern of branching and development of cartilage at various stages of Intrauterine life, Thorax 16:207, 1961.

Campiche, M., Gautier, A., Hernandez, E. I., and Reynold, A.: An electron microscope study of the fetal development of human lung, Pediatrics 32: 976, 1963.

Cudmore, R. E., Emery, J. L., and Mithal, M.: Postnatal growth of the bronchi and bronchioles, Arch. Dis. Child. 27:481, 1962.

Dunhill, M. S.: Postnatal growth of the lung, Thorax 17:329, 1962.

Gluck, L.: Surfactant: 1972, Pediatr. Clin. North Am. 19:325, 1972.

Rossi, F., Pescetto, G., and Reale, E.: Enzymatic activities in human ontogenesis: First synoptic tables in histochemical research, J. Histochem. Cytochem. 5:221, 1957.

Strang, L. B.: The lungs at birth, Arch. Dis. Child. 40:575, 1965.

Thurlbeck, W. M., Benjamin, B., and Reid, L.: Development and distribution of mucous glands in the foetal human trachea, Br. J. Dis. Chest 55:54, 1961.

Wells, L. J.: Development of the human diaphragm and pleural sacs, Contrib. Embryol. 35:107, 1957.

Wells, L. J., and Boyden, E. A.: The development of the bronchopulmonary segments in human embryos of Horizons XVII to XIX, Am. J. Anat. 95:163, 1954.

2 / Resuscitation of the Newborn

GERARD W. OSTHEIMER, M.D.

RESUSCITATION OF A NEWBORN is not an isolated event during parturition. Its necessity is governed by what has happened before conception and during pregnancy. Before conception, the genetic, social, economic and environmental conditions surrounding a woman help to determine the milieu of her subsequent pregnancy. Her prenatal care can be excellent to nonexistent, depending on her economic status, education, personal hygiene and place of residence. One of the greatest problems facing our perinatal health care system is making available and then providing appropriate antenatal and peripartum care. The health care team may or may not be able to provide adequate facilities, equipment, personnel and transportation and have sufficient financial support and educational resources. The consumer may or may not be able to utilize them. Education of the health care consumer should begin as early as possible, preferably in primary school, in order that one may fully utilize the services available.

Peripartum care should be accomplished in a hospital environment with the full range of support facilities available to the parturient and her newborn whenever possible. Obstetric care should include adequate labor areas, trained nursing personnel, fetal monitoring equipment, clinical laboratory, blood bank and fully equipped delivery rooms in which emergency surgery and resuscitation can be performed. Anesthetists should be knowledgeable about the physiologic changes that occur during pregnancy and parturition and be able to provide the full range of analgesia and anesthesia necessary, including major regional blocks and general endotracheal anesthesia for vaginal delivery or cesarean section. Pediatric care should provide a controlled thermal environment in the delivery room, appropriate nursery facilities to care for the normal newborn and transitional care for the ill neonate until transfer to an intensive care center can be accomplished.

The immediate resuscitation of the newborn should be accomplished by the most skilled person in the delivery room, preferably by someone other than the obstetrician who is the primary care physician for the parturient. This can be the anesthetist, pediatrician, delivery room nurse or another obstetrician. A resuscitation rarely is planned; immediate and effective responses are necessary. There is nothing in the immediate resuscitation of the newborn that *only* a physician can accomplish. Statutes may limit who can administer drugs but everyone in the delivery area should be able to clear an airway, administer oxygen by mask and bag and give closed chest cardiac massage (CCCM).

The goal of this chapter is to review the physiologic changes that the neonate undergoes in the transition from intrauterine to extrauterine life; demonstrate why thermal regulation is a very important but often neglected part of caring for the newborn; discuss causes of neonatal depression; and present a straightforward approach to the resuscitation of the newborn, including the prevention and treatment of meconium aspiration.

FETAL AND NEWBORN PHYSIOLOGY

Respiratory System

The fetal lung develops by a budding process from the foregut at approximately 24 days of gestation. By 20 weeks, the airways are lined with epithelium and pulmonary capillaries are developing from the mesenchyme. By 26–28 weeks, the capillaries are close to the developing airways so that oxygen and carbon dioxide exchange can occur, making extrauterine life possible. Surfactant-like material is present in the airway epithelium between 22 and 24 weeks but is not present on the alveolar surface until 26–28 weeks. Steroids administered to the mother facilitate the development of the epithelial cells lining the alveoli and the production of surfactant. The onset of fetal breathing is stimulated by stress (usually hypoxia) and amniotic fluid can be drawn into the lung, as can be demonstrated by meconium aspiration. During vaginal delivery, the chest of the baby is compressed in the vaginal canal by the pelvic floor and much of the fluid in the lungs is expressed by this vaginal "squeeze." The remaining fluid (plasma filtrate and amniotic fluid) is removed from the lungs after birth by lymphatics and capillaries. Premature babies and infants born by cesarean section have increased lung fluid because of the absence of the vaginal "squeeze." Spontaneous respirations usually begin within 1 minute of birth and a rhythmic pattern is established within 2–10 minutes. The rebound of the chest wall from the vaginal "squeeze" helps to fill the lungs with air, and acidosis, hypoxia and hypercapnia stimulate the respiratory center to initiate the onset of rhythmic breathing. Further stimuli to respiration include: cold, tactile stimulation and umbilical cord clamping. Respiratory depression results from severe hypoxia, severe acidosis, central nervous system injury and excessive maternal medication (narcotics, tranquilizers, barbiturates, magnesium sulfate, alcohol and local anesthetics).[1]

Cardiovascular System

Oxygenated blood from the umbilical vein flows into the inferior vena cava and is directed from the right atrium to the left atrium through the foramen ovale and then into the left ventricle. Unsaturated blood flows from the superior vena cava to the right ventricle. This streaming of venous return provides increased oxygenation to the heart and brain. The fetal lung receives less than 10% of the cardiac output because of intense vasoconstriction of the pulmonary capillary bed, which decreases at birth due to increasing pH, oxygenation and lung expansion. The increasing pulmonary blood flow gives increased left atrial pressure that prevents right-to-left shunting of blood through the foramen ovale, which remains patent but functionally closed.

The ductus arteriosus closes after birth on a functional basis in response to increasing levels of oxygen, acetylcholine and parasympathetic nervous stimulation but does not close anatomically for weeks to months, depending on the maturation of the newborn. Peripheral vasoconstriction secondary to a cold environment and the resultant hypoxia and acidosis in the early neonatal period will cause a decrease in pulmonary blood flow due to increased pulmonary resistance. If the pulmonary perfusion pressure increases above systemic arterial pressure, right-to-left shunting will be re-established through the ductus arteriosus. Maintenance of a neutral thermal environment in the stressed newborn is essential to allow cardiovascular adaptation to the extrauterine environment.

THERMOREGULATION

The maintenance of the proper thermal environment is essential to every newborn. They are born wet into an environment that is too cool. Newborns have a large surface area compared to their mass and, therefore, suffer enormous heat losses by evaporation, convection, radiation and conduction. Evaporation is the major cause of heat loss in the delivery room because the baby is born covered with amniotic fluid. Radiation accounts for two-thirds of the heat loss suffered by the neonate in the nursery.

Thermoregulation is a relatively recent innovation in the field of newborn care. In the late 1890s, Budin, a pupil of Professor Tarnier in Paris, reported a striking difference in the mortality of infants weighing less than 2000 gm at birth: If the rectal temperature was less than 32° C, the mortality rate was 98% and if it was over 35° C it was only 23%.[2] Based on these observations, Budin set out to build the first modern incubator. He was assisted by the director of the Paris Zoo and Martin Couney, one of his students who had studied in Germany. This incubator (Fig. 2–1) provided heat, a one-way flow of warm air, additional humidity, freedom of movement and temperature monitoring.

Man is homeothermic—that is, he increases his heat production when exposed to a cold environment to maintain body temperature. Poikilotherms, such as reptiles, cannot increase heat production and their body temperature drifts to that of the environment.

There are two methods of increasing heat production: (1) a physical method of muscle contraction (shivering) used by children and adults and (2) a chemical method used by neonates, referred to as nonshivering thermogenesis.

When the newborn is cold stressed, he increases his oxygen consumption and metabolic activity (Fig. 2–2). Large amounts of norepinephrine are released (in contrast to epinephrine in adults), which activates adipose tissue lipase to break down brown fat (so called be-

Fig. 2–1.—Budin's incubator: *1*, lower door; *2*, copper bottles containing water (these bottles were warmed to provide heat); *3*, unidirectional flow of air; *4*, sponge to provide increased humidity; *5*, thermometer; *6*, cotton clothing; *7*, exhaust orifice; *8*, removable plate glass window.

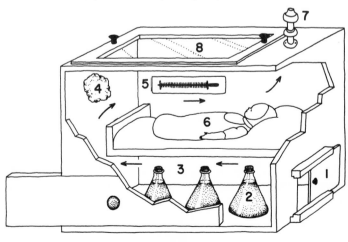

NONSHIVERING THERMOGENESIS

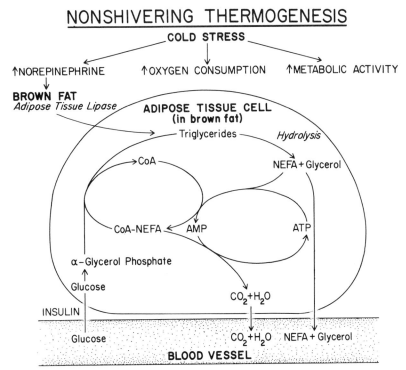

Fig. 2–2. — The clinical and biochemical responses of the newborn to cold stress.

cause of its rich vascular supply) to form triglycerides, which are hydrolyzed to form glycerol and nonesterified fatty acids (NEFA). The NEFA are either oxidized to carbon dioxide and water in the cell or re-esterified with glycerol to form triglycerides. Adipose tissue is not able to phosphorylate the glycerol derived from triglycerides; therefore, re-esterification via the coenzyme A-NEFA complex requires a supply of α-glycerol phosphate derived from glucose that originates outside the cell. Obviously, oxidation is a highly exothermic reaction and Ball and Jungas[3] consider resynthesis of triglycerides to be the same because of ATP utilization in the formation of the coenzyme A-NEFA complex.

Several investigators[4] believe that thermogenesis occurs mainly in the brown fat of the neonate (Fig. 2–3, A and B), which is found at the interscapular mass—the "hibernating gland," the muscles and blood vessels of the neck, the clavicles and axillae, great vessels entering the thoracic inlet and abdominal viscera—especially around the kidneys and adrenals.

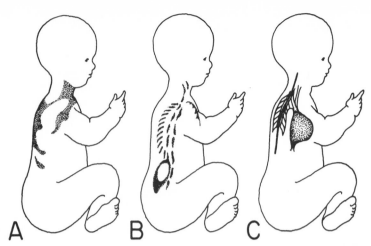

Fig. 2–3. – Sites of brown fat (**A** and **B**) and venous drainage (**C**).

The venous drainage (Fig. 2–3, *C*) from the interscapular adipose tissue joins the drainage of the muscles of the back to form the external posterior vertebral plexus, which drains to the rich venous plexus around the spinal cord, which in turn drains to the jugular or azygos veins, depending on the level – thus supplying heat to the spinal cord and the heart.

We must strive to maintain a neutral thermal environment (32 – 34° C for newborns) at which metabolism (as reflected by oxygen consumption) is minimal yet sufficient to maintain body temperature. Adamson and his co-workers[5] have found that minimal oxygen consumption occurs when the gradient between skin and environmental temperature is less than 1.5° C. In their study, oxygen consumption rose approximately 0.6 ml/kg/min, once the 1.5° C gradient was exceeded. In the newborn, hypothermia may produce metabolic acidosis, hypoxia, hypoglycemia and kernicterus and prolong drug metabolism.

The proper thermal environment can be maintained by a number of radiant heat devices. Dahm and James[6] investigated heat loss in the first 30 minutes after delivery and found that wet infants exposed to room air lost nearly 5 times more heat than those who were dried and warmed. In vigorous infants, promptly drying and wrapping the baby in a warm blanket is almost as effective in decreasing heat loss as placing the baby under a radiant warmer. However, in depressed or immature infants, who may be more asphyxiated or have reduced energy stores, an overhead radiant warmer maintains body temperature while allowing access to the patient during resuscitation (Fig. 2–4).

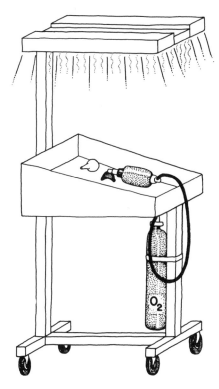

Fig. 2–4.—An overhead radiant warmer with self-inflating resuscitation bag, oxygen and bulb syringe allows resuscitation of newborn while maintaining body temperature.

Miller and Oliver[7] compared the drop in core temperature in term infants under three conditions: Group A had routine delivery room care and bath on admission to the nursery, Group B had the same as A but no bath and Group C had prompt drying and placement in the incubator with an air temperature of 32–35° C. All groups had essentially the same temperature at birth. However, Group A lost 2.5° C in 1 hour, Group B lost 2.0° C in 1 hour and Group C lost 1.0° C in 1 hour. Recovery to normal core temperature (approximately 36° C or 97° F) took 8 hours for Groups A and B whereas Group C recovered in only 3 hours.

Maintenance of a neutral thermal environment is essential in order to give the newborn the best opportunity to establish a strong physiologic foundation from which to combat the other stresses of the new environment.

NEONATAL DEPRESSION

The delivery room care of the "healthy" newborn following a "normal" vaginal delivery includes:

1. Aspiration of the mouth and nose by bulb syringe.

2. Maintenance of normal newborn temperature by drying and placing under a radiant warmer.

3. Routine neonatal identification procedures.

4. Neonatal ophthalmic prophylaxis.

These measures usually are all that is necessary in 90% of the deliveries. However, approximately 10% of newborns will be depressed and this may be totally unexpected. The reasons for neonatal depression can be divided into two categories, maternal and fetal.

Maternal Factors

Drugs administered to the parturient during labor and delivery:

1. Inhalation anesthetics—i.e., 70% nitrous oxide/30% oxygen administration in excess of 15 minutes.

2. Local anesthetics—i.e., excessive absorption of a large mass (concentration X volume) of drug in certain procedures such as paracervical block or direct accidental intravascular injection during paracervical, epidural or caudal block.

3. Parenteral medications—i.e., excessive amounts of narcotics administered to the parturient during labor and delivery for pain relief and the production of amnesia. Also, drugs such as reserpine, magnesium sulfate, ethyl alcohol and lithium have a direct depressant effect on the neonate.

Cardiopulmonary problems:

1. Hypotension—due to the supine hypotension syndrome (aortocaval compression), sympathetic block after major regional anesthesia (epidural, caudal or spinal) or hemorrhage.

2. Hypoxia—due to a low inspired oxygen concentration during general anesthesia secondary to maternal aspiration, faulty gas machines or lung disease.

3. Uterine artery vasoconstriction—due to vasopressors such as methoxamine (alpha stimulators) or local anesthetics.

4. Disease (primary cardiac or pulmonary).

5. Anemia—acute (bleeding) or chronic (due to long-term bleeding or poor nutrition).

Infection—maternal problems, including chorioamnionitis
Labor

1. Cephalopelvic disproportion.

2. Abnormal presentations (breech, brow, face, etc.).

3. Dysfunctional uterine activity.

4. Intrauterine obstetric manipulations.

5. Traumatic delivery.

Uteroplacental factors:
1. Abruptio placenta.
2. Placenta previa.
3. Postmaturity — which is the progressive dysfunction and deterioration of a senescent placenta.
4. Toxemia of pregnancy.
5. Diabetes mellitus.

Fetal Factors
1. Umbilical cord compression (including prolapse).
2. Prematurity.
3. Congenital anomalies.
4. Multiple pregnancy.
5. Meconium staining.
6. Neonatal shock — can occur for several reasons.
7. Neonatal hypothermia.

PRINCIPLES OF NEWBORN RESUSCITATION

A. Airway management.
B. Breathing for the baby.
C. Circulation or maintenance of adequate cardiac output to maintain cerebral oxygenation.

After the birth of the baby's head, the oropharynx and nasopharynx are suctioned with a bulb syringe (Fig. 2–5, A) before the baby's first breath and while the chest still is compressed in the vaginal canal by the pelvic floor (vaginal "squeeze") to prevent aspiration of meconium, blood, debris and mucus into the trachea with the onset of respiration. This procedure may be the most important maneuver in preventing meconium aspiration.[8] The baby then is delivered; the umbilical cord is clamped and cut (Fig. 2–5, B). Further suctioning of the airway is done, if warranted, when the newborn is transferred by the obstetrician to a warmed bassinet that has been placed in a 20° head-down position to facilitate the gravity drainage of liquid material into the oropharynx. A slight lateral tilt of the newborn facilitates the pooling of secretions into one corner of the oropharynx (Fig. 2–5, C). Management of the airway is accomplished by gentle suction with a bulb syringe, not a rubber suction catheter.

Cordero and Hon[9] investigated the effect of nasopharyngeal stimulation by catheter and found that indiscriminate posterior pharyngeal stimulation by catheter may cause cardiac and respiratory arrhythmias of vagal origin. Forty-six neonates were suctioned with a small-diameter nasogastric tube. Seven developed cardiac arrhythmias,

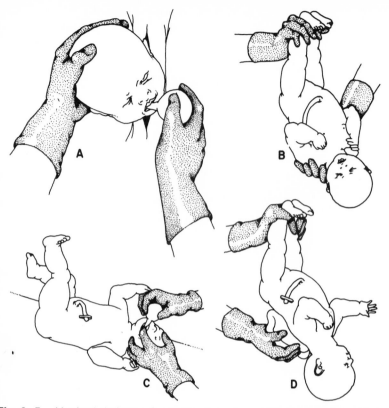

Fig. 2–5. – Vaginal delivery. **A,** suctioning of nasopharynx and oropharynx with bulb syringe, following delivery of the infant's head; **B,** the umbilical cord is clamped and cut; **C,** the infant is placed in a 20° head-down position and suctioned with a bulb syringe; **D,** the infant is thoroughly dried.

including one sinus arrest. Five became apneic. No change in heart rate was noted when a bulb syringe was used in 41 newborns.

Gentle drying of the newborn with a warm, dry towel or slapping of the soles of the feet is all the stimulation needed for the healthy newborn (Fig. 2–5, D). Spanking, cold water showers, jackknifing, "milking" the trachea, dilation of the anal sphincter, alternating hot and cold water baths, rocking beds and excessive rubbing of the back are *condemned* as having no therapeutic value and are potentially harmful.

We now must evaluate the newborn using the Apgar score[10] (Table 2–1). This is a dynamic and continuous assessment applied to the newborn and is recorded at 1 and 5 minutes of life. Virginia Apgar

TABLE 2-1.—APGAR SCORE

SIGN	0	1	2
Heart rate	Absent	Slow (below 100)	Over 100
Respiratory effort	Absent	Slow, irregular	Good crying
Muscle tone	Limp	Some flexion of extremities	Active motion
Reflex irritability (response to catheter in nostril)	No response	Grimace	Cough or sneeze
Color		Blue, pale	Body pink, extremities blue	Completely pink

devised her scoring system in order to focus attention on the newborn during the first crucial minutes of life. The Apgar score is essentially five vital signs: Heart rate, respiratory effort, muscle tone, reflex response and color. There have been some recent attempts to change the total Apgar score from 0 to 8 (leaving out the evaluation of cyanosis). In my opinion, cyanosis is a very graphic sign of oxygenation and peripheral perfusion and should remain in the score.

More sophisticated newborn neurobehavioral testing has been developed to assess the effects of medication on the newborn.[11] This is a great stride forward in assessing subtle differences between drugs or local anesthetics. However, the Apgar score still remains the standard by which all babies are judged.

If the Apgar score is 7–10, no further therapy is necessary except maintenance of the proper thermal environment. If it is 4–6 (moderate depression) without meconium, administer oxygen to the infant by bag and mask and stimulate by slapping its feet or drying the infant with a warm towel. Use low flows of oxygen (less than 5 liters per minute) and maintain a tight mask fit. Brown, Ostheimer, Bell and Datta[12] have demonstrated that high flows of cold, unhumidified oxygen blown on the face of the newborn will cause bradycardia and/or breath-holding in the first few minutes of life. This probably is a response mediated by the vagus nerve after stimulation of the posterior nasopharynx or oropharynx. Intermittent positive-pressure ventilation (IPPV) may be necessary. Careful attention to the heart rate and the infant's attempts at spontaneous ventilation is essential. If the Apgar score is 1–3 (severe depression) or if cardiac arrest has occurred and there is no response to IPPV with 100% oxygen by bag and mask, immediate laryngoscopy, aspiration of the oropharynx and trachea and

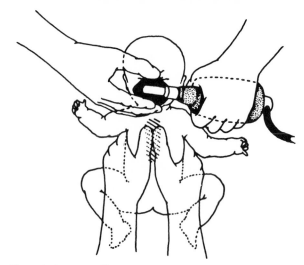

Fig. 2–6. – Closed chest cardiac massage and ventilation by bag and mask.

intubation must be performed concomitantly with closed chest cardiac massage (CCCM). The encircling hands/two thumbs technique over the midsternum at 100 – 120 compressions per minute is the technique of choice for CCCM[13] (Fig. 2 – 6).

One problem that can complicate the ventilation of the newborn is the edema that develops over the occiput of the baby's head (caput) during labor. When the baby is placed supine, the caput can cause flexion of the neck to the extent that the trachea becomes compressed. This problem can be alleviated by elevating the shoulders with a towel or blanket roll so that the neck is hyperextended (Fig. 2 – 7). Often, this maneuver is all that is necessary to help the baby establish an adequate airway and initiate effective ventilation and it makes subsequent laryngoscopy (if necessary) much easier. (The technique of intubation is explained in Chap. 8.)

When the intubation and/or ventilation are done correctly and the

Fig. 2–7. – Hyperextension of the newborn's neck using a towel or blanket roll.

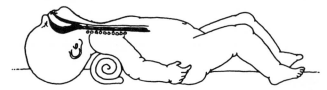

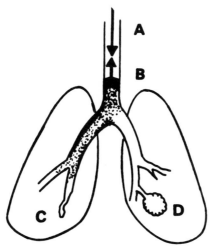

Fig. 2–8.—The stages of expansion of the infant lung. **A,** high positive pressure; **B,** viscous fluid; **C,** collapsed; **D,** expanded.

airway is established, the chest should expand, bilateral breath sounds should be heard and the pulse rate should increase. Equal breath sounds do not guarantee bilateral ventilation, since sounds of aeration are transmitted all over the chest. Always listen over the abdomen to rule out esophageal intubation.

Expansion of the airless, collapsed lung requires higher pressures than those needed to move air into the lung once it has been expanded (Fig. 2–8, A). During the first breath, the newborn develops a negative intrathoracic pressure of about 50 cm H_2O (range −20 to −70 cm H_2O), causing 40–70 ml of air to be drawn into the lung.[14] The newborn must overcome the viscous flow of fluid (plasma filtrate and amniotic fluid) present in the airway (Fig. 2–8, B), the forces of surface tension of the collapsed lung and the elastic forces of the lung (Fig. 2–8, C) and thorax during the first few breaths of life.[15] This first inspiration usually is followed by a cry as the newborn exhales against a partially closed glottis. The first breath may have to be given to the newborn during resuscitation and an inspiratory pressure of 60 cm H_2O or more may be necessary to expand the lungs (Fig. 2–8, D). The first irregular breaths in a spontaneously breathing neonate gradually become more rhythmic and a regular ventilatory pattern usually is established within 10 minutes at about 40 breaths per minute. This regular pattern of ventilation assists the newborn in recovering from the hypoxia, hypercapnia and acidosis that occur in all births. However, poor respiratory patterns in the asphyxiated newborn will cause a slower rate of recovery from the asphyxia of delivery and, in those infants who remain apneic, the hypoxia, hypercapnia and acidosis become severe. Oxygen content falls to near zero in $2\frac{1}{2}$ minutes, carbon dioxide rises at the rate of about 10 torr per minute and pH falls 0.1 pH unit every 3–5 minutes. As a result, there is further depression of the respiratory center, myocardium and peripheral vasculature. If prompt resuscitation is not instituted, central nervous system damage will occur.

In contrast to the acute asphyxial experiments in animals in which depression is instituted at birth, the human newborn has some degree of asphyxia during birth and this can become grossly exaggerated if resuscitation is not initiated immediately after delivery. There is no excuse to abstain from immediate resuscitation when a depressed newborn is delivered.

Gastric aspiration should *not* be done in the first few minutes of life in order to avoid causing any arrhythmias from nasopharyngeal or oropharyngeal stimulation—*unless* there is massive gastric dilation secondary to IPPV with bag and mask or a tracheoesophageal fistula is suspected. Cordero and Hon[9] suggested that after 5 minutes of age, the neonate has become physiologically more stable and will tolerate passage of a nasogastric tube. The passage of a catheter down the nasopharynx through the nose will rule out choanal atresia and will help diagnose tracheoesophageal fistula, duodenal atresia and, perhaps, diaphragmatic hernia.

After the acute resuscitative effort, in which the airway is secured, ventilation is achieved, cardiac output is assessed and, possibly, augmented by closed chest cardiac massage (CCCM), further definitive therapy is indicated if improvement has not been forthcoming. A neonatal care team should transport the child from the delivery area to an intensive therapy room or the special care nursery.

REFERENCES

1. Gregory, G. A.: Resuscitation of the newborn, Anesthesiology 43:225, 1975.
2. Stern, L.: The Newborn Infant and His Thermal Environment, in *Current Problems in Pediatrics* (Chicago: Year Book Medical Publishers, Inc., November, 1970).
3. Ball, E. G., and Jungas, R. L.: On the action of hormones which accelerate the rate of oxygen consumption and fatty acid release in rat adipose tissue in vitro, Proc. Natl. Acad. Sci. 47:932, 1961.
4. Motil, K. J., and Blackburn, M. G.: Temperature regulation in the neonate, Clin. Pediatr. 12:632, 1973.
5. Adamson, K., Jr., Gandy, G. M., and James, L. S.: The influence of thermal

factors upon oxygen consumption of the newborn human infant, J. Pediatr. 66:495, 1965.

6. Dahm, L. S., and James, L. S.: Newborn temperature and calculated heat loss in the delivery room, Pediatrics 49:504, 1972.

7. Miller, D. L., and Oliver, T. K., Jr.: Body temperature in the immediate neonatal period: The effect of reducing thermal losses, Am. J. Obstet. Gynecol. 94:964, 1966.

8. Carson, B. S., Losey, R. W., Bowes, W. A., *et al.:* Combined obstetric and pediatric approach to prevent meconium aspiration syndrome, Am. J. Obstet. Gynecol. 126:712, 1976.

9. Cordero, I., and Hon, E. H.: Neonatal bradycardia following nasopharyngeal stimulation, J. Pediatr. 78:441, 1971.

10. Apgar, V.: A proposal for a new method of evaluation of the newborn infant, Anesth. Analg. 32:260, 1953.

11. Scanlon, J. W., Brown, W. U., Weiss, J. B., *et al.:* Neurobehavioral responses of newborn infants after maternal epidural anesthesia, Anesthesiology 40:121, 1974.

12. Brown, W. U., Ostheimer, G. W., Bell, G. C., *et al.:* Newborn responses to oxygen blown over the face, Anesthesiology 44:535, 1976.

13. Todres, I. D., and Rogers, W. C.: Methods of external cardiac massage in the newborn infant, J. Pediatr. 86:781, 1975.

14. Karlberg, P.: The adaptive changes in the immediate postnatal period with particular reference to respiration, J. Pediatr. 56:585, 1960.

15. Avery, M. E.: Anoxia and Resuscitation, in Cook, R. E. (ed.), *Biologic Basis of Pediatric Practice* (New York: McGraw-Hill Book Company, 1968), Chap. 149, pp. 1448–1452.

3 / Abnormal Respiratory Conditions of the Newborn

BARBARA SCHUCHARDT, R.R.T.

THIS CHAPTER details some of the many diseases that cause pulmonary complications for the neonate. Respiratory distress may be the result of primary lung disease, central nervous system disorders or a variety of congenital malformations. It is the purpose of this chapter to acquaint the reader with some of the more common diseases that cause respiratory distress and to present a method of treatment.

ASPHYXIA NEONATORUM

Asphyxia neonatorum is a term that is used to describe hypoxia, hypercapnia and acidosis in the newborn. All newborn infants present with varying degrees of asphyxia as a result of delivery. The severity of the asphyxia and the probability of it reaching clinically dangerous degrees is a result of numerous extrinsic and intrinsic factors associated with pregnancy, labor and delivery.

During the course of a normal delivery, a fetus may be subject to asphyxia as a result of prolonged or severe contractions, uteroplacental insufficiency, umbilical cord compression and maternal analgesics and barbiturates.

Two parameters that can be monitored and may serve as indicators of fetal distress and asphyxia are the fetal heart rate and fetal scalp blood gases. Intermittent monitoring is limited to auscultation of the fetal heart during the resting phase only. This limitation makes it difficult to detect early asphyxia because it is harder to discern subtle changes in the fetal heart rate that occur immediately postcontraction before the resting phase. Continuous monitoring serves as a better indicator of fetal distress, since it will display decelerations and beat-to-beat variations graphically for more detailed study. This form of monitoring helps pick up subtle alterations in the heart rate before severe asphyxia occurs.

Both of these methods may be augmented by fetal scalp blood gases. These capillary blood gases are drawn in utero during labor and after rupture of the membranes and are useful in diagnosing fetal distress. In data published by Beard *et al.*[1] it has been shown that in the initial stages of labor the fetal pH approximates 7.335 ± 0.052, the PCO_2 41 ± 8.2 mm Hg and the PO_2 23.7 ± 5.6 mm Hg. Later, during the final stages of delivery, umbilical artery blood gases reveal that the pH drops to 7.202 ± 0.045, the PCO_2 rises to 54.9 ± 9.9 mm Hg and the PO_2 falls to 17.2 ± 6 mm Hg. Therefore, any stressful stimuli that alters these values will serve as valuable evidence of fetal distress and asphyxia.

Other factors that frequently are indicative of asphyxia during labor are: passage of meconium (thus, meconium-stained amniotic fluid), fetal bradycardia (less than 100/min) and fetal tachycardia (above 180/min). The asphyxia may be aggravated by a difficult delivery, multiple births, umbilical cord entanglements, cord prolapse and maternal sepsis or hemorrhage.

These infants often have respiratory complications related to the asphyxia. Aspiration of the meconium-containing amniotic fluid is a common complication, especially in term and past term infants (see meconium aspiration, below). The term infants who do not have meconium aspiration pneumonitis usually have tachypnea, increased tidal volume and low PCO_2 (25–30 mm Hg). The etiology of this hyperventilation may be related to hypoxic pulmonary damage, mild aspiration syndromes or asphyxial neurologic damage. Asphyxiated premature infants often develop respiratory distress syndrome (RDS). Cerebral edema often occurs with seizure activity and respiratory depression. Respiratory problems that are due to the neurologic damage usually are indicative of severe brain damage. The recovery of the infant from any of these events varies according to the severity of the asphyxia and its ensuing complications.

RESPIRATORY DISTRESS SYNDROME (RDS); HYALINE MEMBRANE DISEASE (HMD)

The most clinically significant disease entity in the newborn period is hyaline membrane disease. The incidence of the syndrome is about 1 in every 6000 births (Avery[2]) but increases to about 10% in the premature population (Klaus and Fanaroff[3]). Those premature infants most frequently affected are in the range of 1.0–1.5 kg birth weight. Others who are also susceptible are infants of diabetic mothers, the second twin, those delivered by cesarean section and those who have had intrapartum or postpartum asphyxia.

The clinical symptoms usually are present immediately after birth. They include cyanosis in room air, tachypnea (60–120 breaths/min), flaring of the nares, intracostal retractions and an expiratory grunt. The expiratory grunt is the result of exhaling against a partially closed glottis, which maintains pressure across the airways, preventing the alveoli from collapsing. Tachypnea frequently is present, but in those infants most severely affected there is a prolonged grunt that takes as long as 1 second and thus results in a respiratory rate below 60 breaths per minute. The grunting may accompany every exhalation or it may be intermittent. A lessening of the grunting often indicates that the neonate is improving.

Auscultation of these neonates may be difficult, since grunting is the most predominant sound transmitted. If the grunting is minimal, one will note "diminished air entry" and perhaps fine rales bilaterally.

Many of the clinical symptoms associated with this syndrome are also characteristic of other neonatal disorders (e.g., pneumothorax, diaphragmatic hernia and hypovolemia). It is essential to make a differential diagnosis when these symptoms are present. A chest radiograph will aid in making the diagnosis, since there is a classic pattern associated with RDS. This radiologic pattern consists of diffuse bilateral reticulogranular densities (ground glass) and air bronchograms (Fig. 3–1). Cardiomegaly sometimes is present with severe disease.

The histologic findings demonstrate the presence of pink-staining membranes, alveolar atelectasis and dilated alveolar ducts. The hyaline membranes are endogenous in origin and are by-products of blood fibrin and alveolar cells.

The alterations in the functioning of the lung are well defined. The tidal volume is decreased in these neonates and their lung compliance is reduced to approximately one-fifth of normal (Klaus and Fanaroff[3]). Much of the lung is not perfused because of the massive atelectasis. Minute ventilation is increased but effective alveolar ventilation is decreased, the net effect being an increase in the work of breathing. These neonates also have a right-to-left shunt and the ductus arteriosus may remain patent.

The etiology is not clearly understood. The alterations in the lung (e.g., decreased compliance) may indicate that the primary lesion is a decrease or alteration in surfactant. This alteration in surfactant might then initiate a sequence of events that results in progressive atelectasis, respiratory failure, alveolar hypoperfusion and ischemia, ultimately causing alterations in alveolar permeability with the formation of hyaline membranes.

An alternative theory cites intrauterine asphyxia as the primary

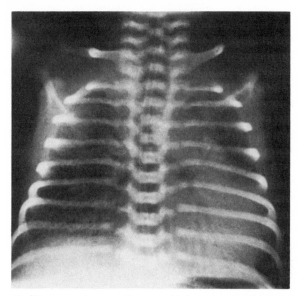

Fig. 3–1.—Hyaline membrane disease. Note ground glass appearance in both lungs and well-defined air bronchograms.

event that initiates a similar sequence of changes beginning with pulmonary vasoconstriction and alveolar hypoperfusion followed by a deficiency in surfactant and an alteration in cell wall permeability, resulting ultimately in the formation of hyaline membranes.

Whatever the mechanism for the potentially life-threatening changes in these neonates, this syndrome responds to various forms of therapy and resolves in many instances. Although the incidence of mortality is quite high, it is constantly being reduced by new forms of treatment.

The initial treatment should include resuscitation if indicated, placement of an umbilical artery catheter and placement of the infant in a neutral thermal environment. Arterial blood gases should be drawn to determine the presence of hypoxia, hypercapnia and acidosis. At birth, the increase in arterial oxygen tension is responsible for the closure of intrauterine circulatory channels (e.g., ductus arteriosus) and a significant decrease in pulmonary vascular resistance. Hypoxia will result in a reopening of the ductus arteriosus and a marked increase in pulmonary vascular resistance (both frequent characteristics of HMD). Acidosis serves to aggravate these changes, and if they are severe or prolonged they may result in a right-to-left shunt via fetal circulatory pathways (e.g., foramen ovale and ductus arteriosus). This return to fetal circulation perpetuates increased pulmonary vascular resistance and hypoxia.

Oxygen administration is beneficial to these neonates, since oxygen is a pulmonary vasodilator. Caution should be used in regulating the fractional inspired oxygen concentration (F_{IO_2}). When the neonate is exposed to high concentrations of oxygen, frequently there is an unexplained disproportionate increase in arterial oxygen tension. The reverse may also be encountered when lowering F_{IO_2}, since vasoconstriction can recur, resulting in an inappropriate fall in the Pa_{O_2} (flipflop). This condition may not be corrected by increasing the infant's F_{IO_2}. Therefore, oxygen concentrations should be altered cautiously. In stable neonates, the F_{IO_2} generally is lowered in decrements of 5% and in those whose conditions are tenuous in decrements of 2%.

The maintenance of these patients in a neutral thermal environment reduces their oxygen consumption and their carbon dioxide production. It is important to note that an infant's sensitive thermal zones are the forehead and the area surrounding the eyes and nose. Cold, unhumidified oxygen delivered to these zones via hood may result in increasing oxygen requirements. Therefore, any oxygen administered to these infants should be warm ($32-34°$ C) and well humidified.

For many of these neonates, supportive therapy and oxygen administration may not be sufficient to ensure survival. These infants generally respond favorably to the application of constant positive airway pressure (CPAP). This pressure replaces the expiratory grunt and serves to stabilize the alveoli, increase the FRC and increase arterial oxygen tensions.

A small percentage of the affected neonates do not respond to CPAP. They are the infants who experience frequent apneas and severe ventilatory compromise (pH < 7.20, Pco_2 > 70 mm Hg, Po_2 < 40 mm Hg in 100% O_2). These neonates require intubation and mechanical ventilation with positive end expiratory pressure (PEEP).

The benefits of oxygen therapy are not without risks. Prolonged breathing of high concentrations of oxygen may result in pulmonary hemorrhage, bronchopulmonary dysplasia and retrolental fibroplasia. The first two are discussed elsewhere in the text.

Retrolental fibroplasia (RLF) seen in premature infants is a result of oxygen toxicity. The toxic effects are dependent on retinal development, length of hyperoxia and the arterial Po_2. Initial hyperoxia (> 100 mm Hg) results in retinal vasoconstriction, which is reversible. Prolonged (several hours) hyperoxia causes growth of new capillaries, which penetrate the retina and may hemorrhage, leading to retinal detachment and blindness. To limit the incidence of this sequela, the arterial oxygen tension in prematures should be kept between 50 and 80 mm Hg and monitored frequently (every hour).

MECONIUM ASPIRATION

The presence of meconium in the amniotic fluid of neonates may be linked to an intrauterine asphyxial episode. Meconium-stained amniotic fluid occurs in 10–20% of all deliveries. In 60% of these neonates, meconium can be aspirated from the trachea, but of this group only about 20–25% will develop respiratory distress (Gregory et al.[4]). Many of the infants who present with meconium staining are postmature (> 290 days). Their skin may be dry and scaly and their nails may be yellow-green as a result of the intrauterine meconium.

Meconium normally is the first stool passed by the newborn. It is thick and very dark greenish brown and is composed of intestinal secretions, bile and cells that have been swallowed in utero. When this meconium is present in the amniotic fluid, it generally is preceded by an episode of fetal distress or bradycardia, which often signals the occurrence of an intrauterine asphyxial episode. Prior to or during delivery, the meconium present in the amniotic fluid may be drawn into the oropharynx and/or trachea. With the initiation of the first breath, the meconium in the pharynx may be inhaled into the lungs.

Since the aspiration of meconium may occur in utero and frequently is associated with fetal asphyxia, the vast majority of these neonates are severely depressed at birth. Their Apgar scores tend to be low, indicating the need for vigorous resuscitation. Positive-pressure resuscitation should be avoided until the airway has been cleared, since the application of this pressure would only distribute the meconium into more airways, resulting in devastating obstruction.

Prompt suctioning (prior to the first breath, if possible) under direct vision, using an endotracheal tube (2.5–3.5 mm) as a suction catheter, should be accomplished by the most experienced person available (Gregory et al.[4]). Suctioning should be carried out by a mouth-to-tube method; a surgical mask should be worn so that inhaling the meconium can be avoided. This procedure then is repeated using a clean endotracheal tube until the airway is clear of meconium. Resuscitation then should be carried out as described in Chapter 2.

Clinically, many of the affected infants are gasping or apneic after delivery. Those who are breathing often are tachypneic and may be cyanotic in room air. The thorax is hyperinflated, and on clinical observation may appear fixed in full inflation. The hyperinflation is produced by a ball-valve mechanism. The meconium in the airways allows air to enter the lung on inspiration but as the airways narrow on exhalation the air is prevented from being exhaled. In 10% of the neonates, this mechanism results in the development of pneumomediastinum or pneumothoraces. On auscultation of the chest, medium rales may be audible.

Radiologically, the chest is hyperinflated, with an increase in density and depression of the diaphragm. There are bilateral areas of fluffy infiltrates and irregularly distributed areas of hyperaeration (Fig. 3–2). A lateral chest film should also be taken, since it may demonstrate the existence of a pneumomediastinum and will demonstrate increased lung volumes with increase in anteroposterior diameter.

The diffusion of gas in the lung is altered by the presence of the meconium. In order to maintain adequate oxygenation, it may be necessary to administer supplemental oxygen or institute mechanical ventilation. These neonates should be kept in a neutral thermal environment to reduce oxygen consumption and carbon dioxide production. Frequent tracheal suctioning and pulmonary hygiene with postural drainage, percussion and vibration to accelerate the clearing of the meconium may be necessary. The stomach should be decompressed to remove any residual meconium and reduce the risk of vom-

Fig. 3–2.—Meconium aspiration syndrome. Note patchy areas of fluffy infiltrate with areas of hyperaeration.

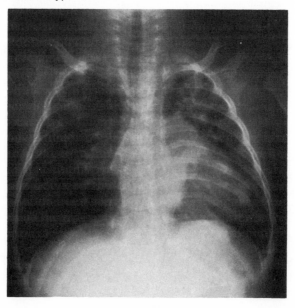

iting and aspiration. Amazingly enough, the lung absorbs the meconium quite rapidly and the neonate's clinical condition may begin to improve within 24–48 hours.

ESOPHAGEAL ATRESIA AND TRACHEOESOPHAGEAL FISTULA

Esophageal atresia with or without tracheoesophageal fistula is a common congenital anomaly. It occurs with varying frequency, but the incidence of the defect is high enough to warrant the careful attention of those who treat newborn infants.

These structural errors occur during the second month of embryonic development. Prior to this time, the esophagus and the trachea are a common channel arising from the foregut. During the second month of embryonic life, the septum, which divides these two structures, is formed. Any interruption in the formation of this septum will result in a fistula between the trachea and the esophagus. After the septum has delineated these two structures, the lumen of the esophagus is obliterated by cellular proliferation but later is recanalized. Any interruption in the recanalization process will result in esophageal atresia (i.e., an esophagus without a lumen).

There are at least seven different variations of this anomaly. The most common type, described by Waterston et al.,[5] is characterized by esophageal atresia with a fistula formed between the distal portion of the esophagus and the trachea above the level of the carina (Fig. 3–3). The second most common variation is characterized by the pure esophageal atresia without fistula formation (Fig. 3–4). The other variations of this anomaly occur with increasing rarity.

At birth, neonates afflicted with these structural abnormalities generally are asymptomatic. However, as oral secretions are produced and accumulated in the esophageal blind pouch, they tend to spill into the trachea via aspiration or via the fistula, if a proximal fistula exists. In addition, aspiration may occur from the stomach across a distal esophagus to the tracheal fistula. The aspiration of fluid tends to produce coughing, choking and cyanosis. If the fistula is small, many infants will remain asymptomatic until they are fed. At this time, they will exhibit severe coughing, choking and cyanosis. They may develop pneumonia as a result of aspiration of saliva, formula or gastric contents. For this reason, infants suspected of having this defect should not be fed orally and their stomach should be decompressed with a catheter attached to continuous suction.

Infants with esophageal atresia not associated with tracheoesoph-

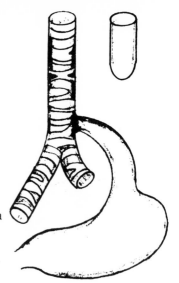

Fig. 3–3.—Diagram of esophageal atresia with a fistula between the esophagus and the trachea.

ageal fistula will not have air in the stomach or intestines and will have copious oral secretions. Those who have a tracheoesophageal fistula will have air in the stomach and intestines as a result of the communication between the trachea and the stomach. If enough air accumulates, the abdomen will become distended and may rupture if the infant has intestinal obstruction.

To determine the existence of esophageal atresia, a catheter (size 10 or 12 French red rubber) may be passed through the mouth or nose until obstruction is met. If the catheter meets obstruction 10–13 cm from the tip of the nose, atresia probably is present. PA and lateral chest films, including the neck, should be obtained with an opaque catheter in place. The catheter will be seen coiled in the pouch when atresia is present. Contrast medium is not necessary in making the diagnosis and is dangerous to the infant.

Prior to surgical correction, these infants should be placed in a warm incubator. They should be positioned on the stomach with the head elevated. This will prevent the aspiration of fluid from the stomach into a distal esophageal fistula.

Aspiration pneumonia is a frequent complication of a tracheoesophageal fistula and many of these infants may exhibit mild to severe respiratory distress as a result of the pneumonia. Arterial blood gases should be drawn to determine hypoxia and/or hypercapnia and oxygen therapy should be initiated if necessary. Many of these neo-

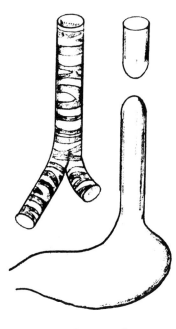

Fig. 3–4. — Esophageal atresia without the fistula.

nates require supplemental oxygen until the pneumonia begins to resolve. To minimize their exposure to increased arterial oxygen tension, their inspired oxygen concentration should be regulated to ensure an arterial Pa_{O_2} of 50–80 mm Hg.

Surgical correction generally is accomplished within the first few days after birth. The repair usually consists of an anastomosis of the two ends of atretic esophagus and a gastrostomy. Postoperative suctioning of the oropharynx should be accomplished cautiously. The suction catheter should be marked with tape so that it will not be passed into the area of the anastomosis and cause trauma to the area.

PULMONARY DYSMATURITY

Pulmonary dysmaturity is a clinical entity first described by Wilson and Mikity[6] in 1960. The disease is characterized by the insidious onset of tachypnea and cyanosis. The neonates affected are premature and generally below 1500 gm birth weight. The disease does not appear to be a result of oxygen toxicity, since many infants diagnosed as having pulmonary dysmaturity have never received supplemental oxygen. It also does not appear to be an extension of RDS, since the onset of pulmonary dysmaturity occurs between 1 and 5 weeks after birth.

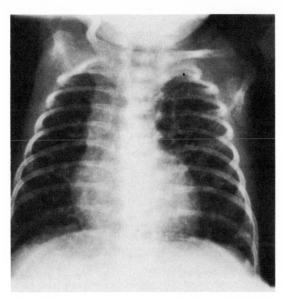

Fig. 3–5.—Wilson-Mikity syndrome. Note the cyst-like foci with lacy pattern of diffuse infiltrate.

The clinical symptoms associated with this entity are tachypnea, cyanosis, dyspnea, wheezing and hyperinflation. The affected infants have a tendency toward cor pulmonale. The respiratory distress associated with the disease and the tendency toward cor pulmonale may affect growth in these infants.

The most consistent diagnostic features of the disease are the radiologic findings. Chest radiographs generally are normal at birth but later reveal cyst-like foci with a lacy pattern of diffuse infiltrates (Fig. 3–5). There is hyperaeration of the lung bases and depression of the diaphragm.

Laboratory data obtained on infants affected with this syndrome are inconclusive concerning any viral, bacterial, fungal or parasitic agent responsible for pulmonary dysmaturity.

The etiology is not clear. The disease may be due to the failure of the alveoli to proliferate, which may account for the lack of alveolar inflation in some parts of the lung and the hyperinflation of alveoli in other portions. The disease appears to have the potential to resolve in those infants who survive and therapy, therefore, is supportive, consisting of supplemental oxygen and treatment of any associated heart failure. The infants who succumb to this entity do so as a result of cardiac or respiratory failure.

APNEA

Apnea is a well-documented occurrence in premature infants. It is an integral portion of periodic breathing, so common in premature infants that it is considered normal (Avery and Schaffer[7]). Periodic breathing is characterized by a series of rapid respirations followed by a short apnea (5–10 sec). This type of respiratory pattern alternates with a normal pattern and generally is not evident until the patient is more than 24 hours of age.

Unfortunately, in premature infants suffering from respiratory insufficiency, apnea is not a benign occurrence. The incidence of severe apnea is quite high (75%) in infants weighing less than 1250 gm and significant (25%) in those weighing 1500 gm or more (Miller et al.[8]).

Mild apnea is not associated with bradycardia, and respirations generally are induced with tactile stimulation. Severe apnea (> 30 sec) does not respond to tactile stimulation and is accompanied by bradycardia (80 beats/min). Severe apnea often requires vigorous resuscitative efforts to initiate spontaneous respirations. In mild apneas lasting 20–30 seconds, the infants generally remain pink and their muscle tone is good. Respiration can be initiated by stroking the neonate's abdomen or slapping the soles of his feet. In those apneas that extend beyond 30 seconds, the infant displays severe cyanosis, bradycardia and the inability to terminate the apnea with sensory stimuli. These infants will require bag breathing with 100% oxygen and cardiac massage. They may even require tracheal intubation, with ventilatory assistance. Since early intervention may abort a severe apneic episode, cardiac and/or respiratory monitors are used for all infants whose gestational age is less than 34 weeks.

The etiology and pathophysiology of apnea are not clear. Since it is seen in increased incidences in very small infants, it may be related to delayed respiratory center development, cerebral dysfunction or brain damage. It is seen with increasing frequency in hyaline membrane disease, pulmonary hemorrhage, severe asphyxia and in infants whose incubator temperatures are above the neutral thermal zone.

Shannon et al.[9] have demonstrated that 2–3 mg/kg of theophylline every 6 hours has been effective in preventing severe apneic episodes in low birth weight infants.

A trial of low-pressure CPAP (2–4 cm H_2O) is also effective in treating recurrent apnea. The mechanism is not well understood but may be attributed to an increase in functional residual capacity and better brain oxygenation.

SPONTANEOUS PNEUMOTHORAX, PNEUMOMEDIASTINUM, PNEUMOPERICARDIUM

Spontaneous pneumothoraces occur in 1–2% of all full-term neonates. These air leaks usually are small. They tend to remain asymptomatic and to resolve without any medical or surgical intervention.

Spontaneous pneumothoraces also occur in the premature newborn. The incidence is decreased (less than 1%); however, these air leaks tend to be more significant and usually are associated with other problems of prematurity. Respiratory distress syndrome and some current forms of therapy appear to be instrumental in an increase in the number of documented pneumothoraces in these infants. Mechanical ventilation, resuscitation and tracheal intubation are also associated with an increased incidence of pneumothoraces.

Macklin[10] described a reasonable and adequate explanation for the occurrence of these air leaks. Increasing intrapulmonary pressure may cause the rupture of weakened or defective alveoli. This free air may travel along the perivascular sheath or interstitial spaces to the hilus of the lung. At this point, the air may enter the mediastinum, causing pneumomediastinum, or may penetrate the pericardium, causing pneumopericardium. This air also tends to form bullae at the hilus of the lung, and increasing intrapulmonary pressure may cause these bullae to rupture and allow air to escape at the hilus between the visceral and parietal pleura, resulting in a pneumothorax.

This type of pneumothorax may be loculated or in communication with the air leak. A loculated pneumothorax is one that is sealed off and may be absorbed without any treatment. This type generally is asymptomatic if small. A spontaneous pneumothorax in communication with an air leak has a chance of increasing in size and producing severe respiratory distress. It may also resolve spontaneously. However, this type responds more favorably to needle aspiration and/or a closed chest tube without subambient pressure.

The clinical symptoms of a significant pneumothorax usually are the onset of irritability or unusual activity and a rapid deterioration in the appearance, with cyanosis, tachypnea and hyperresonance of the chest. There may be diminished breath sounds on the affected side accompanied by an increase in respiratory distress with flaring of the nasal alae and intracostal retractions. A change in the intensity of breath sounds or an alteration in their quality bilaterally may signal the occurrence of a pneumothorax. However, in the premature infant, this expected change in the quality of the breath sounds may not occur, since sound is transmitted readily in the premature infant and breath sounds in the unaffected lung may be transmitted to the affected hemithorax. Careful monitoring of the cardiac impulse may serve as a better indicator of the existence of a pneumothorax, since this type of pneumothorax tends to cause a shift of the mediastinum and a change in the location of the cardiac impulse.

The clinical diagnosis of pneumothorax should be made by lateral and anteroposterior chest radiographs, since this method of diagnosis is the most reliable in this instance (Fig. 3–6). A lateral film will alert the clinician to the presence of a pneumomediastinum that may not be evident on an AP film.

Aspiration of foreign material in the lung, such as meconium, amniotic fluid, blood or cervical mucus, may also play a large role in the development of a pneumothorax in the newborn after delivery. Inflation of normal newborn lungs requires extremely high transpulmonary pressures (in the range of -40 to -100 cm H_2O) to overcome the viscous resistance to the amniotic fluid in the lung. The presence of these foreign substances in the lung may block the airways and prevent the serial openings of some alveoli. As the neonate maneuvers to inflate his lung, he may increase the application of this high transpulmonary pressure in an attempt to open these obstructed alveoli. Prolonged pressure exerted on these fragile alveoli may be enough to cause rupture and a pneumothorax.

Fig. 3–6.—Tension pneumothorax. Note herniation of the pleura across the mediastinum, collapse of the right lung and shift of the mediastinal structure to the left.

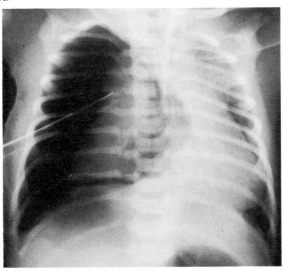

These acute air leaks do not always result in pneumothoraces. As discussed previously, they may dissect along the perivascular sheath to the hilus of the lung and into the mediastinum, resulting in pneumomediastinum, or may find their way into the pericardium, resulting in pneumopericardium. Pneumomediastinum tends to be asymptomatic and resolves without treatment. The only clinical symptom may be the crackle characteristic of this entity or distention of the chest. In some infants, it is seen only on a lateral chest x-ray.

Pneumopericardium is not as benign as pneumomediastinum or pneumothorax. Originally it was considered quite rare, but with the increasing application of positive and negative pressure ventilation, it is being reported with increasing frequency (Brano *et al.*[11]). The air that accumulates in the pericardium may result in cardiac tamponade, evidenced clinically by muffled heart sounds, a drop in systolic pressure, cyanosis and rapid deterioration. Oddly enough, this serious complication may resolve spontaneously and never recur if the amount of air is minimal. It may also be relieved by aspiration of the pericardial air. Although it may be inviting to be nonaggressive in the treatment of this entity in the hope that it may resolve, Brano *et al.* state that infants they treated with pericardiocentesis responded well, and the pneumopericardium did not recur despite continued positive-pressure ventilation.

The diagnosis of all these entities is best made by chest radiographs, since otherwise they may remain undiagnosed and go untreated until they reach clinically significant levels.

The treatment of these entities consists of aspiration of the air and the insertion of a chest tube, if necessary, to re-expand the lung. Vital signs should be monitored as frequently as every 15 minutes and the course of the air leaks should be assessed with frequent chest radiographs. If the pneumothorax or pneumomediastinum is loculated, evacuation of this gas may be enhanced by administering 100% oxygen to the infant for limited periods. The administration of 100% oxygen washes out nitrogen, reducing its partial pressure in the alveolus and the loculated space. This washout also increases the partial pressure of oxygen in the space without a corresponding increase in the capillaries. There is a subsequent alteration in the pressure gradient between the space and the capillaries, hastening the absorption of the air pocket and the recovery of the neonate.

BRONCHOPULMONARY DYSPLASIA

The current trends toward more aggressive therapy in the treatment of severe respiratory distress syndrome in the small premature may be responsible for a previously unrecognized abnormality that affects the neonates recovering from RDS. This sequela has been termed bronchopulmonary dysplasia, since the pathologic and histologic alterations seen in lung tissue closely resemble changes that occur in the adult lung as a result of oxygen toxicity. Northway et al.[12] have attributed the pathologic and histologic alterations in the lung to high inspired oxygen concentrations (> 0.70) in conjunction with continuous positive-pressure ventilation for periods in excess of 6 days.

Stern,[13] however, has reported no occurrence of bronchopulmonary dysplasia with the use of continuous negative-pressure ventilation with high oxygen concentrations. Instead, he implicates endotracheal intubation (unnecessary in negative-pressure ventilation) in conjunction with high oxygen concentrations.

Northway et al. have described four specific radiologic stages in the evolution of this new syndrome:

Stage I occurs during the acute phase of hyaline membrane disease. The chest radiograph demonstrates the classic picture of RDS, with increased opacity, a reticulogranular appearance and the presence of air bronchograms. Pathologically, this stage is identical to hyaline membrane disease. During this stage, the majority of the infants are intubated and are receiving mechanical ventilation with high oxygen percentages.

Stage II occurs 4–10 days after the onset of RDS. Radiologically it is characterized by complete opacification of the lungs. Histologically there is a regeneration of the alveolar epithelium alternating with areas of alveolar emphysema, necrosis and hyaline membranes.

Stage III occurs during the second and third weeks of life and is characterized by radiolucent bullae scattered throughout the lung (Fig. 3–7, A). The chest radiograph characteristic of this stage resembles the classic chest x-ray in pulmonary dysplasia. This stage represents the transition into the chronic phase. Many infants who survive will require continuous supplemental oxygen. They commonly develop cor pulmonale as a result of increasing respiratory distress.

Stage IV is the chronic phase of this disease entity and occurs after 1 month of age. The chest radiograph reveals cystic formations throughout the lung (Fig. 3–7, B). These infants require increasing percentages of supplemental oxygen and display marked respiratory distress, with cyanosis and periods of apnea. The mortality rate as a result of cor pulmonale is 50% in this disease. The administration of oxygen to these infants during this stage is most easily accomplished using a croup tent. Unfortunately, this mode also provides a high degree of isolation to the patient, which may result in maternal deprivation.

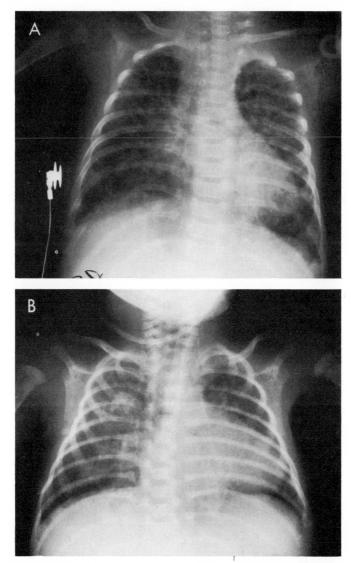

Fig. 3–7.—A, bronchopulmonary dysplasia, stage III. Note early cystic lesions, blurring of the heart border and fine linear radiolucencies, consistent with early interstitial emphysema. **B,** stage IV. Note hyperaeration of the chest with flattening of the hemidiaphragm, pneumonic consolidation in the right upper lobe and the "bubbly" cystic changes of stage IV BPD.

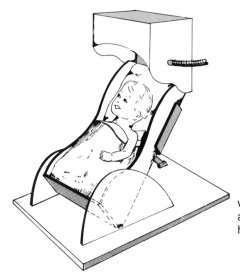

Fig. 3–8.—A hooded chair, which provides a controlled atmosphere of oxygen and humidity.

These infants respond well to being removed from the tent and administered supplemental oxygen with a mask while being cuddled by the parents or staff. The noise level in croup tents is reasonably high, and it is recommended that the infants be removed from this environment frequently. We also utilize an infant hood seat, which enables the infant to receive supplemental oxygen and sit upright, which augments the neonate's labored respirations and enables him to observe his surroundings (Fig. 3–8).

Aggressive pulmonary hygiene is also used as treatment for this disease and many of these infants benefit from aerosol therapy prior to treatment.

The objectives of therapy are to relieve the severe respiratory symptoms with oxygen, humidity and pulmonary hygiene and to control the patient's cor pulmonale until his pulmonary status improves. Perhaps with the increasing application of continuous positive airway pressure, which enables such patients to maintain adequate arterial oxygen tensions at reduced F_{IO_2} levels, there will be a decreased incidence of this debilitating syndrome.

TRANSIENT TACHYPNEA

Transient tachypnea is a syndrome seen in term infants in the newborn nursery. During the first hours of life, these infants exhibit consistently high respiratory rates up to 120 breaths a minute. The infant's blood gases usually are within normal limits and the lungs are free from rales and rhonchi.

Chest x-rays reveal a wet-looking lung with prominent central streaking and possibly an enlarged heart.

It is believed that this syndrome may be a result of slow absorption of amniotic fluid in the lung. It generally clears within 3–5 days and is not associated with any complications or long-term sequelae.

Management consists of cardiopulmonary monitoring and careful observation within the first few hours of life, since it sometimes is difficult to differentiate transient tachypnea from the early stages of hyaline membrane disease.

PULMONARY HEMORRHAGE

Massive pulmonary hemorrhage (MPH) in the newborn has been seen with increasing incidence in recent years (Boothby and deSa[14]). The pathogenesis of this disease is not well defined but is thought to be interstitial or intra-alveolar hemorrhage occurring in two or more lung lobes that are free from infection.

The etiology of this disease is diverse and obscure. MPH has been seen in low birth weight infants and in infants suffering from intrapartum asphyxia, anoxic brain damage and cerebral edema. Boothby and deSa believe that intensive high-concentration oxygen therapy for prolonged periods may be partially responsible for the disease. Pulmonary hemorrhage is also seen as a complication of other disorders of the newborn period (e.g., pneumonia, especially group B beta-streptococcal pneumonia, hyaline membrane disease, aspiration of maternal blood, defective coagulation and hypothermia).

More recent studies conducted by Cole et al.[15] indicate that many of these infants are suffering from acute left ventricular failure, which results in an increase in pulmonary capillary pressure, resulting in the swift movement of hemorrhagic fluid into the alveoli. They attribute the left ventricular failure to the high incidence of asphyxia, with concurrent acidosis and hypoxia seen in these neonates.

The clinical symptoms noted by Cole et al. include peripheral vasoconstriction, bradycardia and apnea, or gasping respirations several minutes prior to the occurrence of the hemorrhage. In infants who were intubated, the bloody fluid pours through the endotracheal tube, completely occluding it. In the infants who were not intubated, this fluid was found pouring from the vocal cords into the oropharynx. Many of these infants require vigorous resuscitation and aspiration of the secretions in the airway. Frequent aspiration is required, since many of the infants continue to hemorrhage. Blood gases drawn as the hemorrhage occurred indicated a marked metabolic acidosis (base deficit − 15 to − 19 mEq/l) (Cole *et al.*[15]).

Mechanical ventilation frequently is required for these patients, but it generally is not successful. Positive end expiratory pressure (PEEP) may result in improvement, as may prolonged inspiratory times and reversed inspiratory-expiratory ratios (Reynolds[16]). The mortality rate in this disease is high.

DIAPHRAGMATIC HERNIA

This congenital condition results from the incomplete fusion of the embryonic diaphragm. In the eighth to tenth week of gestation, the diaphragm is formed, separating the thoracic cavity from the abdomi-

Fig. 3–9. — Diaphragmatic hernia. Note the abdominal contents in the left chest with a shift of the mediastinal structure to the right; also note paucity of bowel gas pattern in the abdomen.

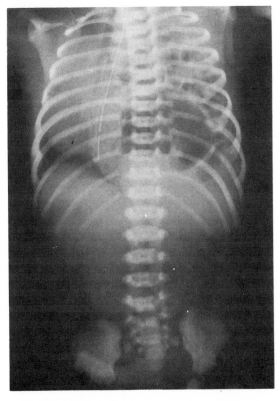

nal cavity. During this same time, the embryo is undergoing major gastrointestinal development. As a result of an incomplete fusion of the components of the diaphragm, the stomach and intestines may herniate into the thoracic cavity. The most common site of herniation is through a posterolateral defect at the foramen of Bochdalek. This defect accounts for approximately 80% of the left-sided hernias. There is a lower incidence of right-sided hernias (see Chap. 1).

The presence of these abdominal organs in the thoracic cavity results in a hypoplastic (underdeveloped) or compressed (after development) lung on the affected side. The extent of the herniation will determine the degree of pulmonary compromise. Most of the neonates affected exhibit respiratory distress at birth, with cyanosis, flaring of the nasal alae and severe retractions.

The diagnosis may be made by a chest roentgenogram (Fig. 3–9). The affected hemithorax will contain air-filled loops of bowel or the stomach, and the presence of these organs may result in a displacement of the heart toward the unaffected side.

The treatment is an immediate reduction of the hernia by withdrawing the viscera from the chest and surgical correction of the congenital defect. The "hypoplastic" lung, caused by loops of bowel being in the chest, will gradually expand in a week or two. Although low-pressure intermittent positive-pressure breathing (IPPB) may be indicated, aggressive attempts at expanding the lung quickly should be avoided.

CHOANAL ATRESIA

Choanal atresia is a congenital anomaly characterized by a failure of adequate development of the nares, with blockage of one or both nares by a membranous or bony closure. Since infants are obligate nose breathers, those afflicted with a bilateral obstruction generally will exhibit respiratory distress shortly after birth. These infants may be cyanotic and have severe intercostal, substernal or suprasternal retractions.

Infants with unilateral obstruction may remain completely asymptomatic. However, the insertion of a nasogastric tube into the infant's only patent nostril may cause him to have respiratory distress. If gastric decompression is necessary in these cases, an orogastric tube should be used. If a physician suspects choanal atresia, the definitive diagnosis may be made by instillation of contrast medium into the nares, and a lateral skull x-ray will demonstrate the obstruction. The immediate form of treatment should be the insertion of an oral airway. The airway may be secured by adhesive tape or twill tape wrapped around the airway and tied behind the patient's neck. Many of these infants are more comfortable in the prone position, since this opens the airway by allowing the tongue to fall forward.

The patient's condition influences the need for immediate surgical correction. The infants who display severe respiratory compromise must be repaired immediately. The infants who are asymptomatic may be corrected whenever the physician believes that it is appropriate. Surgical correction consists of perforation of the membranous or bony obstruction. Short pieces of endotracheal tubes or catheters then are inserted into the nares to keep them patent while they heal. This procedure should be done in the operating room by trained surgeons.

CONGENITAL LOBAR EMPHYSEMA

The incidence of congenital lobar emphysema is low. Those neonates afflicted with this anomaly exhibit extreme respiratory distress. They may be cyanotic and dyspneic, with rapid, labored respirations. Intercostal retractions, suprasternal indrawing and flaring of the nasal alae are quite common.

On physical examination, the affected hemithorax usually is hyperresonant, with diminished air entry on that side accompanied by an expiratory wheeze. The mediastinum frequently is displaced toward the unaffected hemithorax.

Congenital lobar emphysema occurs most frequently in the left upper lobe, but it has been reported to occur in the right middle lobe and the right upper lobe. The lower lobe on the affected side generally is compressed and atelectatic and the emphysematous lobe herniates into the anterior mediastinum and results in mediastinal shift.

The pathogenesis of this defect is not clearly defined. The defect may be a result of softer than normal cartilaginous rings that allowed air to enter the lobe on inspiration but collapsed on expiration and trapped the air. This collapse or narrowing of the bronchus during expiration may be responsible for the expiratory wheeze so commonly heard. The presence of mucus or a fold of skin in the airway that acts as a check valve may also be responsible for the anomaly.

Since the clinical symptoms of this entity closely resemble spontaneous pneumothorax, a chest radiograph should be obtained to make the diagnosis.

The treatment consists of surgical resection of the affected lobe, with a chest tube in place for re-expansion of the remaining lung lobes. Some infants are not treated but followed closely, and in several cases the emphysematous lobes have resolved. On follow-up radiologic examinations, these resolved lobes appear translucent. The prognosis for neonates who are afflicted with this anomaly is quite good and there generally is no recurrence of the emphysema.

REFERENCES

Cited References

1. Beard, R., *et al.:* pH of foetal capillary blood as an indicator of the condition of the fetus, J. Obstet. Gynaecol. Br. Commonw. 74:812, 1967.
2. Avery, M.: *The Lung and Its Disorders in the Newborn Infant* (2d ed.; Philadelphia: W. B. Saunders Company, 1968).
3. Klaus, M. H., and Fanaroff, A. A.: *Care of the High Risk Neonate* (Philadelphia: W. B. Saunders Company, 1973).
4. Gregory, G. A., Ketterman, J. A., Phibbser, H., Tooley, W. H., and Hamilton, W. K.: Treatment of the idiopathic respiratory distress syndrome with continuous positive airway pressure, N. Engl. J. Med. 284:1333, 1971.
5. Waterston, D. J., Bonham-Carter, R. E., and Aberdeen, E.: Congenital tracheo-oesophageal fistula in association with oesophageal atresia, Lancet 2:55, 1963.
6. Wilson, M. G., and Mikity, V. G.: A new form of respiratory disease in premature infants, Am. J. Dis. Child. 99:489, 1960.
7. Avery, M., and Schaffer, A. J.: *Diseases of the Newborn* (3d ed.; Philadelphia: W. B. Saunders Company, 1971).
8. Miller, H., Behrle, F., and Smull, N.: Severe apnea and irregular respiratory rhythms among premature infants, Pediatrics 23:676, 1959.
9. Shannon, D. C., Felicita, G., and Stein, I.: Prevention of apnea and bradycardia in low-birthweight infants, Pediatrics 55:589, 1975.
10. Macklin, C.: Transport of air along sheaths of pulmonic blood vessels from alveoli to mediastinum, Arch. Intern. Med. 64:913, 1939.
11. Brano, Y. W., Pitts, M., and Cassady, G.: Neonatal pneumopericardium, Am. J. Dis. Child. 130:393, 1976.
12. Northway, W. H., Rosan, R. C., and Porter, D. Y.: Pulmonary disease following respiratory therapy of hyaline membrane disease: Bronchopulmonary dysplasia, N. Engl. J. Med. 276:357, 1967.
13. Stern, L.: The use and misuse of oxygen in the newborn infant, Pediatr. Clin. North Am. 20:447, 1973.
14. Boothby, C. B., and deSa, D. J.: Massive pulmonary hemorrhage in the newborn, a changing pattern, Arch. Dis. Child. 48:21, 1973.
15. Cole, V., Norman, I., Reynolds, E., *et al.:* Pathogenesis of hemorrhagic pulmonary edema and massive pulmonary hemorrhage in the newborn, Pediatrics 51:175, 1973.
16. Reynolds, E. O.: Effects of alterations in mechanical ventilator settings on pulmonary gas exchange in hyaline membrane disease, Arch. Dis. Child. 46:152, 1971.

Suggested Readings

RESPIRATORY DISTRESS SYNDROME

Banerju, C. K., Girling, D. J., and Wigglesworth, J. S.: Pulmonary fibroplasia in newborn babies treated with oxygen and artificial ventilation, Arch. Dis. Child. 47:509, 1972.

Berg, J. J., Pagtakhan, R. D., Reed, M. H., Langston, C., and Chernick, V.: Bronchopulmonary dysplasia and lung rupture in hyaline membrane disease — influence of continuous distending airway pressure, Pediatrics 55:51, 1972.

Boston, R., Geller, F., and Smith, C.: Arterial blood gas tensions and acid-base balance in the management of respiratory distress syndrome, J. Pediatr. 68:74, 1966.

Chernick, V.: Continuous distending pressure in hyaline membrane disease: Of devices, disadvantages and a daring study, Pediatrics 52:114, 1973.

Chernick, V., and Vidyasagar, D.: Continuous negative chest wall pressure in hyaline membrane disease: One year experience, Pediatrics 49:753, 1972.

Dewhurst, C. J., Dunham, A. M., Harvey, D. R., and Parkinson, C. E.: Prediction of respiratory distress syndrome by estimation of surfactant in the amniotic fluid, Lancet 1:1475, 1973.

Hawker, J. M., Reynolds, E. O., and Taghizadeh, A.: Pulmonary surface tension and pathological changes in infants dying after respirator treatment for severe hyaline membrane disease, Lancet 2:75, 1967.

Hawks, J. M., Reynolds, E. O. R., and Taghizadeh, A.: Pulmonary surface tension and pathologic changes in infants dying (with) after respiratory treatment for severe hyaline membrane disease, Lancet 2:75, 1967.

Joshi, V. V., Mandavia, S. G., Stern, L., and Wiglesworth, F. W.: Acute lesions induced by endotracheal intubation, Am. J. Dis. Child. 124:646, 1972.

Miller, M. H.: The roentgenographic course and complications of hyaline membrane disease, Pediatr. Clin. North Am. 20:381, 1973.

Prod'hom, L. S., et al.: Care of the seriously ill neonate with hyaline membrane disease and with sepsis (sclerema neonatorum), Pediatrics 53:170, 1974.

Stahlmann, L., Hedwall, G., Dolanski, E., Fanelius, G., Burko, H., and Kirk, V.: A six year follow-up of clinical hyaline membrane disease, Pediatr. Clin. North Am. 20:433, 1973.

ESOPHAGEAL ATRESIA

Clatworthy, W. H.: Esophageal atresia: Importance of early diagnosis and adequate treatment illustrated by a series of patients, Pediatrics 16:22, 1955.

Grow, J. B., and Neerken, A. J.: Esophageal atresia and tracheoesophageal fistula, JAMA 152:1614, 1953.

Kappelman, M. M., Dorst, J., Haller, J. A., and Stambler, A.: H-type tracheoesophageal fistula, Am. J. Dis. Child. 118:568, 1969.

PULMONARY DYSMATURITY

Burnard, E. D.: The pulmonary syndrome of Wilson and Mikity, Pediatr. Clin. North Am. 13:999, 1964.

Krauss, A. N., Klain, D. B., and Auld, P. A. M.: Chronic pulmonary insufficiency of prematurity (CPIP), Pediatrics 55:55, 1975.

Thibeault, D. W., Grossman, H., Hagstrom, J. W. C., and Auld, P. A. M.: Radiologic findings in the lungs of premature infants, J. Pediatr. 74:1, 1969.

APNEA

Perlstein, P., Edwards, H., and Sutherland, J.: Apnea in premature infants and incubator-air temperature changes, N. Engl. J. Med. 282:461, 1970.

PNEUMOTHORAX, PNEUMOMEDIASTINUM, PNEUMOPERICARDIUM

Chernick, V., and Avery, M. E.: Spontaneous alveolar rupture at birth, Pediatrics 32:816, 1963.

Kirkpatrick, B. V., Felman, A. H., and Eitzman, D. V.: Complications of ventilator therapy in respiratory distress syndrome: Recognition and management of acute air leaks, Am. J. Dis. Child. 128:496, 1974.

Leonidas, J. C., and Rhodes, P. G.: Pneumoperitoneum in ventilated newborns, Am. J. Dis. Child. 128:677, 1974.

Lubchenco, L. O.: Recognition of spontaneous pneumothorax in premature infants, Pediatrics 24:996, 1959.

Markarian, M., and Ablow, R. C.: Neonatal pneumopericardium, Pediatrics 47:634, 1971.

Mikity, V. G., and Taber, P.: Complications in the treatment of the respiratory distress syndrome, Pediatr. Clin. North Am. 20:419, 1973.

Miller, R. D., and Hamilton, W. K.: Pneumothorax during infant resuscitation, JAMA 210:1090, 1969.

BRONCHOPULMONARY DYSPLASIA

Nash, G., Blennerhassett, J. B., and Pontoppedan, J.: Pulmonary lesions associated with oxygen therapy and artificial ventilation, N. Engl. J. Med. 276: 368, 1967.

Philip, A. G. S.: Oxygen plus pressure plus time: The etiology of bronchopulmonary dysplasia, Pediatrics 55:44, 1975.

TRANSIENT TACHYPNEA

Avery, M., Gatewood, O., and Brumley, G.: Transient tachypnea of newborns, Am. J. Dis. Child. 111:380, 1966.

PULMONARY HEMORRHAGE

Ceballos, R.: Aspiration of maternal blood in the etiology of massive pulmonary hemorrhage in the newborn infant, J. Pediatr. 72:390, 1968.

Chessells, J. M., and Wigglesworth, J. S.: Secondary hemorrhagic disease of the newborn, Arch. Dis. Child. 45:539, 1970.

McAdams, A. J.: Pulmonary hemorrhage in the newborn, Am. J. Dis. Child. 113:255, 1967.

DIAPHRAGMATIC HERNIA

Butler, N., and Claireaux, A. E.: Congenital diaphragmatic hernia as a cause of perinatal mortality, Lancet 1:659, 1962.

Carter, R. E., Waterston, D. J., and Aberdeen, E.: Hernia and eventration of the diaphragm in childhood, Lancet 1:656, 1962.

CONGENITAL LOBAR EMPHYSEMA

Holzel, A., Bennett, E., and Vaughan, B. F.: Congenital lobar emphysema, Arch. Dis. Child. 31:216, 1956.

White-Jones, R. H., and Temple, L. J.: Congenital lobar emphysema, Arch. Dis. Child. 29:248, 1954.

4 / Radiologic Findings in Newborn Respiratory Disease

BERNARD BLUMENTHAL, M.D.

THE EVALUATION of the chest roentgenogram of the newborn must be done in a systematic manner. To be evaluated are: chest configuration, lung infiltrates, pulmonary vasculature, heart size and configuration, mediastinal position, liver size, catheter and tube position, abdominal gas pattern and bone structure. With repetition, this systematic scanning of the roentgenograms will become automatic.

The shape (configuration) of the newborn's chest is basically that of a truncated cone with two concave impressions on the base of the cone. In the lateral projection, the ribs should slope gently downward from back to front. The diaphragms should be well rounded in both projections (Fig. 4 – 1).

When the lungs are overaerated, the cone configuration is lost; the anterior chest wall begins to parallel the spine and the lateral chest wall angles begin to diverge. The diaphragmatic domes are depressed, flattened or even inverted. The upper ribs no longer slope downward anteriorly but are horizontal.

With underaeration, the chest volume is noticeably decreased and the diaphragms are elevated. The anterior chest wall may become concave. The ribs slope sharply downward.

In the normal newborn, if one searches carefully, the pulmonary vessels can be seen as sharply defined structures all the way out to the chest wall. With minimal pulmonary infiltrates, the outlines of the fine peripheral vessels are lost and the vessels fade into the background. With increasing severity, the infiltrates become patchy or fluffy areas of lung opacification. The entire lung or large anatomic lung segments may become completely opacified (consolidated).

The pulmonary vasculature is difficult to evaluate in the newborn because of the small size of the vessels and because of the rapid changes in the pulmonary circulation in the first several days of life.

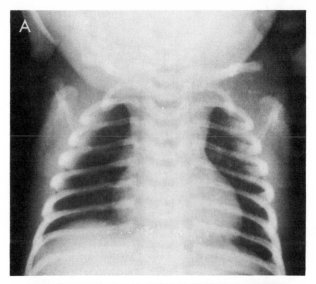

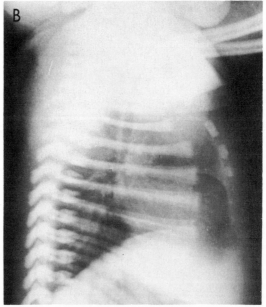

Fig. 4–1.—Normal newborn chest: AP **(A)** and lateral **(B)**. Note the triangular shape of the chest, the rounded configuration of the diaphragms, the downward slope of the ribs and the prominent triangular right lobe of the thymus gland.

Once the change from fetal to infantile hemodynamics is made (about 72–96 hours of life), one should be able to make out three to five pulmonary vessels in the medial aspect of both lung bases as seen through the heart. These vessels should taper gently and should disappear as they cross beneath the diaphragm.

The size of the heart is difficult to evaluate in the first day of life because of the rapidly changing cardiovascular dynamics. After the first day of life, the transverse diameter of the heart should not exceed 60% of the transverse diameter of the lungs on an inspiratory film.

The cardiac and thymic outlines generally are inseparable, making evaluation of cardiac configuration difficult. The shape of both the heart and thymus changes with respiration and the cardiac cycle. With stress, the thymus will shrink dramatically. Either lobe of the thymus may extend to the diaphragm; however, the right lobe usually terminates at the horizontal fissure.

In the frontal roentgenogram, the mediastinum should be in the midline. Unilateral change in the volume of one hemithorax will cause a shift in the position of the mediastinum. The mediastinum will shift away from an area of increased volume and toward an area of decreased volume.

The liver is well seen in neonates because of the relatively large volume of gas present in the bowel. Liver size can be just as easily evaluated by palpation; however, clinical assessment can be thrown off by high or low position of the right diaphragm. Although there are no standards for liver size in the neonate, serial observations are valuable, especially in the early detection of right heart failure.

Umbilical vascular catheters are used for monitoring of blood gases, blood sugar, acid-base balance and central venous pressure. They are also used for the infusion of blood, fluids and electrolytes and for exchange transfusions. The position of these vascular catheters must be carefully assessed radiographically.

The ideal umbilical venous catheter position is in the inferior vena cava just below the entrance of the cava into the right atrium or in the right atrium itself. The optimal position of the umbilical arterial catheter is in the descending aorta between the fourth and eleventh thoracic vertebral body or in the abdominal aorta between the second and third lumbar vertebral bodies. The gross anatomy of the major arteries and veins and their connections with the umbilical vessels are shown in Figure 4–1.

The position of the endotracheal tube should be carefully noted in both the frontal and lateral radiographs of the chest. The division of the trachea into right and left main bronchi in the newborn occurs at about the level of the fourth thoracic vertebral body. Ideally, the tip of the endotracheal tube should be between the second and third thoracic vertebral bodies. If the tip of the tube slips into one of the main bronchi, the opposite lung usually will collapse.

Occasionally the endotracheal tube will be inadvertently passed into the esophagus. In this situation, the stomach and bowel will become massively distended with air and the tube can be seen to lie behind the normally air-filled trachea.

The upper abdomen usually is included in the chest radiographs of the newborn, allowing evaluation of the bowel gas pattern. The stomach of the neonate usually fills with air immediately after birth. The air should reach the rectum in 6–8 hours. When bowel obstruction is present there is progressive gaseous distention of the bowel down to the point of obstruction.

A gasless abdomen is seen in certain types of esophageal atresia, diaphragmatic hernia and midgut volvulus.

Air free in the peritoneal cavity may be seen in the supine frontal views, but usually special views of the abdomen are needed to demonstrate the full extent of the pneumoperitoneum. Pneumoperitoneum most commonly is due to neonatal gastric perforation but will be seen whenever any portion of the bowel is perforated or as a rare sequela to pneumomediastinum.

Last, the bony structures of the thorax, neck and skull should be scanned. Gestational age of the infant can be estimated by the appearance of the tooth buds or, more accurately, by the length of the thoracic spine. A bell-shaped configuration of the thorax may be seen in the infant with central nervous system damage or in the overly sedated infant.

The ribs and spine should be scanned for congenital anomalies that may be associated with serious organ anomalies. The proximal humeri may be abnormal in congenital syphilis and intrauterine viral infections.

Generalized increased or decreased bone density may be seen in certain rare congenital (hereditary) bone diseases.

HYALINE MEMBRANE DISEASE (HMD)

The lungs of the infant with hyaline membrane disease are small, i.e., underaerated. The degree of underaeration correlates with the severity of the disease. The conical configuration of the chest is accentuated; the "cone" becomes short and squat. The diaphragms are elevated and the downward slope of the ribs becomes more acute.

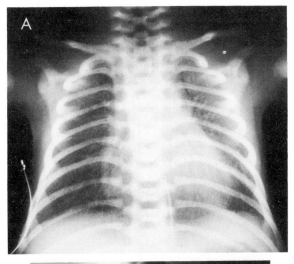

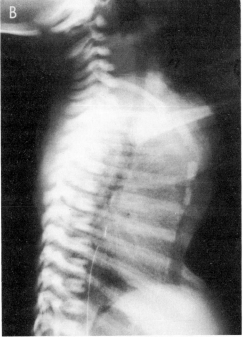

Fig. 4–2.—Hyaline membrane disease: AP **(A)** and lateral **(B)** chest. Lung volume is less than normal. The thorax is narrow and the heart appears to be enlarged. There is a fine, diffuse granular pattern of density over the lungs.

The pattern of lung density in HMD varies with the severity of the disease from a faint finely granular to a finely lacy to a complete "white-out" with a prominent air bronchogram (Fig. 4–2).

As the HMD resolves, the lungs tend to clear from peripheral to central and from upper to lower and the lung volume increases to normal. Complete resolution of the radiographic findings of mild to moderate HMD may take as long as 2–3 weeks.

One of the common complications of HMD is persistent patency of the ductus arteriosus. With resolution of the HMD and decreasing pulmonary vascular resistance, the patent ductus manifests itself by increasing heart size, prominence of the pulmonary vessels and increasing liver size (Fig. 4–3). These changes are apparent radiographically some time before the infant exhibits clinical evidence of congestive heart failure.

Occasionally, an extremely ill infant with HMD will develop patchy, shifting areas of diffuse lung opacification representing areas of pulmonary hemorrhage. This event usually is preterminal and may be accompanied by cerebral hemorrhage.

The use of mechanical respirators to sustain infants with HMD may lead to the "air-leak phenomena" of bronchial dilatation, interstitial emphysema, pneumomediastinum, pneumothorax, pneumopericardium, pneumoperitoneum and cervical emphysema. These phenomena occur in a predictable sequence; the entire sequence may not be seen in every affected infant, since each radiograph depicts only a small fraction of a second of the infant's life. With increased end expiratory pressure and prolongation of the expiratory phase of respiration, the small central airways and alveoli become progressively distended. Radiographically, the dilated airways are seen as multiple uniform central bubbles of air that never exceed 1.5 mm in diameter.

With increasing airway pressure, air may leak from a weakened alveolus into the supporting structure of the lung (the interstitium), giving rise to large irregular streaks and bubbles of air that may extend to the periphery of the lung. The involved lung increases in volume due to "inflation" of the interstitium (Fig. 4–4).

The interstitial air will follow the vessels back to the mediastinum, giving rise to a pneumomediastinum. Air in the mediastinum usually is confined to a small area immediately above and anterior to the heart. The usual "occupant" of this compartment, the thymus, is displaced upward and outward by the air, giving rise to the "spinnaker" sign in the frontal view of the chest (Fig. 4–5). Occasionally, the mediastinal air may extend beneath the lung, between the pleura and the diaphragm. This is not part of a pneumothorax and is distinguished

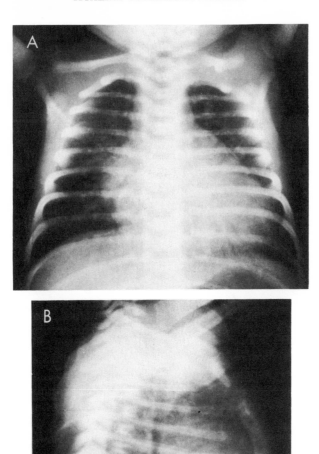

Fig. 4–3.—Patent ductus arteriosus: AP **(A)** and lateral **(B)** chest. The heart is enlarged and the pulmonary vessels are very prominent.

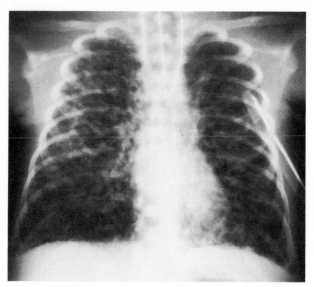

Fig. 4–4. — Pulmonary interstitial emphysema: AP chest. The lung volume is markedly increased. There are multitudes of large irregular streaks and bubbles of air in the lung interstitium. The chest tube on the left was used to decompress a pneumothorax.

from a pneumothorax by the way the air conforms to the curvature of the diaphragm without extending over the lateral and medial aspects of the lung.

If the peripheral air leak continues, the pneumomediastinum may progress to pneumothorax, pneumopericardium, cervical emphysema or pneumoperitoneum.

Pneumothorax is the consequence of escape of air from the mediastinum into the pleural space. It causes collapse of the lung on the involved side and, with increasing volume, may compress the lung on the unaffected side. The lung of the infant with HMD is too stiff to totally collapse as a result of air in the pleural space. Consequently, small early pneumothoraces frequently are overlooked. The radiographic signs of a small, early pneumothorax in the frontal view are: (1) increased volume of the involved side with widening of the spaces between the ribs, flattening of the diaphragm and shift of the mediastinum (heart) away from the involved side and (2) increased sharpness of the marginal outline of the heart and mediastinum on the involved side. This latter phenomenon is due to the interposition of the anterior accumulation of pleural air between the lung and the heart border.

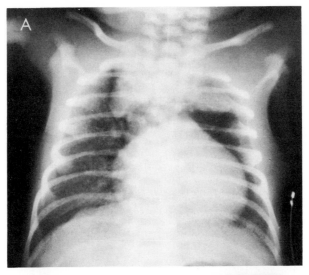

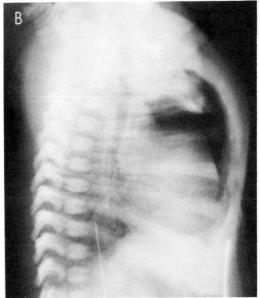

Fig. 4–5.—Pneumomediastinum: AP **(A)** and lateral **(B)** chest. Note the air above and anterior to the heart outlining the sail-shaped thymus gland (the spinnaker sign).

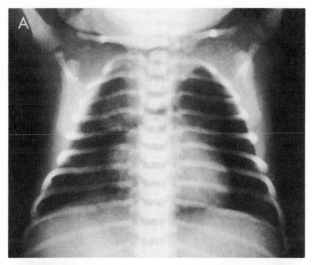

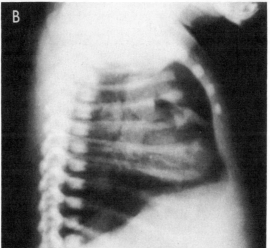

Fig. 4–6.—Subtle left pneumothorax and pneumomediastinum: AP **(A)** and lateral **(B)** chest. The pneumothorax on the left is causing an increase in volume of the left hemithorax and is accentuating the left heart border. In the lateral view, the air in the mediastinum outlines the normally hidden thymus gland.

The pleural air first accumulates anteriorly because the infant is supine and air rises (Fig. 4–6). In the lateral view, the pneumothorax is seen as a lucent strip interposed between the anterior chest wall and the lung.

As the volume of the pneumothorax increases, the air is seen to to-

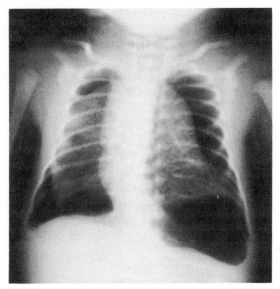

Fig. 4–7.—Bilateral tension pneumothoraces: AP chest. Thoracic volume is increased and the lungs are surrounded by free air. The stiff diseased lungs cannot totally collapse.

tally surround the lung. There is increasing shift of the mediastinum, with consequent compression collapse of the uninvolved lung, with disastrous consequences (Fig. 4–7).

In rare instances, air in the mediastinum may enter the pericardium, causing compression of the heart. The radiographic appearance of pneumopericardium is distinctive; a crescent of air will be seen extending around and *beneath* the heart (Fig. 4–8).

Pneumomediastinum may extend upward along the trachea, esophagus and vessels into the neck and even into the facial soft tissues. This cervical and facial emphysema is of no clinical significance but the infants so affected have a bizarre clinical and radiographic appearance.

The mediastinal air may also decompress along the aorta, vena cava and esophagus into the peritoneal space. The resulting pneumoperitoneum causes some problems: (1) the consequent elevation of the diaphragm further compromises lung volume and (2) pneumoperitoneum from air leak must be differentiated from that due to a bowel perforation, which is a surgical problem. Although not 100% diagnostic, the pressure of air *and fluid* in the peritoneum is characteristic of a bowel perforation.

Some infants who survive HMD and air-leak complications may

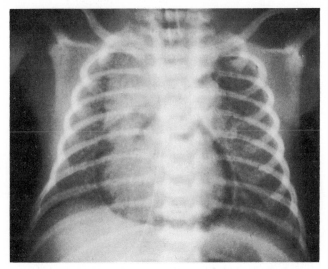

Fig. 4–8.—Pneumopericardium: AP chest. Note the halo of air completely surrounding the heart; this occurs only in pneumopericardium.

develop a form of long-lasting lung disease known as bronchopulmonary dysplasia (respirator lung disease). These infants initially exhibit the classic radiographic findings of HMD (1–3 days), followed by increasingly dense, granular infiltrates that tend to obliterate cardiac and diaphragmatic margins. From 10 to 20 days of age, the pattern of abnormality changes to one of small cyst-like areas in the otherwise opaque lungs. Beyond 1 month of age, the survivors demonstrate a lace-like pattern of interspersed strands of increased density and irregular lucent, cyst-like areas accompanied by generalized increased lung volume. The end stage lung disease may be accompanied by an enlarged heart, probably due to persistence of the ductus arteriosus. The children who develop respirator lung disease may become "respiratory cripples."

MECONIUM ASPIRATION SYNDROME

The aspiration of meconium-contaminated amniotic fluid can occur in any newborn with moderate or severe fetal distress but is most common in the postmature and other small-for-gestational-age neonates. Fetal hypoxia induces gasping, which sucks the meconium-contaminated amniotic fluid into the tracheobronchial tree. The tenacious, viscous, meconium particles then cause diffuse bronchial obstruction. Some airways are totally blocked, causing collapse

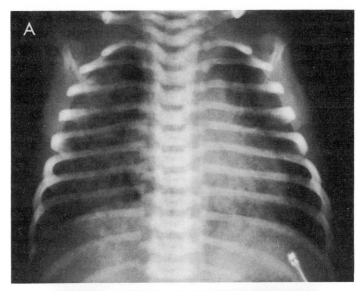

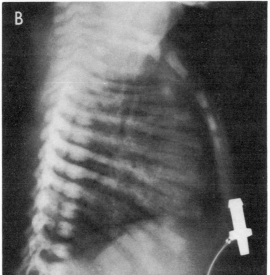

Fig. 4–9.—Meconium aspiration syndrome: AP **(A)** and lateral **(B)** chest. The lung volume is increased. There are coarse asymmetric infiltrates throughout both lungs. This pattern may be described as "ropy."

(atelectasis) of the alveoli distal to the block; other airways are partially occluded, causing distal overaeration.

The radiographic picture of meconium aspiration usually is that of an over-all increase in lung volume (overaeration) accompanied by varying amounts of asymmetrically distributed, coarse, patchy lung infiltrates (Fig. 4–9). The severity of the overaeration usually parallels the infant's respiratory distress.

Mild cases of meconium aspiration clear rapidly in 24–72 hours whereas the more severe cases may take 1–2 weeks to clear completely. Infants with meconium aspiration syndrome may develop air-leak phenomena without the assistance of respirators.

NEONATAL PNEUMONIA

The neonate may acquire pneumonia in utero (transplacental or ascending infection), during delivery or postnatally. The causative agent may be bacterial, viral, fungal, protozoan or chemical.

The radiographic findings in pneumonia are increased lung volume (overaeration) and asymmetric pulmonary infiltrates (Fig. 4–10). The infiltrates may vary in severity from fine, almost invisible accentuation of the lung markings to dense patches of fluffy density to total consolidation of part or all of the lung.

Although the chest radiograph is the most reliable means for detecting pneumonia, the radiographs are of no value in determining the causative agent. Only appropriate bacteriologic and virologic tests can identify the particular causative organism.

TRANSIENT TACHYPNEA OF THE NEWBORN (WET LUNG SYNDROME)

Transient tachypnea of the newborn (TTN) is caused by delayed resorption of normal fetal lung fluid. The affected infants are deprived of the full force of the thoracic "squeeze," which during vaginal delivery normally forces up to one-third of the fetal fluid from the lungs. The lung fluid then must be resorbed by pulmonary capillaries and lymphatics.

The radiographic findings in TTN are increased lung volume, fine diffuse pulmonary infiltrates, prominence of the pulmonary vessels, fluid in the lung fissures and slight enlargement of the heart (Fig. 4–11). The radiographic abnormalities gradually resolve in 3 days. This clearing trend usually can be seen in the first 12–18 hours of life.

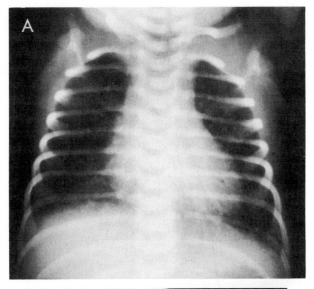

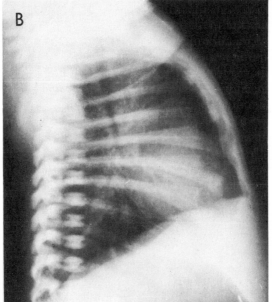

Fig. 4–10.—Pneumonia: AP **(A)** and lateral **(B)** chest. The lung volume is increased and there are fine patchy infiltrates throughout both lungs.

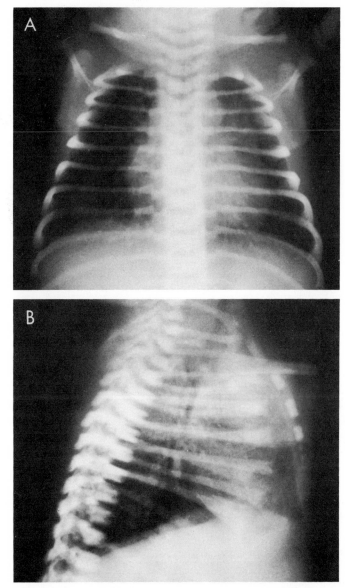

Fig. 4–11.—Transient tachypnea of the newborn (wet lung syndrome): AP **(A)** and lateral **(B)** chest. The lung volume is increased, the pulmonary vessels are prominent, there is fluid in the lung fissures and the heart is slightly enlarged.

SELECTED REFERENCES

Caffey, J.: *Pediatric X-ray Diagnosis* (7th ed.; Chicago: Year Book Medical Publishers, Inc., 1978).

Singleton, E. B., and Wagner, M. C.: *Radiographic Atlas of Pulmonary Disorders in Children* (Philadelphia: W. B. Saunders Company, 1971).

Swischuk, L. E.: *Radiology of the Newborn and Young Infant* (Baltimore: The Williams & Wilkins Company, 1973).

Wesenberg, R. K.: *The Newborn Chest* (New York: Harper & Row, 1973).

5 / Pharmacology for Respiratory Care of the Newborn

BRUCE R. PARKS, JR., PH.D.

DRUGS, with the notable exception of the antibiotics, exert their effects through the alteration of physiologic processes. These effects can be either beneficial or harmful and are the result of some change brought about in the individual being treated.

In order for a drug to have an effect, it must reach the location at which it can influence homeostatic mechanisms. To be of clinical value, drugs must also be eliminated once the desired action has occurred. These things are accomplished through the processes of absorption, distribution, biotransformation and excretion.

The newborn is unique in several respects in relation to his exposure to and handling of pharmacologic agents. In utero, the fetus is the indirect recipient of drugs and of their effects, which usually are intended for the maternal organism. Postnatal acquisition of drugs by the neonate must be with cognizance of the rapid physiologic and biochemical changes occurring in the developing organism.

PLACENTAL TRANSFER

Pharmacologic Principles

The placenta serves as an organ of both absorption and elimination for the fetus. Although physical intermixing of maternal and fetal blood does not occur, the two circulations are in such close approximation that rapid exchanges are possible. Both endogenous and exogenous agents cross the placenta and the transfer is not unidirectional.

The human placenta is of the villous hemochorial type. Nutrient-poor fetal blood enters the placenta by two umbilical arteries at the chorionic plate. These vessels successively divide into smaller and smaller branches until they form capillaries at the tip of fetal villi.

Maternal blood, thought to be spurted from spiral arteries into the intervillous space, flows upward to the chorionic plate, then back down to the decidua basalis and drains out of the uterine vein. Three layers separate fetal and maternal blood: the fetal trophoblast, connective tissue and the endothelium of fetal capillaries. An exchanging molecule must traverse these tissues as it passes from maternal to fetal plasma.

Several mechanisms are involved in placental transport:

1. Simple diffusion appears to be the primary mechanism by which substances cross the placenta. The transfer occurs in the direction of a concentration gradient; e.g., from an area of higher concentration to an area of lower concentration. The respiratory gases oxygen and carbon dioxide are transported in this manner, as are smaller ions, fatty acids and most drugs.

2. Facilitated diffusion also occurs down a concentration gradient, but at a faster rate than could be accounted for by a simple diffusion process. This mechanism is important for the transfer of glucose and other carbohydrates.

3. Active transport is an energy-requiring process by which substances can be transported against a concentration gradient. Amino acids, water-soluble vitamins and larger ions are transferred in this manner.

4. Bulk flow plays a minor role and involves the passage of substances through pores in the membranes.

5. Pinocytosis is a process by which substances are transferred across membranes in small vesicles. In humans, immune globulins appear to be transported in this manner.

6. Breaks in the placental architecture may allow the transfer of fetal red cells, which under certain conditions can lead to erythroblastosis fetalis.

Factors influencing permeability of the placenta to drugs may be related to physicochemical properties of the drug itself or to intrinsic properties of the placenta.

Membranes are lipoprotein in nature; therefore, compounds with high lipid solubility pass through them most rapidly. Drug molecules tend to penetrate biologic membranes more rapidly in their un-ionized state.

Although transfer of drugs occurs primarily through the membrane itself and not through pores, molecular size or weight will affect the transfer. In general, drugs with a molecular weight of less than 600 rapidly traverse the placenta whereas the placenta is relatively impermeable to those with a molecular weight of greater than 1000.

Transfer of highly lipid-soluble drugs appears to be proportional to placental blood flow. Anything that decreases placental blood flow, such as uterine contractions during labor, therefore will inhibit the transfer of drugs to the fetus.

Metabolism of drugs by the placenta has been demonstrated in vitro. Its significance in humans is not fully understood.

Placental thickness is also a determinant of transfer. With increasing length at gestation, the placenta becomes thinner, allowing for more ready passage of substances.

TERATOLOGY

Teratology in its simplest form refers to the production of congenital malformations by exogenous substances such as drugs or environmental agents. Congenital malformations result from an interaction between environmental and genetic factors, such as maternal infection, radiation and drug administration. The origin of the vast majority of congenital malformations, however, is as yet unexplained.

Four basic teratologic principles govern the possible occurrence of congenital malformations: the nature of the responsible agent and its accessibility to the fetus, the developmental state of the embryo or fetus, the level and duration of its dosage and the genetic make-up of the individual.

The timing and duration of exposure will determine the type of expected malformation. During the preimplantation period, which in humans usually is assumed to be the first 2 weeks following conception, there usually is an "all-or-none" response to an insult. Either the blastocyst is killed outright and expelled or no detectable damage occurs.

During the organogenetic period, the state of embryonic development is crucial with respect to the type of malformation produced. The central nervous system is at its greatest sensitivity at 15–25 days of gestation, the cardiovascular system at 20–40 days and the limbs at 24–46 days.

Organogenesis is essentially complete by 8–10 weeks. After this period, the fetus is at risk for the same drug-induced adverse effects as can be induced in adults.

Several agents can induce the same type of malformation, and one drug can induce more than one type. The genetic make-up modifies environmental influences so that the final response differs among species, strains and individuals. This explains why teratogenic potential is not always discovered in animal models and, conversely, why teratogenicity in animals does not always cause the same result in humans.

The teratogenic dose of a particular agent may be difficult to determine. It lies between the amount that causes a temporary impairment and one that causes fetal death. Teratogenicity generally, but not always, follows a dose-effect relationship. The total dose and length of exposure must also be considered. Repeated dosage can result in changes whereas a single exposure may not. This is exemplified by the production of a cluster of defects known as the fetal alcohol syndrome.

DRUGS ADMINISTERED DURING LABOR AND DELIVERY

The other major time at which the fetus is exposed to drugs that may represent a hazard is during the intrapartal period. Drugs administered for maternal comfort may be transferred to the fetus, which, after delivery, is dependent on its own immature or compromised processes for metabolism and excretion. It is particularly important to recognize when an infant's symptoms may be the result of a self-limited intoxication and not due to hypoxic-ischemic or traumatic events.

During the labor and delivery process, the baby is exposed to a wide variety of drugs that may affect him. Much dependence is placed on the Apgar score, which has proved to be an extremely valuable tool. However, those insults that lower the Apgar score must be potent depressants and less gross or delayed effects may be missed.

Anesthesia and analgesia during labor and delivery are provided for maternal comfort. Both direct and indirect effects on the fetus must be considered when drugs are administered for this purpose. Systemic analgesics and anesthetics may have both direct and indirect effects whereas local anesthetics usually have only direct effects. It should be borne in mind that many factors may cause problems in the newborn. It is unusual to unequivocally prove that a specific drug has influenced the neonate.

Sedatives are used during the early first stage of labor to promote tranquility in the anxious patient. The drugs most commonly used for this purpose are the barbiturates. All are highly lipid-soluble molecules that easily penetrate membranes.

The brain receives a greater proportion of the cardiac output in utero than in newborn life, suggesting that relatively more drug might reach the fetal cerebral cortex when given during labor. Barbiturate obstetric sedation may cause poor sucking responses in infants for up to 4 days.

Neither pentobarbital nor secobarbital used in an intramuscular dosage of 100 mg will have significant effect on the ventilatory state of the mother. The correlation between maternal sedation and the clinical condition of the newborn does not suggest that these agents have a profound depressant effect on the normal newborn. In fetal and neonatal asphyxia, however, their additive effects could result in prolonged recovery from central nervous system depression.

Cesarean section with general anesthetics usually includes induction with a thiobarbiturate. The most commonly used agent is thiopental. This drug rapidly traverses the placenta, being detectable in fetal blood within 45 seconds. Despite its rapid passage across the placenta, thiopental in a single dose of 4 mg/kg is associated with the delivery of neonates with good Apgar scores.

All narcotics can produce some degree of fetal and neonatal depression. Fetal depression has been demonstrated by the onset of bradycardia following maternal administration of morphine. Neonatal effects are seen as respiratory depression, myosis, absence of reflexes and hypotonia.

One of the most widely used drugs for labor discomfort is meperidine. This drug is a synthetic narcotic once thought to be less depressant than morphine. However, when both drugs are given under similar conditions and at equianalgesic doses there is very little difference in the neonatal depression produced.

Meperidine rapidly crosses the placenta. The umbilical vein achieves 70% of the maternal level within 30 seconds following intravenous administration. Maternal/fetal equilibrium is reached within minutes. Normeperidine, meperidinic acid and normeperidinic acid, which are maternal metabolites, also cross the placenta. Biotransformation in the fetal liver may take up to 2–3 hours.

When administered intramuscularly to the mother between 1 and 3 hours prior to delivery, meperidine depresses the newborn. No significant lowering of Apgar scores occurs, however, if the meperidine is given less than 1 hour before delivery. This possibly can be explained on the basis that metabolic products of meperidine are more depressant on the neonate than is the parent compound.

In an effort to avoid this delayed depression, the drug may be given intravenously at the onset of a uterine contraction. Drugs administered by this route remain in a bolus for one or two circulation times. This creates local areas of high concentration, thus increasing the rate of transfer across permeable membranes, as discussed earlier. If the bolus of drug reaches the uterus at the peak of its contraction, uterine circulation is momentarily occluded, thus allowing the drug to distribute more evenly throughout the maternal circulation and decreasing the concentration presented to the placenta when the uterus relaxes and its blood flow is restored.

Pentazocine is a potent analgesic that is not currently subject to narcotic control. Although it has been used during labor, there are conflicting reports as to its depressant effects on the neonate, and its safety in pregnancy is not yet fully documented. Its possible advantages include a lesser emetic effect than meperidine and a reduced rate of placental transfer, although the latter is not certain.

Regional anesthesia for delivery has become the method of choice. This involves the local administration of two major types of anesthetics. The esters have a relatively slow onset of action, a short duration with poor tissue penetration and cross the placenta poorly. The amides have a rapid onset, prolonged duration and good tissue penetration. The latter type are the drugs most commonly used.

Maternal hypotension can be caused by regional block leading to placental insufficiency. Adequate maternal positioning and hydration usually can prevent this effect.

Excessive transplacental passage resulting in fetal toxicity is possible. All local anesthetics cross the placenta and detectable fetal plasma levels have been measured within 30 seconds of maternal administration.

Clinical manifestations of local anesthetic toxicity in the neonate include: seizures, bradycardia (observed most frequently), hypotonia, apnea and mydriasis. Although the CNS effects are similar to those seen with hypoxia, an early onset suggests local anesthetic poisoning.

Prompt resuscitation and maintenance of adequate ventilation are of paramount importance, since hypoxia usually poses the greatest threat to the infant's survival and prognosis for normalcy. Drug elimination can be promoted by forced diuresis. In the event of renal failure, gastric lavage and exchange transfusion provide alternatives. Treatment of local anesthetic seizures consists of the cautious use of anticonvulsants. The use of potent drugs is best avoided, as the intoxication generally is of a self-limiting nature.

One other drug used in labor deserves discussion, as it can exert profound effects on the newborn. Magnesium sulfate is used in the treatment of toxemia. It readily crosses the placenta and equilibrates between fetal and maternal blood. Clinical manifestations of hypermagnesemia in the newborn are evidenced by hypotonia, hyporeflexia, hypotension and respiratory depression. Magnesium is slowly excreted by the newborn, plasma concentrations requiring as long as

72–96 hours to become normal. Calcium is a physiologic antagonist in adults; however, its benefits in the newborn are not conclusively established.

RESUSCITATION

The primary effort in resuscitation should be aimed at establishing and maintaining adequate respiration. For this, oxygen is the drug of choice. It will not be further discussed in this chapter, as its uses have been covered elsewhere in this text.

Plasma Volume Expanders

Many preterm infants are volume depleted at birth secondary to in utero asphyxia. Hypovolemia is corrected by the use of various solutions, the required volume of which may be very large.

Whole blood, cross-matched against the mother's blood, should be used if sufficient warning is available. In an emergency, placental blood can be used. The placenta is cleaned with an iodine solution and blood withdrawn from the umbilical artery or vein into a syringe containing at least 1 unit of heparin for each milliliter of blood taken. The potential problem of sepsis militates against using this technique as a routine procedure.

Colloidal solutions may be used as blood substitutes. Salt-poor albumin is used frequently. This solution is available in a 25% strength and should be diluted to approximately 5% and given at a dose of 1 gm/kg of body weight. Plasma protein fraction or 5% human serum albumin may be administered at a dose of 10 ml/kg.

Isotonic crystalloids can be used as volume expanders. Sodium bicarbonate and saline solutions have been used. They do not remain in the vascular spaces as well as colloids and the production of hypernatremia must be considered.

Narcotic Antagonists

Neonatal depression as the result of maternal narcotic administration can be alleviated by the use of a narcotic antagonist. Nalorphine and levallorphan are partial agonists. This means that in the absence of narcotics, these drugs will themselves cause respiratory depression in the infant.

More recently, naloxone has been released for use in the neonate. This agent is a pure antagonist. It has a rapid onset and a short duration of action. It has the additional advantage of reversing the effects of pentazocine, which is not true of the partial agonists.

Naloxone can be administered intravenously or intramuscularly in a dose of 0.01 mg/kg of body weight. If no result is apparent, it may be repeated within 2 minutes.

Other Agents

The metabolic component of acidosis is corrected by sodium bicarbonate. For significant acidosis when adequate ventilation has been established, 2–3 mEq/kg sodium bicarbonate may be given slowly through an umbilical arterial catheter. The commercially available preparation must be diluted with several volumes of sterile water to reduce its osmolality.

Bradycardia that persists despite good ventilation frequently responds to calcium. This is given as calcium gluconate, 100 mg/kg over 5–10 minutes. Improved heart rate is the desired response; if the heart rate falls, the calcium gluconate should be discontinued immediately.

Unresponsive asystole in the asphyxiated is treated with 1–3 ml of a 1:10,000 solution of epinephrine. The drug can be given intravenously or by intracardiac injection.

NEONATAL PHARMACOLOGY

Pharmacologic Principles

The newborn no longer is perceived as a miniature adult. Indeed, neonates cannot even be considered as a homogeneous population. Pharmacologic intervention in the newborn should be undertaken with an understanding of the basic differences in developmental stage, body composition and body size.

As mentioned at the beginning of the chapter, the efficacy and safety of any drug are dependent on four basic processes — absorption, distribution, biotransformation and excretion. These processes are influenced by physiologic and anatomic development within the infant.

For a drug to reach its site of action it must first be absorbed. This requires its passage across several barriers. Several factors, such as the nature of the drug and its route of administration, influence the rate of absorption.

Drugs administered by the oral route in the newborn generally are well absorbed. However, alterations in both the rate and quantity of drugs absorbed by active processes may occur. The oral route may be useful in some neonates, but because of the nature of the disease process (e.g., vomiting, diarrhea), this route is not commonly used.

Parenteral administration of therapeutic agents frequently is used. Subcutaneous administration is limited due to the restricted volumes that can be administered without compromising the blood flow to overlying skin and variation in absorption because of poor or impaired circulation to peripheral areas. This is of particular concern in ill babies with thermal instability.

To a somewhat lesser extent, the drawbacks listed above also apply to intramuscular injections. However, the intramuscular route has been shown by experience to provide adequate drug concentrations in the circulation for the treatment of disease.

The absorption of drugs through the skin of the newborn occurs to a larger extent than in older patients. This is due to the immaturity of the stratum corneum in neonates. Consideration must be given to the systemic absorption of agents intended primarily for topical effects. This is especially important in infants undergoing phototherapy, where heat from the lights causes an increased blood flow to the skin.

The initial phase of absorption is accomplished by the intravenous injection of drugs. The agents enter the circulation directly and there is no concern about delayed or incomplete absorption. Although most drugs can be given by this means, some either cannot or must be given with great caution. Knowledge of the nature of the agent and the composition of the dosage form is necessary to allow for the safe use of this route of administration.

The absorptive process leads to the presence of the drug in the circulation. The series of events leading to the passage of drugs across membranes and out of the intravascular space is termed distribution.

The pattern of a drug's distribution is dependent on the physicochemical properties of the agent and physiologic conditions within the patient. The initial distribution of a drug is closely related to the blood flow to a specific tissue. The final distribution is determined by many factors, as discussed earlier.

Drugs that are absorbed into the circulation are bound to plasma proteins, especially albumin, to varying extents. That part of the drug that is protein-bound does not take part in pharmacologic effects. This may be considered as an internal reservoir of the drug and any changes in plasma protein concentration may have a significant influence on the distribution and effect of the drug.

Endogenous substances such as bilirubin are also bound to albumin. This assumes practical importance when drugs are administered to newborns, because some drugs compete with the bilirubin for binding sites on the albumin. Some drugs, therefore, are contraindicated in newborns because of their ability to displace bilirubin, which then can gain access to the brain, where it has a toxic effect.

Most drugs are highly lipid soluble and thus are reabsorbed at the renal tubules. Their elimination, therefore, requires a transformation to a more water-soluble form. These biotransformations are enzyme-catalyzed processes that occur primarily in the liver.

The activity of many of these enzymes is low in the newborn and the achievement of adult values takes varying lengths of time. This then becomes the rate-limiting step in the process of elimination and in part accounts for the prolonged half-life seen with some drugs in the neonate.

Many pathways of excretion exist in the body, but renal excretion is the dominant route. Drugs, either unchanged or metabolized, are eliminated principally in the urine.

As with other organs, consideration must be given to the stage of anatomic and physiologic development of the newborn kidney. Renal blood flow and glomerular filtration rates are only approximately 30% of adult values. Tubular secretion, although not as well characterized as the other indices of renal function, also appears to be greatly diminished in the newborn. The differences in kidney functions are more pronounced in the preterm infant. Very rapid maturational changes may occur in the first few days of life.

Dosage regimens for drugs in newborns cannot be empirically derived. They must be based on the interplay of the foregoing processes. The size of the dose is determined to a large extent by the inherent ability of the immature organism to bring about the biotransformation of a drug. The dosage interval is dependent on the rate at which the developing kidney can excrete the drug.

Specific Groups of Drugs

Infections are common in the newborn period, especially in infants who are otherwise compromised. These infections frequently are of bacterial origin, although specific causative agents are not always isolated.

The penicillins comprise a group of drugs that are effective against most gram-positive organisms and some gram-negative ones. These drugs have been used for many years and there is broad experience with them in the therapy of neonatal infections.

Adverse reactions to the penicillins are almost unknown in the newborn. Seizures, however, have been observed when very high levels of penicillin are present in the cerebrospinal fluid.

Penicillin G is the prototype of this group of drugs and has been used most extensively in newborns. Penicillin G is excreted as the unchanged drug in the urine. It is the rate of excretion, therefore, rather than biotransformation that controls serum levels.

Both birth weight and postnatal age have been shown to correlate directly with the clearance of penicillin from the plasma. Thus, both the total daily dose and the dosage interval change with increasing postnatal age.

Penicillin G usually is administered as a 15–30-minute intravenous infusion but may be given intramuscularly. Twenty-five thousand units/kg are administered every 12 hours for infants less than 1 week of age and every 8 hours for infants older than 1 week. For patients with suspected or confirmed meningitis, the dosage is increased two- or threefold.

Ampicillin is a semisynthetic penicillin that has a broader antibacterial spectrum than penicillin G and is effective against some gram-negative bacteria. It is handled by the body in the same manner as penicillin G.

The suggested dose of ampicillin is 24 mg/kg administered at the same intervals as penicillin G. The dosage must be increased in meningitis.

Some bacteria have become resistant to penicillin due to the development of an enzyme that inactivates penicillin. These organisms are treated with semisynthetic penicillins that are resistant to the penicillinase. These agents are indicated only when suspected or proved penicillinase-producing organisms are found.

Two drugs of this class have been most extensively used in the newborn—methicillin and nafcillin. These drugs are very similar in action and differ primarily in dosage requirements.

Methicillin is given as a 25 mg/kg dose every 12 hours for infants less than 2 weeks of age, every 8 hours for infants less than 2000 gm and 2 weeks to 1 month of age and every 6 hours for infants greater than 2000 gm and older than 2 weeks.

Nafcillin is administered in a 20 mg/kg dose every 12 hours for infants less than 1 week of age and every 8 hours thereafter.

In both instances, the intramuscular route is preferred, although the drugs can be given as a 15–30-minute intravenous infusion.

Monitoring of infants to whom these drugs are administered is advisable. Nephrotoxicity has been reported with the use of methicillin, but may be age-related, as this has not been reported in neonates.

Neonatal sepsis frequently is the result of a mixed infection or due to gram-negative organisms. For this reason, the initial treatment often is the combination of a penicillin and one of the aminoglycosides, a group of drugs that includes kanamycin, gentamicin, streptomycin and neomycin. These potent drugs act by inhibiting protein synthesis in bacteria. They are not absorbed to any extent from the gastrointestinal tract and, therefore, usually are given by the parenteral route.

The toxicity of aminoglycosides is related to their effect on the eighth cranial nerve, involving either or both the vestibular and cochlear branches, or damage to the kidney. If severe enough, this could lead to hearing loss, vertigo or proteinuria and azotemia. The limiting factor appears to be the total dose administered rather than the duration of treatment.

Most of the experience in newborns with these drugs has been with kanamycin and gentamicin. These agents both appear to be effective and safe for routine use in newborns.

Kanamycin* may be given in a dose of 7.5 mg/kg for infants less than 1 week of age and less than 2000 gm, 10 mg/kg for others. The dosage interval is every 12 hours for infants less than 2000 gm and all infants less than 1 week of age. For infants weighing more than 2000 gm and older than 1 week, the interval is decreased to every 8 hours.

Gentamicin* is given in a dose of 2.5 mg/kg every 12 hours for infants less than 1 week of age and every 8 hours for infants older than 1 week.

The preferred route for both these drugs is intramuscular. However, they may be cautiously infused intravenously.

Two newer members of the aminoglycoside family have been marketed recently—tobramycin and amikacin. There is limited clinical experience with these two drugs in the newborn. They probably are best reserved for situations in which pathogens have shown susceptibility to these drugs and resistance to kanamycin or gentamicin.

Chloramphenicol exhibits a broad spectrum of antimicrobial activity. It is bacteriostatic by inhibition of protein synthesis in both gram-positive and gram-negative bacteria, *Rickettsia* and *Chlamydia.*

The toxicity of chloramphenicol is exemplified by the so-called gray baby syndrome. This is a syndrome of cardiovascular collapse. It is believed to be the result of high levels of unconjugated drug when excessive dosages are used. With proper appreciation of its pharmacokinetic properties, however, chloramphenicol can be used in neonates.

The suggested dose for infants is 25 mg/kg. This can be given as a

---

*These dosages are not necessarily recommended by the manufacturer.

single daily dose or divided into several doses. The drug can be given as an intravenous infusion or by mouth.

This drug should be reserved for the treatment of infections caused by pathogens that are resistant to the aminoglycosides or that do not respond to therapy after an appropriate time.

Neonates undergoing chloramphenicol therapy should be closely monitored for early signs of the gray baby syndrome. These signs include vomiting, poor sucking, respiratory distress, abdominal distention and diarrhea, all of which may be difficult to distinguish from the underlying disease.

Respiratory problems in the newborn period are best treated with ventilatory support. There are, however, two drugs that are used primarily for their ability to improve oxygenation in carefully selected cases.

In patients with elevated pulmonary arterial pressure or refractoriness to mechanical ventilation, tolazoline has been utilized with mixed results. Following administration of the drug, a dramatic rise in Pa_{O_2} may occur in some cases; however, the response is not always predictable.

Tolazoline exerts its effects primarily through alpha adrenergic blockade, but may have a direct nonadrenergic relaxant effect on vascular smooth muscle. It also bears a chemical relationship to histamine.

Potential complications arising from tolazoline in the newborn are not known with certainty but may be anticipated from the chemical and pharmacologic properties of the drug. The histaminic effects may lead to gastric bleeding. Alterations in renal blood flow may result in oliguria, which may be difficult to distinguish from the decreased urinary output produced by severe hypoxemia.

Since there is limited clinical experience with tolazoline and the indications for its use are not clearly delineated, its unrestricted use is to be proscribed.

A not infrequent problem encountered in neonatal intensive care units is apnea and bradycardia. Although the long-term consequences of apnea on the central nervous system are not fully defined, treatment is desirable.

The xanthines have been demonstrated to be effective in the treatment of apnea. The most widely used drug of this class is theophylline, although caffeine has been tried with some success also.

Theophylline appears to exert its effect by a direct stimulation of the respiratory center in the medulla. In addition, it has a cardiotonic action and the most common side effect, tachycardia, is an extension of this effect.

Theophylline can be administered by any of several routes, including rectal, oral and intravenous. Rectal administration may result in incomplete or erratic absorption and therefore is not the preferred route.

There is a wide variability in the pharmacokinetics of the drug in newborns. This makes determination of dosage and frequency of administration difficult. The use of this drug is best reserved for those situations in which serum levels of theophylline can be measured. This now is a relatively simple process requiring a minimum of blood sample. Safe serum levels have not yet been precisely defined, but side effects are uncommon in the usual therapeutic range of 10–20 μg.

It is the effect of the base that is responsible for its beneficial results in the treatment of apnea. Theophylline is marketed in a variety of salts and the pure base. If any of the salts is used, it is imperative to know the theophylline content and base the dose on this rather than the total amount of the drug-salt complex.

In general, theophylline is well tolerated. The previously cited problems with tachycardia usually can be controlled by skipping a dose or reducing the dose. Theoretically, there could be changes in cerebral blood flow, the consequences of which are not known.

The optimal duration of therapy is not known. There does not appear to be a good correlation between duration of treatment and response.

CONCLUSIONS

Perinatal pharmacology is a relatively new and rapidly expanding field. No longer is it acceptable to simply use drugs empirically. Consideration must be given to the changes in the developing organism that modify responses to therapeutic agents.

REFERENCES

Abouleish, E.: The placenta and placental transfer of drugs at term, Pa. Med. 78(5):56, 1975.

Abrahamsen, A. M., Grendahl, H., and Müller, C.: Hemodynamic effects of tolazoline, Acta Med. Scand. 190:199, 1971.

Ahokas, R. A., and Dilts, P. V.: Assessing narcotics and their antagonists, Contemp. OB/GYN 5:55, 1975.

Bednarek, F. J., and Roloff, D. W.: Treatment of apnea of prematurity with aminophylline, Pediatrics 58:335, 1976.

Cohen, S. N., and Ganapathy, S. K.: Drugs in the fetus and newborn infant, Clin. Endocrinol. Metab. 5:175, 1976.

Cohen, S. N., and Ganapathy, S. K.: Pharmacology in Evans, H. E., and Glass, L. (eds.), *Perinatal Medicine* (New York: Harper & Row, 1976).

Davi, M. J., Sankaran, K., Simons, K. J., Simons, F. E. R., Seshia, M. M., and Rigallo, H.: Physiologic changes induced by theophylline in the treatment of apnea in preterm infants, J. Pediatr. 92:91, 1978.

Dodson, W. E.: Neonatal drug intoxication: Local anesthetics, Pediatr. Clin. North Am. 23:399, 1976.

Gerhardt, T., Bancalari, E., Cohen, H., and Rocha, L. F.: Use of naloxone to reverse narcotic respiratory depression in the newborn infant, J. Pediatr. 90:1009, 1977.

Goetzman, B. W., Sunshine, P., Johnson, J. D., Wennberg, R. P., Hackel, A., Merten, D. F., Bartoletti, A. L., and Silverman, H. N.: Neonatal hypoxia and pulmonary vasospasm: Response to tolazoline, J. Pediatr. 90:617, 1976.

Gregory, G. A.: Resuscitation of the newborn, Anesthesiology 43:225, 1975.

McCracken, G. H., and Helson, J. D.: *Antimicrobial Therapy for Newborns* (New York: Grune & Stratton, 1977).

McDonald, J. S.: Preanesthetic and intrapartal medications, Clin. Obstet. Gynecol. 20:447, 1977.

Mirkin, B. L. (ed.): *Perinatal Pharmacology and Therapeutics* (New York: Academic Press, 1976).

O'Brien, T. E., and McManus, C. E.: Drugs and the human fetus, U. S. Pharmacist 2:36, 1977.

Ralston, D. H., and Shnider, S. M.: The fetal and neonatal effects of regional anesthesia in obstetrics, Anesthesiology 48:34, 1978.

Scanlon, J. W.: Obstetric anesthesia as a neonatal risk factor in normal labor and delivery, Clin. Perinatol. 1:465, 1974.

6 / Transportation of the High-Risk Infant

MARVIN D. LOUGH, R.R.T.

NEONATAL MORTALITY RATE is significantly lower where neonatal intensive care units are available.[1,2,3] The creation of these specialized care centers has precipitated the development of a system for conveying the ill infant from the community hospital to the regional center. It is an accepted fact that the uterus is the ideal "transport incubator" when the mother has been identified as a high-risk mother. I concede that the mother should be transferred to a high-risk maternal center whenever possible. This chapter will discuss transporting those infants who develop distress following a seemingly normal prenatal and perinatal period.

The transportation of a sick infant is a complex act requiring the coordination of several members of the health care team. Once the referring physician has requested a transfer, the coordinative effort should come from the referral center. Usually the referral center will have at least one physician with a particular interest in infant transfer who will oversee the preparation and management aspects of the transfer. This physician and his highly skilled team will travel to the community hospital, become acquainted with the infant's clinical history, examine the infant and provide therapy prior to departure. The team that accompanies the physician should consist of at least one nurse and one respiratory therapist whose major professional activities are devoted to the care of the high-risk infant.

Although the decision to transfer has been made, the referring hospital personnel should make every effort to stabilize the condition of the infant while waiting for the transport team to arrive. The precarious condition of the infant can be stabilized or even improved by using basic principles of newborn care, such as prevention of heat loss, maintenance of an airway, appropriate oxygen therapy and correction of acid-base disorders. Evaporative heat loss can be prevented by thoroughly drying the infant immediately after birth. The infant then should be placed in a preheated incubator or under a radiant heat warmer. When these devices are not available, a hot water bag or ordinary desk lamp will help. The hot water bag and lamp must be carefully monitored, as accidental burns may develop due to overheating.

Maintenance of a clear airway is of paramount importance. All meconium-stained infants should be fully inspected with a laryngoscope and thoroughly suctioned immediately after delivery. Repeated suctioning may be necessary if upper airway obstruction persists. Metabolic acidosis and hypoxic brain damage can be caused by oxygen deprivation. Therefore, when there is unavoidable doubt as to the oxygen requirements, it is less hazardous to err on the side of possible hyperoxygenation. Blood gas analysis should be done whenever possible. If these determinations are not available, oxygen in sufficient amounts to relieve all signs of hypoxia should be provided. When available, a snugly fitting oxygen hood should be used to supply warmed humidified oxygen. If a hood is not available, a common household funnel or Dixie Cup can be placed near the infant's face until the transport team arrives.

The biochemical response during asphyxia is the conversion from aerobic oxidation of glucose to anaerobic glycolysis in response to hypoxia, with the accumulation of lactate and the development of metabolic acidosis. In addition, respiratory acidosis can occur if there is cord compression during delivery, acute placental insufficiency or airway obstruction at birth. Whenever possible, pH and blood gas values should be obtained. If pH and blood gas values are not available, one can make an arbitrary correction of the probable acidosis by using 3 mEq/kg of sodium bicarbonate intravenously for infants greater than 2 kg and 4 mEq/kg for infants less than 2 kg.

Table 6–1 is a list of items that the referring hospital should have

TABLE 6–1.–CHECK LIST OF ITEMS FOR
DELIVERY AT REFERRAL HOSPITAL

1. Maternal and cord blood specimens
2. Patient identification
3. All available x-rays
4. Laboratory results
5. Bacteriologic studies
6. Patient's chart
7. Parental consent
8. Telephone number of referring physician
9. List of drugs infant received
10. Maternal history

ready for the transport team to take with them on their departure. Once the transport team arrives, the care of the infant should be turned over to the transport officer and his team. The team will remain only long enough to make a quick clinical appraisal and to stabilize the infant's condition. After the infant has been placed in the transport incubator and his condition has been stabilized, a short visit with the mother before departure will help to allay some of her fears about the transport and the nature of the care her infant will receive at the center.

TRANSPORT VEHICLES AND EQUIPMENT

Ambulance and Vans

Vehicles used for infant transport range from a standard ambulance to jet aircraft.[4] The simplest form of ground transportation is the hearse type of ambulance, a transport incubator and a tackle box. This system is adequate for short trips (50 miles or less). The privately owned ambulance will come to the center, pick up the transport incubator and the transport team. A small tackle box of drugs and equipment listed in Table 6–2 provides the team with adequate supplies for short-distance transports. A proper contract should be worked out with the ambulance company in order to ensure the availability of an ambulance 24 hours a day. Preliminary tests should be made to ensure that the transport incubator is compatible with the power sources in each ambulance that the company owns. Most ambulances are equipped with an inverter that transforms the 12-volt direct current into 110-volt alternating current. However, even if it has a frequency of 60 cycles per second, similar to standard hospital current, it usually has a square wave characteristic and is not suitable for devices other than a simple lamp. Therefore, it is recommended that the transport incubator be operated directly from the 12-volt DC battery of the ambulance. The receptacle, usually a cigarette lighter, should be adapted with wiring and fuses that will operate at 20 amperes.

A more sophisticated ground transport system has been developed by The University of Iowa General Hospitals.[5] This unit is basically an intensive care nursery on wheels (Fig. 6–1). This van provides a nursery 6′ × 10′ × 6½′. The van is heated, air-conditioned, well lighted and equipped with two incubators (one stationary, one transport), oxygen, suction and monitoring. This ground unit is designed for trips within a 120-mile radius.

As with any system there are potential problems associated with ground transport units. The most persistent, realistic and frustrating

TABLE 6-2.—SUPPLIES FOR
SHORT-DISTANCE TRANSPORTS

QUANTITY	ITEM
1	Laryngoscope handle with premature infant blade (Miller 0)
	Fore-clear endotracheal tubes, sizes 3.0, 3.5 and 4.0 mm
1	Universal endotracheal tube adaptor
1	Breathing bag
1	Set of small Bennett circle masks
2	10 or 12 1/2 ml syringes, sterile with #20 needle
5	3 ml syringes, sterile, with #22 needle
5	Three-way stopcocks, sterile
1	Umbilical catheterization set and extra catheters
2	#5 F single-holed catheters
2	#5 and #8 F feeding tubes
3	Stopcock plugs (needle caps)
2	Tuberculin syringes with #26 needle
2	30 ml amp. sterile distilled water
2	30 ml amp. sterile saline
1	10 ml heparin, sterile. 1000 units/ml
2	50 ml vials sodium bicarbonate
1	50 ml vial 50% glucose
1	1:1000 aqueous adrenalin
	Valium
	6 feet of latex tubing
1	Scissors, nonsterile
2	Hemostats, nonsterile
	Scotch tape or equivalent
3	Vial files—sharp
	Dextrostix
	Suction catheter with rubber tubing
	Tape measure
	Disposable gloves
	Specimen tubes
	Alcohol sponges
	Preparation tray with amphyl
	Intensive care record sheet
2	Glass 3 ml syringes for artery sticks
2	#23 scalp needles
1	#21 scalp needle
	Rubber bands
	Lancets
2	Receiving blankets
	Stethoscope

problem, over which we have no control, is traffic conditions within a large city. An ambulance driver with a good knowledge of city streets will minimize the delay created by traffic congestion. Another real problem with ground transport is weather conditions, particularly during the winter season in the northern states. The transport coordinator always should check with the ambulance company to make sure that

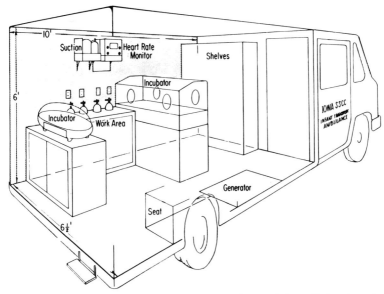

Fig. 6–1.—Layout of infant transport van. (From Baker, G. L.: Am. J. Dis. Child. 118:743, 1969. Copyright 1969, American Medical Association. Reprinted by permission.)

the ambulances have been properly winterized so as to prevent unnecessary delay prior to or during transport.

Although there are disadvantages to the ground system, it also has several advantages. In a unit that is properly balanced with a heavy-duty chassis, the ride is relatively smooth, which makes for better monitoring conditions. The ambulance can also come to a complete stop if emergency procedures are required. Ground vehicles in general have better lighting, more precise temperature control and more working space than air vehicles.

Helicopters and Fixed-Wing Aircraft

When the distance and travel time become impractical for ground transport systems, air travel must be utilized. Helicopters and fixed-wing aircraft are valuable in areas where the neonatal intensive care center is greater than 100 miles from the referring hospital. Many centers that accept referrals from a 5–7-state area have developed air transport systems.[4, 6] Due to the cost of the aircraft, the centers usually contract service with a private company or make arrangements with a military reserve that has such aircraft available.

The obvious advantage to helicopter transport is the drastic de-

TABLE 6-3.—EFFECTS OF ALTITUDE ON
AMBIENT AND ALVEOLAR OXYGEN

ALTITUDE	ATMOSPHERIC PRESSURE (mm Hg)	PARTIAL PRESSURE OF OXYGEN (mm Hg)		
		Ambient	Alveoli	Blood
Sea level	760	159	105	100
2000	707	148	97	92
6000	609	127	84	79
10,000	523	109	74	69
20,000	349	73	40	35
30,000	226	47	21	19

crease in transport time. However, there are several factors that must be overcome before air transport systems are used. The vibration levels in a helicopter are considerably greater than those of ground vehicles. Excessive vibration makes it difficult to observe the adequacy of ventilation, and auscultation is virtually impossible. Therefore, since the helicopter cannot "pull over," the newborn must be stabilized before leaving the referring hospital. Solid-state monitors with self-contained power supplies are necessary for monitoring vital signs because of the internal vibration and fluctuating power supplies of the aircraft.

A serious complication associated with aircraft transport is the rapid change in atmospheric pressure at higher altitudes, leading to unrecognized hypoxia, pneumothorax complications and abdominal distention. An altimeter should be kept in the cabin and oxygen concentrations varied according to altitude (Table 6-3).

Good radio communication should be established with both the referring and the receiving hospitals. This will expedite the rendezvous with the connecting ambulance and permit communication to the center for emergency consultations.

Before instituting any transport system, several "dry runs" should be made in order to familiarize the team with the vehicle and equipment and to ensure that no one suffers from motion sickness.

Transport Equipment

The basic unit is a portable incubator with unrestricted visibility (Table 6-4). The incubator must be equipped with an oxygen supply, self-contained power supply and precise temperature control. Additional equipment can be added to meet the requirements of the transporting team (Fig. 6-2). Figure 6-3 shows a self-contained system developed at Stanford University. Although this unit is expensive, it is

TABLE 6-4.—CHARACTERISTICS OF TRANSPORT INCUBATORS

	OHIO	AIR-SHIELDS	CAVITRON
Dimensions H × W × D (inches)	28 × 44 × 22	35 × 42 × 18	28 × 36 × 18
Weight (lb)	165	122	180
Battery type	Lead-acid	Gelled electrolyte	Gel cell
Mattress size (inches²)	190	220	225
Warm-up time (minutes) (21.5° C to 33° C)	25	37	18
Interior sound level (dBA)	52	52	Ambient
Maximal leakage current (uA)	32	30	<100

completely equipped with precise temperature control, unrestricted visibility, self-contained power supply and solid-state monitors for temperature, blood pressure, heart rate, respiratory rate and inspired oxygen. This unit is also equipped with a ventilator, aspirator and Holter infusion pump.

The importance of properly functioning equipment cannot be over-emphasized. All transport equipment should be checked and recorded by the respiratory therapist on each shift.

Fig. 6–2.—Transport incubator with therapy and monitoring equipment added.

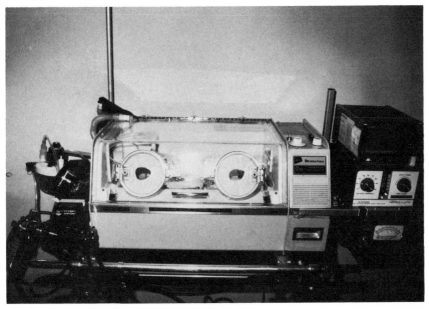

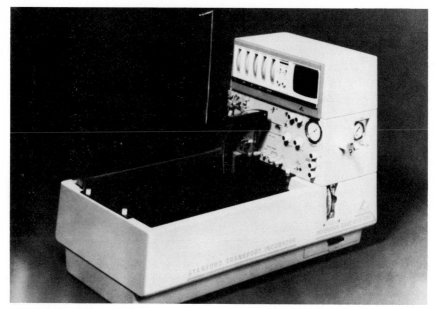

Fig. 6–3. — Self-contained transport system with patient care and monitoring equipment built in.

Practical Hints:

1. There is a striking difference in voltage and amperage when AC current-operated equipment is powered from an inverted DC battery supply. Failure to appreciate this difference can result in equipment malfunction or failure. This factor is magnified when a motor (infusion pump) or a digital timing (ventilator) circuit is involved. A self-contained power supply should be used whenever possible or all AC-operated equipment should be checked for accuracy prior to transport usage.

2. All transport vehicles, particularly helicopters, have increased levels of vibration. Therefore, solid-state monitoring equipment should be used whenever possible. Tube-type circuitry is not only larger but draws more current and can sustain mechanical damage to the cathode or filament from increased levels of vibration.

3. The heating mechanism of the transport incubator consumes the greatest amount of current from the power supply. The amount of heat required to maintain neutral thermal temperature can be minimized by using a double-walled incubator. The double wall will help to insulate the incubator and at the same time prevent heat radiation from

TABLE 6–5.–ESTIMATING OXYGEN
NEEDS DURING A TRANSPORT

CYLINDER SIZE	CUBIC FEET	LITERS	DIMENSIONS	DURATION FACTOR
E	22	624	4¼ × 30	0.28
G	187	5295	5½ × 55	2.41
H	244	6909	9 × 55	3.14

the infant. If the transport incubator does not have a double wall, a small clear plastic shield can be placed over the infant to create the "thermos bottle" effect.

4. Most transport incubators provide space for an "E" cylinder of oxygen. To avoid running out of oxygen during a trip, there should be at least 1.5–2 times the calculated requirement. Table 6–5 provides details to help in estimating oxygen needs during a transport. If the team is starting with a partially filled tank, an estimate of the remaining gas can be calculated using the following formula:

$$\frac{\text{Duration of flow}}{\text{in minutes}} = \frac{\text{gauge pressure (psi)} \times \text{factor (from Table 6–5)}}{\text{liter flow}}$$

As an example, let us estimate the remaining oxygen in an E cylinder that has 900 psi. If we intend to use 5 liters/minute, the factor from Table 6–5 for an E cylinder is 0.28. Therefore:

$$\frac{900 \times 0.28}{5} = 50 \text{ minutes}$$

If space is a problem, a liquid oxygen supply can be used. A liquid oxygen system stands 27″ high, is 24″ in diameter, weighs 68 lb and contains 13,000 liters of gaseous oxygen. Although the partial pressure of oxygen varies with altitude, the functioning of the system itself is not affected. Liquid oxygen systems are not intended to be used with equipment requiring 50 psi driving force.

5. Constant positive airway pressure and mechanical ventilation often are part of the therapy during transport. A fluidic type of ventilator (see Fig. 10–25) provides continuous flow that may be time-cycled for automatic ventilation with or without positive end expiratory pressure. It may also be used to provide continuous positive airway pressure. This unit is controlled by miniature pneumatic logic elements that do not require any electrical power. This is a distinct advantage, since the voltage and waveforms of the electrical supply vary on most transport units.

6. Above all, some method of protecting the infant from injury should be provided without rigidly immobilizing limb movement. Sudden acceleration, deceleration or a drop in altitude can cause the infant to slide into the incubator walls.

In the past, transport vehicles have been used only to transport injured and/or sick patients from one location to another. Recent advances in vehicle design and medical technique now enable treatment to begin and continue during the transport process.

REFERENCES

1. Perinatal mortality of the province of Quebec: Reports of study committee, 1967 and 1968. Government of Province of Quebec.
2. Scott, K. E.: Report of the committee on maternal and perinatal health of the province of Nova Scotia, Nova Scotia Med. Bull. 49:81, 1970.
3. Rawlings, G., *et al.*: Changing prognosis for infants of very low birth weight, Lancet 1:516, 1971.
4. Shepard, K. S.: Air transportation of high-risk infants utilizing a flying intensive-care nursery, J. Pediatr. 77:148, 1970.
5. Baker, G. L.: Design and operation of a van for the transport of sick infants, Am. J. Dis. Child. 118:743, 1969.
6. Harris, B., *et al.*: Aeromedical transportation for infants and children, J. Pediatr. Surg. 10:719, 1975.

7 / Newborn Respiratory Care Procedures

MARVIN D. LOUGH, R.R.T.

ONE MUST CONCEDE that infants are not just little adults. Therefore, many respiratory care procedures are unique to the infant. Also, the equipment necessary to perform these unique procedures is either specifically designed or carefully modified. This chapter will discuss some of these procedures as they pertain to respiratory care of the sick newborn infant.

THERMOREGULATION

Since the physiology of temperature control in infants is discussed in Chapters 2 and 8, this section will deal with equipment and technique of thermoregulation.

Incubators √

The most commonly used device for environmental control of the infant is the single-walled incubator (Fig. 7–1). This device will provide precise control of temperature, oxygen, humidity and an isolated or filtered gas environment.

Air and/or oxygen enter the unit through a microfilter. The air is heated to the proper temperature as it passes through a heating coil. High relative humidity (75–90%) is achieved as the warm air passes over the water in the humidity reservoir. Due to the slight positive pressure maintained inside the incubator hood by the air-circulating system there always is a tendency for air inside the hood to flow to the outside, thus ensuring a high degree of isolation.

Heat Shield

The single-walled incubator is an efficient method of keeping the infant warm by convection, but because the temperature of the plastic walls cannot be controlled, radiant heat loss from the infant will occur. If the nursery is cool or if the incubator is placed near a cold window

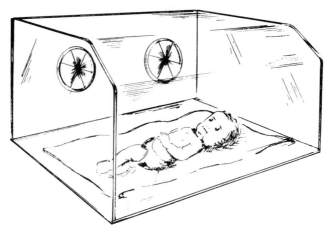

Fig. 7–1.—A single-walled incubator for the control of temperature, oxygen and humidity.

or wall, the infant will radiate heat to the cold incubator walls and it will be virtually impossible to maintain a neutral thermal environment. When a small clear plastic heat shield is placed over the infant inside the single-walled incubator (Fig. 7–2), the warm incubator air will heat the plastic wall of the shield to the same temperature as the air within the incubator. The infant then will radiate only to the warm inner plastic wall, as radiant waves from the infant (2–9 μ) will not penetrate the plastic wall of the heat shield.

Fig. 7–2.—A single-walled incubator with an inner heat shield that prevents the radiation of heat from the infant to the cold outer wall of the incubator.

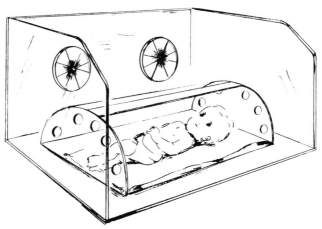

Radiant Heat Panels

Radiant heat panels provide another method of controlling the core temperature of the infant. However, some concern about the use of these devices stems from potential hazards and the lack of information regarding possible effects of the device.[1, 3, 5, 6, 8, 11-15, 17] Until some of the questions about safety and the effects of infrared radiation on newborn infants can be answered, one might consider sacrificing the convenience of radiant warmers for a more proved method of controlling thermoneutrality.

OXYGEN THERAPY

In general, oxygen is delivered to the infant in one of four ways: (1) hood, (2) bag and mask, (3) continuous positive airway pressure and (4) mechanical ventilation. This section will deal with oxygen delivery by hood and bag and mask only, since continuous positive airway pressure and mechanical ventilation are discussed in detail in Chapters 9 and 10, respectively.

Hood

The simplest and most efficient way to deliver an oxygen-enriched atmosphere to a spontaneously breathing infant is with a clear plastic hood placed over the infant's head. Air and oxygen proportional controllers allow for the delivery of oxygen (21 – 100%) through a cascade

Fig. 7–3.—An oxygen hood with controlled temperature, humidity and oxygen.

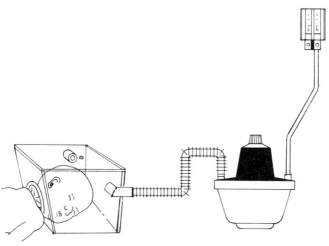

humidifier to the oxygen hood (Fig. 7–3). The air-oxygen mixture must be humidified and warmed to the same temperature as that of the incubator air, which should be in the range of thermal neutrality. The concentration of environmental oxygen should be analyzed and recorded every hour or when the FI_{O_2} has been altered.

Bag and Mask Therapy

In general there are two types of bag and mask systems commonly used for the resuscitation of the newborn infant—flow-inflating and self-inflating. The flow-inflating system utilizes a 0.5 or 1 liter thin-walled rubber anesthesia bag and a round face mask with a rubber air-filled rim. Proper pressure and inflation of the bag can be obtained by varying either the flow of gas or the pressure relief valve. The mask, when applied to the face, should avoid the eyes and have a small but definite leak around the mask in order to prevent rebreathing of carbon dioxide and to act as a pressure "pop-off."

Self-inflating Systems

Unlike the flow-inflating bag, the self-inflating bag does not require a source gas. The recoil characteristics of this bag allow for reinflation following a manual deflation. This is a distinct advantage, since a source of compressed gas is not always available. Table 7–1 lists the characteristics of 5 commonly used self-inflating bags. Some of the problems associated with the self-inflating bag and mask systems are (a) varying and unknown concentration of oxygen, (b) the "feel" for bagging is lost due to the recoil characteristics of the bag and (c) the safety release valve often is limited to less than 40 cm H_2O.

Complications arising from the use of bag and mask therapy include pneumothorax, corneal lacerations, pressure necrosis from the mask and a dependence on assisted ventilation. Although bag and mask therapy often is used as a resuscitative measure, it can also be used as an alternative to respirator therapy.[7]

EXTERNAL CARDIAC MASSAGE

Whenever cardiac massage is indicated, it should be started promptly and maintained at a constant rhythm of 100–120 compressions per minute. The sternum should be compressed 1.5–2.0 cm with each stroke. Two techniques of massage currently are acceptable.

The first technique (Fig. 7–4) is to use the tips of the index and middle finger. These two finger tips are positioned over the infant's nipple and brought straight across the chest to the sternum. For maximal effectiveness, the infant should be lying supine on a firm surface.

TABLE 7–1.–CHARACTERISTICS OF SELF-INFLATING BAGS

BAG	APPROXIMATE VOLUME (full)	OXYGEN RESERVOIR	MAXIMUM FI_{O_2}	PRESSURE RELIEF
Hope	730 ml	Sleeve	100%	40 cm H_2O
Penlon	250 ml	Tube	100%	Fixed leak
Ambu (Pediatric)	500 ml	Tube	100%	None
Laerdal (Infant)	240 ml	Tube	100%	35 cm H_2O
AIRbird (Pediatric)	500 ml	Tube	90%	None

The alternative method (Fig. 7–5) is the two-thumb technique. The thumbs should be placed on the middle third of the sternum. Both hands then should encircle the infant's chest. Care must be taken to compress with the thumbs and not push upward on the infant's back with the fingers.

The effectiveness of cardiac massage is monitored by the presence of a carotid or femoral pulse.

TRACHEAL INTUBATION

Intubation of the trachea seldom is an emergency procedure. Bag and mask breathing is more than adequate until steps have been taken to ensure that all necessary equipment is working properly and the correct tubes have been obtained.

One can expect to find the anatomy of the infant unlike that of the

Fig. 7–4. – Two-finger technique of external cardiac massage.

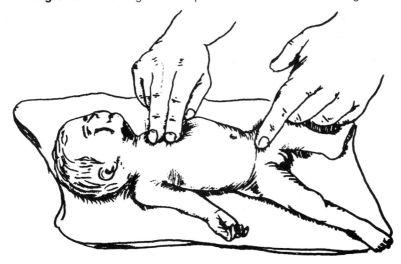

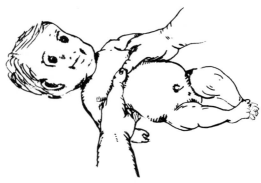

Fig. 7–5. – Two-thumb technique of external cardiac massage.

adult, the epiglottis being soft and folded ("omega [Ω] shaped"), the glottic chink being higher and anterior (level of C-1) and the tongue being relatively large and bulky.

Procedure

The infant should be held so that his head is slightly extended into a "sniffing position" and his shoulders flat to prevent arching of the back. Grasp the laryngoscope handle between the thumb and the first finger of the left hand. The blade then is inserted near the midline and moved to the left side of the mouth, gently deflecting the tongue. Stabilize the infant's head by grasping the chin with the second and third fingers of the left hand. Gently advance the blade into the vallecula, anterior to the epiglottis (Fig. 7–6). At no time is an attempt made to pick up the epiglottis directly with the laryngoscope blade. The soft, fragile tissue of the epiglottis is easily traumatized and prone to edema and hemorrhage. Gently lift the jaw and tongue upward while using the small finger of the left hand to apply pressure over the hyoid bone to move the larynx posteriorly and expose the vocal cords. Insert the endotracheal tube alongside the laryngoscope, not down the barrel of the blade. Insert the tube between the cords and approximately 2 cm beyond. The laryngoscope blade then is carefully withdrawn while the position of the tube is maintained by the right hand. The tube now is connected to 100% oxygen and the infant is ventilated (40–60 times/min at 20–25 cm H_2O pressure). The maximal allowable time for any one attempt is 30 seconds or until bradycardia or hypotension occurs. If intubation has not been accomplished within this criteria, the infant should be ventilated with 100% oxygen for at least 2 minutes before a second attempt is made.

Correct placement of the tube can be verified by (a) listening to both

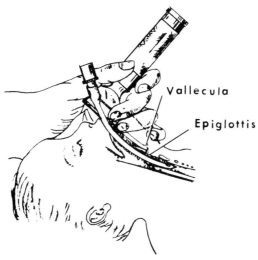

Vallecula

Epiglottis

Fig. 7–6.—Position of bronchoscope and endotracheal tube during endotracheal intubation.

sides of the chest for equal breath sounds, (b) listening over the stomach to be sure that the tube is in the trachea, not the stomach and (c) symmetric chest movement with inspiration. Of course, the best verification is by x-ray.

Practical Points for Tracheal Intubation

ENDOTRACHEAL TUBES. — Endotracheal tubes should be made of nontoxic polyvinyl chloride that will conform to the trachea when warmed to body temperature. They should be sterile, tissue-implant tested and radiopaque to facilitate localization. There are basically two types of tubes used for infant intubation. The more popular tube has the same internal diameter over its entire length with a Murphy eye at the tip. The Cole tube has a shoulder between the narrow tracheal portion and the remainder of the tube. This design is to prevent accidental cannulation of the mainstem bronchus and to decrease the resistance to air flow. Although the Cole tube is easier to insert, which makes it useful for emergencies, it has been associated with laryngeal dilation when used for extended periods.[2]

Endotracheal tubes should fit snugly within the trachea while allowing for a small air leak between the tube and the glottis when positive pressure is applied. Table 7–2 provides data to assist in determining the inside diameter (ID) and length of endotracheal tubes suitable for use in infants. Endotracheal tubes should be cut to length and

TABLE 7-2.—DATA FOR DETERMINATION OF INSIDE
DIAMETER AND LENGTH OF ENDOTRACHEAL TUBES

	FRENCH SIZE	INTERNAL DIAMETER	ORAL LENGTH	NASAL LENGTH	15-MM ADAPTER (mm internal diameter)
Premature < 1000 gm	12	2.5	7.5	10	3
Premature > 1000 gm	14	3.0	8.0	11	3
Newborn 5000 gm	16	3.5	8.5	13	4
2–24 weeks (5–7 kilos)	16–18	3.5–4.0	10.0	15	4

the 15-mm adapter should be in place before insertion. To prevent an increase in air-flow resistance, the 15-mm male connector must be as large as, if not larger than, the internal lumen of the tube. This can be accomplished by dipping the end of the tube, after it has been cut to length, into boiling water and allowing it to become soft before inserting the oversize connector.

LARYNGOSCOPE HANDLE AND BLADE.—The most commonly used laryngoscope for the intubation of the infant is the medium-sized handle with a Miller "0" blade. Before attempting intubation, one should be sure that the battery power is sufficient to produce a white light. The Miller "0" blade (75 mm in length) is specifically designed for premature infants. The Miller "1" or the Wis-Hipple infant blade, both 100 mm in length, can be used for near-term or full-term infants.

TUBE FIXATION.—Once the tube has been inserted to the predetermined distance, securing the tube is of major importance. After drying the mouth and upper lip, paint the cheekbones, upper lip and endotracheal tube with benzoin. After the benzoin has become tacky, place a piece of ½-inch adhesive tape on the right cheekbone and draw it across the upper lip and press it firmly to the skin. Continuing, wrap the tape firmly around the tube (2 revolutions) in a counterclockwise direction. Take the excess tape and secure it to the left cheekbone. Using a second strip of tape, begin on the left cheekbone and reverse the procedure, wrapping the tape in a clockwise fashion. Common adhesive tape, as opposed to waterproof adhesive tape, adheres better to polyvinyl chloride endotracheal tubes when moistened with saliva or nasal secretions.

NASOTRACHEAL INTUBATION.—Under most circumstances, oral intubation is preferable. Although fixation of the tube may be easier via the nasal route, trauma and necrosis to the nasal septum suggest that it be an elective procedure and should be used sparingly.

The method of nasotracheal intubation is essentially the same as oral intubation, with a few exceptions. The tube is inserted through one nostril into the pharyngeal space before the cords are visualized. After the cords are visualized, in the same manner as with oral intubation, a McGill forceps is used to direct the tube into the larynx. Nasotracheal tubes should be cut approximately 20% longer.

TEACHING MODEL FOR INTUBATION. — Four-week-old kittens serve as excellent teaching models for endotracheal intubation of the neonate.[9] The kitten should be anesthetized with about 40 mg of ketamine, injected into the triceps muscle. Ketamine will take effect in about 5 minutes and leaves the laryngeal reflex intact. The anatomy of the kitten is very similar to the infant, with the exception of a slightly larger, broader epiglottis. The kitten can be intubated using a 3.0-mm tube and a Miller "0" laryngoscope blade. The kitten will be awake and well in less than 1 hour.

INDWELLING CATHETERS

The use of indwelling umbilical arterial catheters is the preferred method of obtaining blood for the assessment of oxygen requirement of the newborn. With this type of catheter in place, repeated samples of blood can be withdrawn for blood gas analysis and a direct measurement of arterial pressure can also be assessed.

Procedure

Umbilical artery catheterization is best performed on an open table using proper surgical precautions. Neutral thermal conditions should be maintained using an overhead radiant warmer whereas oxygen requirements can be met with an oxygen hood or a simple bag and mask.

A 3.5 for infants < 1500 gm or a 5.0 for infants > 1500 gm French catheter should be marked according to location desired (Fig. 7–7). The catheter should be soft, have a rounded tip with an end hole, transparent and have a radiopaque line. The catheter is connected to a three-way stopcock and filled with sterile heparinized saline (1 unit of heparin to 1 ml of sterile saline).

The umbilical cord is cut, leaving a stump of 1–1.5 cm. The stump and surrounding area are cleansed with an antiseptic solution and a "circumcision drape" placed over the stump. The arteries are small, constricted, thick-walled vessels located at about 4 and 8 o'clock (Fig. 7–8). The artery to be used is teased open with a forceps or small obturator. The catheter is inserted into the lumen and gently advanced. It is common to meet resistance slightly below the abdominal wall,

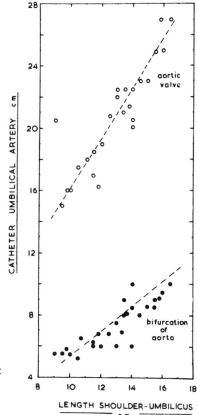

Fig. 7–7. — Graph that demonstrates the relationship between the distance from the shoulder to the umbilicus and the length of the catheter needed to reach the aortic bifurcation and/or aortic valve. (Modified from Dunn, P. M.: Localization of the umbilical catheter by post-mortem measures, Arch. Dis. Child. 41:69, 1966.)

where the vessel turns suddenly downward, and at the junction of the hypogastric artery (5–6 cm). Gentle sustained pressure on the catheter usually will relax the artery and allow the catheter to advance. If gentle pressure is not successful, 0.1–0.2 ml of 2% lidocaine (without epinephrine) can be injected in an attempt to relieve vasospasm. If resistance persists, catheterization of the other artery should be attempted. The catheter can be held in place by a pursestring suture around the cord stump (see Fig. 7–8). The catheter may safely be placed either on the lower thoracic aorta between the ductus arteriosus and the celiac artery or in the lower abdominal aorta between the inferior mesenteric artery and the aortic bifurcation. Once the catheter is in place, the position should be confirmed immediately by x-ray.

When no longer needed, slowly withdraw the catheter to allow the artery to constrict and tie off the vessel with a silk suture.

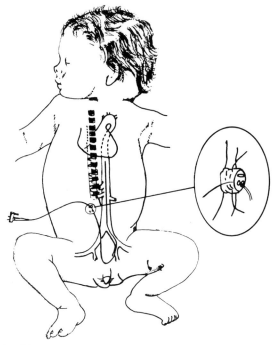

Fig. 7–8.—Position of umbilical artery catheter and an exploded view of umbilical cord showing position of umbilical arteries.

HELPFUL HINTS.—After the catheter is in place, palpate the femoral pulse. Occasionally, the femoral artery will go into spasm, causing blanching or cyanosis of the extremity. Reflex vasodilation may be attempted by warming the contralateral extremity. The catheter should be removed if prompt improvement in circulation is not observed.

Since indwelling catheters offer little resistance to the flow of electrical current, all electrical equipment used around the infant should be checked for leakage of current and adequate grounding (less than 100 microamperes).

Temporal and Radial Artery Puncture

An alternative to umbilical artery catheterization is radial or temporal artery puncture.

The techniques of temporal and radial artery puncture are very similar. A heparinized 23-gauge butterfly infusion set and a 1-ml syringe is used to collect the blood. The frontal or parietal branch of the superficial temporal artery is located by palpation (Fig. 7–9). The skin then is cleansed with an antiseptic solution. With the bevel side of the

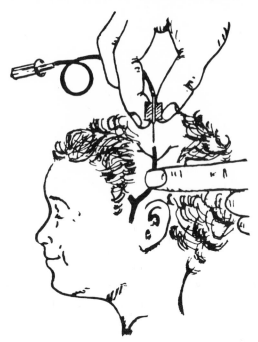

Fig. 7—9. — Technique of temporal artery puncture.

needle up, the artery is entered in the direction opposite to the blood flow. As the needle enters the artery, a spontaneous flow of blood will fill the tubing. Connect the syringe to the infusion set and collect the sample. After the sample has been collected, remove the needle and apply pressure to the site for at least 5 minutes.

The radial artery is punctured in a manner similar to the temporal artery. After the syringe and butterfly have been heparinized, palpate the radial artery just proximal to the transverse wrist crease. Puncture the skin at about a 35° angle and gently insert the butterfly until a pulsatile flow of blood enters the tubing (Fig. 7–10). Connect the 1-ml syringe and collect a sample. The needle then is removed and pressure applied for a minimum of 5 minutes.

PHYSIOLOGIC MONITORING

All physiologic monitoring devices have three basic components. An understanding of the basic principles of these components will facilitate accurate biomedical measurements. The physiologic signal to be measured either is directly available or is obtained by the transfor-

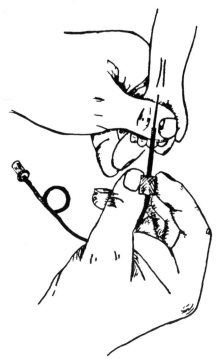

Fig. 7–10. — Position of the hand and wrist for radial artery puncture.

mation of a biophysical event into an electrical signal (transducer). This signal is conditioned (e.g., amplified, filtered) and displayed (e.g., recorder, oscilloscope, meter) (Fig. 7–11).

Transducers

A transducer is a device that senses a biophysical event and transforms it into an electrical signal. Although there are many types of transducers, I will limit my discussion to electrodes, pressure, temperature and gas concentration. As far as this text is concerned, I will include electrodes as a transducer, since it is necessary to measure signals at the skin resulting from electrical activity within the body (i.e., ECG, body impedance). A resistive transducer is a device whose

Fig. 7–11. — The three basic components of a biophysical monitoring system.

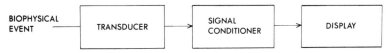

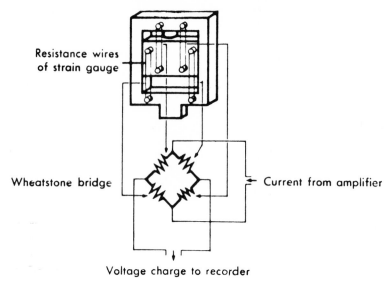

Resistance wires of strain gauge

Wheatstone bridge

Current from amplifier

Voltage charge to recorder

Fig. 7–12. — Resistive displacement transducers.

resistance changes in proportion to some physical quantity. A thermistor used for temperature control and/or monitoring is one form of resistive transducer. A strain gauge pressure transducer (Fig. 7–12) probably is the most common kind of resistive transducer for monitoring devices. The principle of operation of the resistive transducers involves the measurement of the changes in current, through a thin wire, which has a constant voltage supply. As a pressure is applied to a strain gauge, the physical characteristics (increase in length and decrease in diameter) of the thin wire change the resistance to the flow of current. This change in resistance can be quantitated to reflect the amount of pressure applied to alter the physical characteristics of the thin wire. When properly calibrated, the change in resistance will be proportional to the change in pressure. The electrical signal generated will be conditioned and displayed.

Conditioning Equipment

Biophysical events are very difficult to measure because of the weak electrical signals generated by the transducer. The signal generated by the transducer therefore must be amplified to be compatible with the display device. An amplifier is a device that is designed to increase the power level of the signal to be amplified. Another form of signal conditioning is discrimination between the biophysical event and extraneous signals. Signal filters are used to reject or "filter out" interference signals and undesired noise from the environment. Signal-conditioning equipment is also used to combine or relate the outputs of two or more transducers. In essence, the purpose of the signal conditioning is to process the signals from the transducers in such a way that they will be meaningful when displayed.

Displays

It often is necessary, or at least desirable, to record the biophysical event for later use (graphic pen recorder) while at the same time having a visual display (analog or digital meter) for immediate evaluation. An oscilloscope often is used to evaluate size and shape of the event being recorded. Long-term storage for permanent records or data analysis is best achieved by recording on magnetic tape or disks.

Using the three basic components (transducer, signal conditioners and displays), one can construct a system for monitoring many physiologic parameters of the newborn infant.

Impedance Monitors (Apnea and Heart Rate)

Apnea monitoring is achieved by several different methods (air mattress, nasal thermistor, radar). The most common apnea monitors use the technique of impedance pneumography to measure respiration activity by sensing the resistivity changes due to the movement of air into and out of the lung. The product of a constant high-frequency current and the thoracic impedance changes produces a voltage that changes with each respiration. If respiration ceases and the voltage

Fig. 7–13.—Block diagram for impedence pneumonography utilizing biopotential skin electrodes for monitoring of heart rate and respiration.

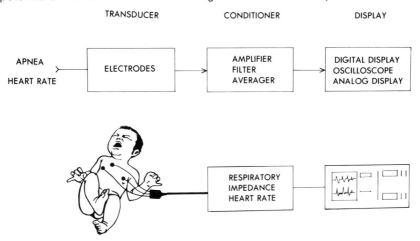

does not change over a preselected period, an audible alarm will sound. Heart rate can also be obtained from the impedance pneumograph at the same time. Splitting the signal and sending part of it through a high-pass filter (signal conditioner) will filter out all low-frequency signals (respiratory impedance) and permit the higher-frequency signal (heart rate) to reach the display (Fig. 7–13).

Pulmonary Function (Tidal Volume, Respiratory Rate, Minute Volume)

Pulmonary function studies in general are difficult to obtain in infants because of the lack of cooperation. However, some respiratory parameters can be measured and these provide useful data. Tidal volume, respiratory rate, minute volume and inspiratory-expiratory ratio can be measured using a pneumotachygraph (Fig. 7–14). A closely fitting face mask is used to provide an airtight seal between the infant's face and the pneumotachygraph. The pneumotachygraph consists of a fine-mesh screen that provides a known pressure difference as the air flows through it. Since the pressure difference is directly

Fig. 7–14.—Block diagram of instrumentation for monitoring tidal volume, respiratory rate and minute volume using a pressure differential transducer that produces electrical signals proportional to flow.

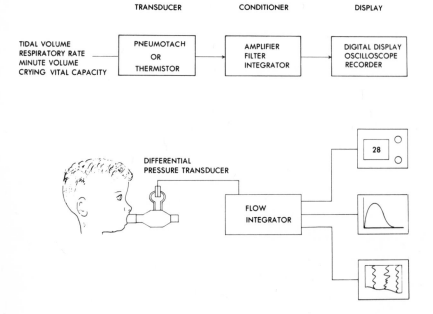

proportional to the flow, and flow is volume per unit of time, volume itself is the integral of flow. Respiratory rate and inspiratory-expiratory ratios can be calculated by estimating the portion of time devoted to inspiration, expiration and combined inspiration-expiration. The more standard pulmonary function tests usually are not performed on ill infants because the trauma imposed usually is greater than the benefit reaped.

Environmental Temperature Monitoring

The necessity for precise environmental temperature control is discussed in Chapters 2 and 8. The device most commonly used to control and monitor precise temperature is a thermistor. Thermistors are variable resistance devices formed into disks, rods and glass beads. Cooling the thermistor will register a reduction in resistance; likewise, heating the thermistor will register an increase in resistance. The change in the resistance will be displayed as a change in temperature (Fig. 7–15).

Blood Pressure Monitoring

The use of indwelling arterial catheters in sick infants has become common practice in recent years. These catheters provide a means of coupling the vascular pressure to an external transducer for the direct measurement of intra-arterial blood pressure. A strain gauge transduc-

Fig. 7–15. – The instrumentation for measuring temperature utilizing a thermistor whose resistance varies with the temperature.

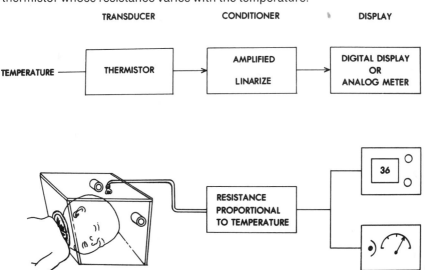

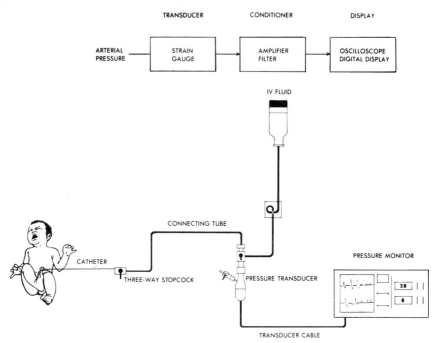

Fig. 7–16. — Block diagram for the instrumentation necessary for the direct measurement of aortic pressure in the newborn infant utilizing a strain gauge transducer.

er is attached to a catheter that has been properly placed and confirmed by x-ray. The signal-conditioning system consists of an amplifier, filter and an averaging circuit that looks at several systolic-diastolic waveforms and displays the average (Fig. 7–16). Often an infusion pump is incorporated into the system for fluid infusion and to maintain a patent catheter.

Expiratory Gas Analysis

Monitoring of expiratory gas as a means of assessing the pulmonary status is not common with the newborn infant because the high sample flow rate of the conventional gas analyzers is not compatible with the small tidal volume of the infant. It is, however, possible to make direct measurements of alveolar gas tension with a mass spectrometer.

A mass spectrometer is an apparatus that separates a stream of charged particles (ions) into a spectrum according to their mass-to-charge ratios and determines the relative abundance of each type of ion present. Medical mass spectrometer systems include the following elements: a sample inlet assembly, an ionization chamber, a dis-

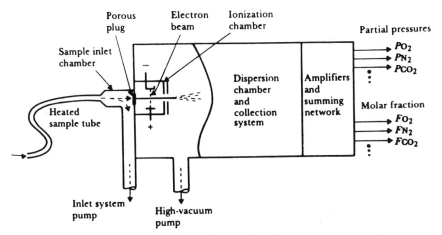

Fig. 7–17. — The essential components of a mass spectrometer.

persion chamber and an ion-detection (collector) system (Fig. 7 – 17).

The sample inlet assembly consists of a heated or unheated capillary tube (approximately 0.25 mm ID) and a sample inlet chamber. Gas is drawn through this system by a rotary pump that reduces the pressure in the inlet chamber to about 10–20 mm Hg (1.3 – 1.7kPa) absolute. A small amount of gas in the inlet chamber leaks by diffusion through a porous plug into the ionization chamber, which, along with the dispersion chamber, is evacuated to approximately 10^{-7} mm Hg (10^{-5}Pa) by a high-vacuum, high-capacity pump. A stream of electrons traveling between a heated filament and an anode bombard the gas entering the ionization chamber and cause the molecules to lose electrons, thereby producing positive ions. These are focused into a beam and accelerated by an electric field into the dispersion chamber, where the ion beam is sorted into its components on a molecular mass basis. The separated ion beams fall on the collector system, which produces an output signal for display.

The technology for moving small tidal volumes (10 – 15 ml) long distances through tubing and manifolds has not been developed; therefore, multiple patient scanning with one mass spectrometer is not suitable for respiratory monitoring in the newborn intensive care areas.

Transcutaneous Oxygen Monitoring

The knowledge gained in the past decade about the risks associated with both hyperoxia and hypoxia has made the clinician aware that partial pressure of oxygen in the arterial blood should be monitored on a regular basis. At present, the most reliable method for this assess-

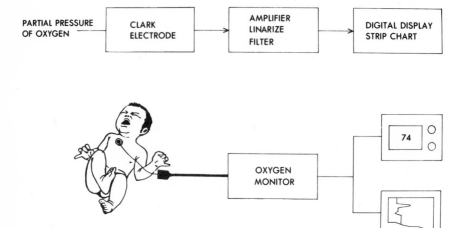

Fig. 7–18. — Instrumentation for the measurement of cutaneous Po_2 by heated oxygen sensor.

ment is periodically withdrawing a small sample of arterial blood from an umbilical catheter and analyzing it with the appropriate equipment. Since such measurements provide data that are relevant only to the time of sampling, changes that occur between samples will not be detected.

The development of a transcutaneous oxygen sensor, which utilizes the phenomenon that oxygen diffuses through the skin, makes possible second-by-second recordings of blood oxygen levels. Active vasodilation of the cutaneous vessels is achieved by warming the metallic parts of the sensor to a temperature (42–45° C) that is higher than normal body temperature. Oxygen diffuses from the arterialized capillaries through the skin and is measured by electrochemical reduction (Clark electrode). The signal is amplified, conditioned and displayed, usually on a digital meter as well as a strip chart recorder (Fig. 7–18).

CHEST PHYSIOTHERAPY

Chest physiotherapy is an accepted method of assisting the normal clearing mechanisms of the tracheobronchial tree in children and adults. Finer and Boyd[4] recently have demonstrated its effectiveness in infants with respiratory distress.

Removal of secretions from the bronchi is facilitated by the force of

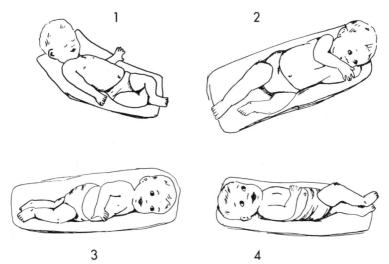

Fig. 7–19.—Positions for chest physiotherapy: *1,* the anterior segment of the upper lobes is drained in a supine position at a 30° upright angle. *2,* drain the apical segment of the right lung while the infant lies on his left side at a 30° upright angle. *3,* the posterior segment of the right upper lobe is drained in a prone position with the right side elevated 45°. *4,* drain the anterior segment of the upper lobe in a supine position.

gravity in various positions and by percussion, sometimes called "clapping." The lung congestion and the infant's tolerance will dictate the need for postural drainage alone, postural drainage with percussion and/or postural drainage with percussion and vibration. Figures 7–19 and 7–20 illustrate the various positions for proper drainage of the upper, middle and lower lobes of the infant.

The infant should be placed in a position such that the segment being drained is uppermost and the major airway leading out of the segment is pointed downward.

Percussion or clapping over the thorax in the area of the segment being drained will facilitate the movement of secretions from smaller airways into larger ones. Since the adult hand usually is larger than the infant's thorax, a small plastic medicine cup attached to the clinician's finger will provide effective percussion with a cupping action.

Vibration is applied to the chest wall, over the affected area, during the expiratory phase. Vibration is a fine shaking motion, which is achieved by tightening all the muscles of the arm and shoulders.

All loosened secretions must be removed, via suctioning, following each treatment.

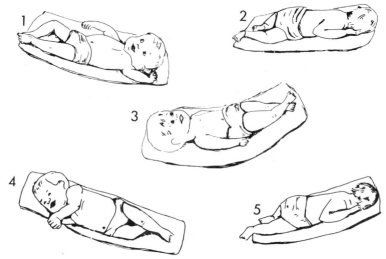

Fig. 7–20.—*1*, the right middle lobe is drained at a 15° head-down angle with a 45° rotation to the left. To drain the lingula, rotate to the right. *2*, the superior segment of the lower lobes drains in a prone position. *3*, drain the anterior basal segments of the lower lobes at a 30° head-down position. *4*, the basal segments of the lower lobe are drained at a 30° head-down position while the infant is lying on the side. *5*, the posterior basal segments of the lower lobes are drained at a 30° head-down prone position.

TRANSILLUMINATION

Transillumination via fiberoptic probe has been used successfully for the diagnosis of pneumothorax in infants.[10] This procedure is performed with the overhead nursery lights turned out, but total darkness is not necessary. With the infant in a supine position, the probe is placed superior and then inferior to the nipple on both sides of the chest. If either side of the chest transilluminates more than the other, several spots at varying distances from the sternum should be transilluminated. If abnormal air collections are present in particular areas of the infant's chest, the transillumination will be greater in those areas. Unless there is a drastic difference between the transillumination of several locations on the infant's chest, a confirming chest radiograph should be taken before needle aspiration or chest tube placement is performed.

Transillumination of the extremities for the purpose of arterial blood sampling is an easily performed technique with a high degree of success.[16] With the room lights dimmed, the probe is placed against the extremity directly opposite the arterial site to be sampled (Fig.

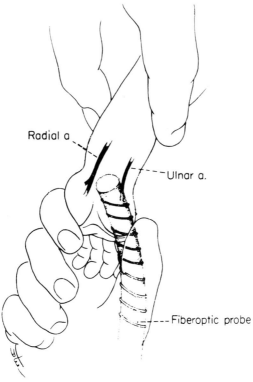

Radial a.

Ulnar a.

Fiberoptic probe

Fig. 7–21.—Position of the hand and wrist and the fiberoptic probe for radial artery puncture.

7–21). Anatomic landmarks and the artery to be sampled are easily visualized. The artery appears as a pulsating linear structure with indistinct edges due to pulsation. Transillumination of the sampled artery should be repeated 24 hours later to confirm visible pulsation at the puncture site.

REFERENCES
1. Al-Salihi, F. L., and Curran, J.: Airway obstruction by displaced eye mask during phototherapy, Am. J. Dis. Child. 129:1362, 1975.
2. Branstater, P.: Dilation of the larynx with Cole tubes, Anesthesiology 31:378, 1969.
3. Committee on Environmental Hazards: Infant radiant warmers, Pediatrics 61:113, 1978.
4. Finer, N. N., and Boyd, J.: Chest physiotherapy in the neonate: A controlled study, Pediatrics 61:282, 1978.
5. Fleishman, A.: Letter to the editor, J. Pediatr. 91:984, 1977.

6. General Hospital and Personal Device Panel, Washington, D.C., Aug. 23–24, 1976.
7. Gruber, H. S., and Klaus, M. H.: Intermittent mask and bag therapy: An alternative approach to respirator therapy for infants with severe respiratory distress, J. Pediatr. 76:194, 1970.
8. Harris, F., and Smith, C. F.: More on apnea resulting from obstruction of nares by an eye shield, J. Pediatr. 90:995, 1977.
9. Kisling, J.: The kitten as a teaching model for intubation of the human neonate, Respiratory Care 21:1243, 1976.
10. Kuhns, L. R., et al.: Diagnosis of pneumothorax or pneumomediastinum in the neonate by transillumination, Pediatrics 56:355, 1975.
11. Lucey, J. F., and Hewit, J.: Photopharmacology and Bilirubin, in Goresky, C. A., and Fisher, M. M. (eds.), *Jaundice* (New York: Plenum Publishing Co., 1974), pp. 276–277.
12. *Medical Device Amendments of 1976*, Pub. L. No. 94–295, 90 Stat. 539 (1976).
13. Segal, S., and Hale, D. R.: Inactivation of infant thermal control by hospital paging system. Read before the Canadian Paediatric Society, Montreal, 1977.
14. Sliney, D. H., and Frazier, B. D.: Evaluation of radiation hazards, Appl. Optics 17:1, 1973.
15. VanPelt, W. F., Payne, W. R., and Peters, R. W.: *A Review of Selected Bioeffects Thresholds for Various Special Ranges of Light* (Rockville, Md.: Bureau of Radiological Health, Food and Drug Administration, 1973).
16. Wall, P. M., and Kuhns, L. R.: Percutaneous arterial sampling using transillumination, Pediatrics 59:1032, 1977.
17. Wu, P. Y. K., and Hodgman, J. E.: Insensible water loss in preterm infants: Changes with postnatal development and non-ionizing radiant energy, Pediatrics 54:704, 1974.

8 / Nursing Care of the Sick Neonate

DONNA deMONTERICE, R.N., M.N.
AND
ROSANNE GUGINO-TOUFEXIS, R.N., M.S.

OVER THE PAST 10 YEARS, the role and responsibility of the neonatal nurse have become increasingly specialized and complex. This chapter will present an overview of the basic nursing care of the neonate in relation to temperature regulation, feeding and monitoring. Special nursing considerations relating to the infant requiring respiratory support are also discussed.

BASIC CARE OF THE SICK NEONATE

Thermal Regulation

The ability to regulate an infant's thermal environment and to protect the infant from cold stress is dependent on a thorough understanding of the principles of heat production and the mechanisms of heat loss. Although the nurse is in an ideal position to control the thermal environment of the infant, it is essential that all professionals involved in the infant's care be aware of how failure to adhere to these principles can affect the entire hospital course of the infant, from his initial respiratory status to his later ability to gain weight. This section will discuss heat production in the neonate, the mechanisms of heat loss, the consequences of cold stress and, finally, the clinical application of these principles.

HEAT PRODUCTION.—It is well established that the newborn is a homeotherm; he strives to maintain his temperature within a narrow normal range despite the temperature of the environment. Heat that is lost to the environment must be replaced. The adult human can utilize shivering and voluntary muscle activity in order to produce heat, but these mechanisms are ineffective in the neonate. The primary mechanism that the neonate utilizes to produce heat is a chemical process—

nonshivering thermogenesis through the metabolism of brown fat. This process is discussed in detail in Chapter 2. This metabolic process requires additional oxygen and calories and is a limited compensatory mechanism. Infants with inadequate energy stores or those who are limited in the utilization of oxygen will, because of their respiratory disease, be unable to compensate for heat that is lost to the environment.

MECHANISMS OF HEAT LOSS.—Newborn infants are more prone to the loss of heat from the core of the body to the surface of the body because of their large surface area-to-mass ratio and because of the absence of an insulating layer of fat. Heat loss from the surface of the body to the environment is controlled by four physical principles:

Radiation is the loss of heat from the body to surrounding cooler, solid objects. The nude infant in an incubator loses heat to the cooler walls of the incubator. The amount of heat that is lost in this way is controlled by the temperature gradient between the incubator walls and the room temperature. As the difference between the temperature of the incubator walls and the room increases, the amount of heat that is lost by the infant also increases.

Evaporation is the loss of heat through the changing of moisture from a liquid to a gas state on the body surface.

Conduction is the loss of heat to a cooler, solid surface that is in direct contact with the body.

Convection is the loss of heat through the movement of air currents across the body.

Radiation and convection are the primary modes of heat loss in cool environments, evaporation becoming the primary mode of heat loss in warmer environments.[1] Radiation and conduction can also be used as modes of heat gaining, as they represent the transfer of heat from a warm object to a cooler one.

Understanding these modes of heat loss is the basis for the prevention of hypothermia in the neonate, which is discussed in detail later in this section.

CONSEQUENCES OF COLD STRESS.—Minimal cold stress can produce hypoxia and hypoglycemia due to the increased utilization of oxygen and glucose during the metabolism of brown fat. Acidosis and also inhibition of surfactant production are other consequences of cold stress.[2]

With severe or prolonged cold stress, neonatal cold injury can occur. The infant, usually of low birth weight, has a bright red color, is lethargic, feeds poorly and is cold to the touch. Other physical findings are bradycardia, slow respirations and central nervous system depression.[3]

Clinical application.—The goal of the nursing care of the neonate in relation to thermal regulation is the prevention of any of the manifestations of cold stress.

Neutral thermal environment.—The infant in an incubator is maintained in a neutral thermal environment, ". . . that range of thermal environment in which a baby with a normal body temperature has a minimal metabolic rate and can maintain a constant body temperature. . . ."[4]

The neutral thermal environment for an individual baby is based on the infant's weight at birth and his age, the temperature range becoming cooler with advancing age. There is no one appropriate environmental temperature for all babies. Although complete tables are available,[5] it is useful in clinical practice to have the figures for each particular weight category available; these then can be placed on the incubator next to the thermometer (Fig. 8–1). This gives the nurse a

Fig. 8–1.—The NTE chart is used as a reference point for establishing incubator temperature.

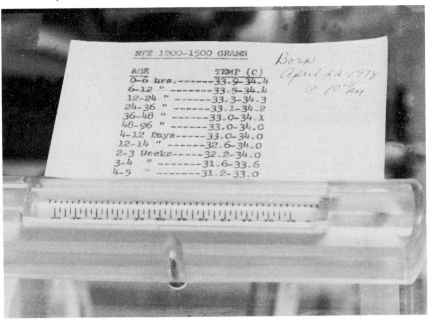

constant reference point in her assessment of the thermal environment of the infant.

In general, smaller infants require higher environmental temperatures to maintain a body temperature of 36.5° C. The smaller and younger infant tolerates only a very narrow range of environmental temperature without becoming heat or cold stressed. With increasing age, the infant will tolerate a wider range of environmental temperature. Smaller infants usually need to be kept in the higher range of neutral thermal temperature. If an infant is having apnea, it is best to maintain him in the lower range of the neutral thermal environment.

Special neutral thermal environment considerations. — Maintenance of the incubator air temperature in the range that is appropriate according to the Scopes chart does not ensure that the infant is in an optimal thermal environment. Cool incubator walls create a heat gradient within the incubator. The baby will lose heat by radiation to these cooler surrounding walls. The amount of heat lost through this route will depend on the room temperature and also on the placement of the incubator within the room. A cool room or the presence of a cool window next to the incubator will result in radiant heat loss that makes strict use of neutral thermal environment charts difficult.

Fig. 8–2. — Heat shields are used to minimize radiant heat loss in low birth weight infants.

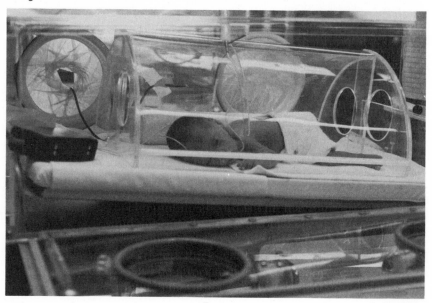

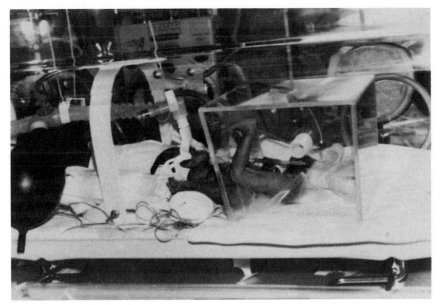

Fig. 8–3. – Plastic oxygen hoods can be used as a heat shield when the small infant requires assisted ventilation.

One solution, suggested by Hey and Monnt,[6] is the use of a clear plastic heat shield inside the incubator. The walls of the heat shield are warmed by the air in the incubator, which is warmer and more stable than room temperature (Fig. 8–2). The baby radiates heat only to the wall of this inner chamber. The heat shield is most appropriate for the baby under 1200 gm who is at high risk for radiant heat loss. The use of a heat shield is impractical for infants who require respiratory assistance. An oxygen hood may be used over the lower body of these infants to help protect them from radiant heat loss (Fig. 8–3).

The use of oxygen hoods, CPAP and ventilators in the treatment of respiratory disease adds another consideration in the maintenance of neutral thermal environment. The temperature of the gas that is delivered to an infant via a hood or by nasal CPAP should be within 0.5–1.0° C of the temperature in the incubator. Particularly in the case of the oxygen hood, this will prevent cold stress due to the stimulation of the temperature receptors of the face.[7] The temperature of the gas delivered via an endotracheal tube should be close to body temperature. This will compensate for the loss of warming that usually takes place in the upper airways.

Servo-control.—Another method of thermal regulation that has been utilized is servo-control. Servo-control is based on the use of the infant's temperature to regulate the temperature of the environment. The desired skin temperature signals the incubator to generate more heat until the infant's temperature is corrected. Although this appears to be a logical way to control an infant's thermal environment, many authors[8, 9] believe that its disadvantages negate the ease with which servo-control operates.

A major disadvantage of servo-control is that the infant's temperature is lost as a measure of his well-being. Without careful observation of the incubator temperature, thermal instability, often an early sign of complications such as sepsis, will not be noticed.

Other hazards of servo-control relate to the position of the skin probe. A probe that is not securely placed will be interpreted by the incubator as a lowering of the skin temperature and could result in the infant becoming overheated. If the infant should inadvertently be turned onto the probe, the incubator temperature will lower in response to the warmth produced by the mattress against the probe. This will produce cold stress in the infant, although the temperature probe still may register a normal temperature. The use of bilirubin lights necessitates that the probe be covered by aluminum foil to ensure an accurate reading.

Servo-control can be used successfully, but it requires extensive education of the nursing staff regarding the hazards involved and the need for continuous careful observation of the infant and his environment.

Radiant heater.—The radiant heater can also be utilized for temperature control of the neonate. The radiant heater is an overhead device that can be regulated by servo-control. The amount of heat generated is controlled by a skin probe that monitors the infant's temperature. Problems with the radiant heater include convective heat loss and increased insensible water loss when used for extended periods. Radiant warmers are best used for acute situations, such as in the delivery room[10] or treatment room when access to the patient is important. Radiant warmers are also very helpful in preventing heat loss during routine nursery procedures, such as blood drawing and bathing.

Common Problems

Although cooling commonly presents a hazard for the neonate, overheating is also an important consideration. Excessively warm environments increase the infant's metabolism and consequently oxygen and caloric requirements. The neonate has difficulty dissipating heat, and hyperthermia inevitably results. If unrecognized or untreated, hyperthermia can result in death. The most common ways an infant becomes overheated are through the use of phototherapy, through exposure to sunlight and malfunction of servo-control probes.

PHOTOTHERAPY. — The use of bilirubin lights may necessitate lowering the incubator temperature out of the neutral thermal range, especially in larger infants. When the lights are discontinued, a heat source is lost and the nurse must again place the infant in his appropriate neutral thermal environment.

GREENHOUSE EFFECT. — The greenhouse effect can occur when the baby in an incubator is placed near a sunny window. The short wavelengths of the sun pass through the incubator wall. Within the incubator, the short wavelengths are converted to long-wave radiant emission, which does not pass through the plastic walls of the incubator.

SERVO-CONTROL PROBES. — Servo-control probes that become loose can lead to the infant being overheated. The incubator will increase its heat output in response to the cooler temperature of the probe.

Assessment of Body Temperature

It is obvious from the preceding discussion that body temperature is only one of the factors that need to be evaluated in the assessment of the infant's thermal environment. To monitor the neonate's body temperature, axillary or skin readings are preferred over rectal temperatures. The skin temperature will more quickly reflect cold stress; changes in the rectal temperature will occur only after the infant already has been stressed. It must be remembered that a "normal" body temperature does not ensure that the infant is in a neutral thermal environment; the body temperature will remain normal as long as the infant is able to increase his metabolism and replace the heat that is being lost. Constant surveillance of the infant and his environment is necessary to prevent heat loss.

Prevention of Heat Loss

In addition to protecting the infant from heat loss while in the incubator, it is essential that he be protected during times when he might be out of the incubator; for instance, during transport to the nursery or to other areas of the hospital and during routine nursery procedures. It is helpful to anticipate the possibility of heat loss by again viewing the ways in which heat is lost by the body.

Evaporative heat losses can be prevented by drying the infant immediately after birth and by keeping the linen under the infant in an incubator dry. Bathing a critically ill neonate probably is unnecessary. When bathing is done, the low birth weight infant should be left in the incubator or a radiant warmer should be used.

Radiant heat losses can be prevented during transport by the use of transport incubators. If the infant is transported in a crib, a plastic swaddling bag[11] or clothing and blankets can be used.

Low birth weight infants should not be taken out of incubators for any reason unless they are dressed and wrapped in a blanket. If the incubator door is open for any length of time and a radiant warmer is not available, the infant should be covered with a blanket. Ensuring that the incubator is not placed near a cold window and that the room temperature remains stable will also help to prevent radiant heat loss.

Conductive heat loss can be prevented by covering potentially cold surfaces before the infant is placed on them. Scales, x-ray plates and examining tables are the most common sources of conductive heat loss.

Convective heat loss can be prevented by avoiding the placement of infants in drafty areas or near air conditioning outlets. Keeping incubator portholes closed will prevent drafts from crossing the infant's body. Use of cold O_2 over an infant's face also results in convective heat loss, as the infant's face is particularly sensitive to temperature changes.[12]

Treatment of Hypothermia

Although we have stressed the importance of prevention of heat loss, it obviously will not always be possible to avoid hypothermia. The treatment of hypothermia involves:

1. Warming the baby slowly, keeping the ambient air temperature no more than 1.5° C higher than the body temperature to minimize further metabolic stress.[13]

2. Observing the infant carefully for apnea, which has been seen during rapid rewarming.

3. Checking the infant's temperature every 15 minutes and adjusting the incubator temperature accordingly.

4. Avoiding the use of hot water bags and other devices that warm by conduction. These probably are not necessary and carry with them the potential for heat stress and burning.

5. Withholding nipple feeding of any baby who is cold stressed, because of the increased risk of aspiration.

CATEGORIZATION BY GESTATIONAL AGE

In order to understand the problems of the newborn, it is helpful to have a firm grasp of how newborns are classified by weight and gestational age. Since the 1960s,[14] newborns have been classified by gestational age into three major categories: preterm, term and post-term. The preterm infant is defined as any infant born before 37 weeks of gestation. The term infant is one with a gestational age of 38–42 weeks and the post-term, or postmature, infant is born after 42 weeks of gestation. The classifications bear no absolute relation to birth weight. Neonates are also classified according to weight. The newborn whose birth weight is below the 10th percentile for a corresponding gestational age is classified as small for gestational age (SGA). Newborns presenting between the 10th and 90th weight percentile at a given gestational age are classified as appropriate for gestational age (AGA). Those whose birth weights are above the 90th percentile for their given gestational age are termed large for gestational age (LGA).

Each newborn, therefore, is assigned two categories: either SGA, AGA or LGA and also either preterm, term or post-term. Mortality and morbidity rates are different for each group of neonates. Each group is at risk to develop somewhat similar sets of problems and subsequent growth patterns. Table 8–1 outlines major conditions that may be present in the high-risk groups. The nurse, in doing her assessment of the

TABLE 8–1.—PROBLEMS THAT MAY
EXIST IN HIGH-RISK NEWBORNS

PRETERM PROBLEMS	POST-TERM PROBLEMS
RDS	Neonatal asphyxia
Hypoglycemia	Meconium aspiration
Hypothermia	Intrauterine death
Hyperbilirubinemia	
Anemia	
SGA PROBLEMS	LGA PROBLEMS
Intrauterine infection	Hypoglycemia
Hypoglycemia	Birth trauma
Major malformations	
Polycythemia	
Perinatal asphyxia	
Aspiration	
Hypothermia	

newborn, screens for these problems in the early neonatal period and identifies infants who will require therapy for resolution of problems that have been detected.

DETERMINATION OF GESTATIONAL AGE

Gestational age of the newborn can be determined through a combination of milestones that occur during pregnancy and physical and neurologic assessment of the newborn. The pregnancy landmarks most commonly utilized are: date of last menstrual period, appearance of fetal heart tones, quickening and uterine size. When these landmarks have not been adequately observed or documented during the prenatal course, increased reliance on sophisticated technologic advances such as ultrasound and amniocentesis may be necessary to assess growth patterns and maturation of the infant in utero. After birth, however, there are many methods that combine physical characteristics and neurologic responses of the newborn to determine the gestational age.

The most common formats used are those developed by Dubowitz et al.[15] and those developed by Amiel-Tison.[16] These scales involve detailed scoring of physical criteria such as breast tissue, ear cartilage, foot creases and nipple formation, and also critical scoring of the infant's neuromuscular development. Both examinations are most reliable within the first 3 days after birth. These can be performed by nurses or physicians who are trained in their use. The categorization of the infant by gestational age and size complements data from the prenatal and intrapartum course in providing a basis for nursing care. Based on this information, many respiratory and metabolic problems of adaptation may be anticipated and promptly corrected in the early neonatal course.

FEEDING THE NEONATE

Feeding the critically ill neonate presents several problems to his caretakers: the need to replace losses that occur naturally through the urine, stool and skin; to supply the requirements for metabolism and growth and yet avoid the hazards that the use of the gastrointestinal tract presents. Other dilemmas are deciding what to feed, in what quantities and with what frequency.

Intravenous Feeding

The initial route for feeding the critically ill neonate is the intravenous one. There is evidence that early intravenous feeding can affect the mortality of the small, high-risk premature infant.[17] Using this route, the infant's maintenance fluid requirements can be achieved readily. Fluid requirements will vary depending on the infant's size, age, activity and degree of illness. Excessive loss of fluid through the normal routes will also alter fluid requirements. Infants under 1 kg require approximately 100 ml/kg on the first day of life and approximately 140–200 ml/kg/day thereafter.[18] Larger infants require proportionately less fluid.

Intravenous solutions consisting of 10% glucose are adequate for the first 24 hours of life; electrolyte solutions are necessary after that. Additional glucose may be necessary, depending on the infant's serum glucose level.

Intravenous hyperalimentation may be necessary to supply calories and protein and to prevent the breakdown of body protein for energy. This is necessary when the gastrointestinal tract will be unavailable for feeding for long periods because of severe respiratory disease. Hyperalimentation may be given through a peripheral intravenous line if diluted solutions are used. The use of full-strength hyperalimentation requires the use of a central line that is placed in a high-flow area such as the superior vena cava or the subclavian vein. The provision of more calories is thought to improve the infant's ability to survive severe illness.[19] It is estimated that infants require 50–100 cal/kg/day in the first week of life and 110–200 cal/kg/day during active growing periods.[20] Recently, the use of fat emulsion solutions (Intralipid) has made it possible to provide essential fatty acids and an additional nonosmotic source of calories by peripheral infusion.

Nursing Responsibilities

Nursing responsibilities in the area of fluid administration include assessment of fluid balance, maintenance of the prescribed rate of flow and detection of complications in the therapy. Assessment of fluid balance is best accomplished through observation and recording of the intake and output and through weighing the infant. Infants under 1200 gm, who are prone to large insensible water losses, and infants who have had extensive surgery should be weighed twice a day. Urine output can be measured by weighing disposable diapers before and after the infant has voided. Plastic urine collectors may cause skin breakdown and should be used only if exact measurements of urine are needed.

The small premature infant does not tolerate large fluctuations in his fluid intake. There never should be attempts to "catch up" the infant's fluid intake if it falls behind the prescribed amount by using large boluses of fluid. The use of infusion pumps helps to overcome this problem by allowing the administration of small amounts of fluid at a fairly even rate. Infusion sets with a small chamber or buret always should be used when administering intravenous fluids to infants. Filling the chamber with no more than the prescribed amount of fluid for 1 or 2 hours helps to prevent accidental fluid overloading of the infant.

Parenteral fluid intake should be measured and recorded every half hour. The calculation of the amount of fluid that should have been infused is also recorded to provide a baseline. This process allows the nurse to intervene quickly to prevent errors in fluid administration.

The IV site should be evaluated every hour for signs of infiltration. This is particularly important when concentrated glucose solutions (over 5%) or medications are being infused; infiltration of these solutions into the tissue can cause necrosis, sloughing and scarring.

Infants receiving 10% glucose or hyperalimentation solutions should have routine Dextrostix determinations done to detect hyperglycemia or hypoglycemic reactions. Urine Labstix and Clinitest determinations will detect spilling of sugar excreted in the urine, which could produce an osmotic diuresis. Urine specific gravity is also useful in determining the adequacy of the therapy and neonatal kidney function.

Intravenous solutions and administration sets should be changed daily. Hyperalimentation solutions provide excellent growth medium needed for bacteria. Extreme care must be used in handling the container and the tubing while they are being assembled. To eliminate debris and microorganisms, a micropore filter (0.2 m) should be used. To further protect against contamination, the hyperalimentation line should not be used for intravenous medications.

Gavage Feedings

Once the infant has begun to recover from his respiratory illness, feeding via the gastrointestinal tract can begin. Oral feeding should be avoided in the premature infant and any infant with rapid respirations because of the greatly increased risk of aspiration. The preterm infant (less than 34 weeks of gestation) has not yet developed the ability to coordinate sucking and swallowing or a "gag reflex." The full-term infant who is breathing rapidly (> 60 breaths per minute) will have difficulty coordinating sucking and swallowing. In these infants, gavage feeding is indicated.

A variety of methods of gavage feeding have been utilized in the past, among them nasogastric, orogastric, nasoduodenal and nasojejunal. The nasoduodenal and nasojejunal methods bypass the stomach and therefore eliminate the risk of vomiting and aspiration. These methods are not without risk; they carry the difficulties of tube placement and possible complications, such as perforation.[21]

Nasogastric feeding with an indwelling tube has been utilized since 1951[22] and can be used safely if attention is paid to careful tube placement, securement and assessment of tube position before each feeding. The nasal route presents the hazard of respiratory distress, since infants are obligate nose breathers. For this reason, a small size tube (5 Fr) should be used and care should be taken in taping the tube so that the tape does not cover the naris. Oral tubes may be used but cannot be secured stably and need to be carefully rechecked before feeding.

The distance the tube should be inserted depends on the size of the infant. To determine the correct distance, measure from the nose to the front of the ear and down to the xiphoid process.

Tube placement must be checked after the tube is inserted and secured and before each feeding. If the tube were inadvertently placed in the trachea, the infant would respond with cyanosis, restlessness and coughing. A more likely possibility than the tube being in the trachea is that the tube is midway up the esophagus and not in the stomach. This would put the infant at risk for regurgitation and aspiration. Position can be assessed by listening over the stomach with a stethoscope while instilling 0.5 – 1.0 ml of air through the tube. The air can easily be heard as it enters the stomach. If the end of the tube is in the esophagus, the sound will be diminished and distant. If there is any question as to tube placement, the tube should be removed and reinserted.

Stomach contents are aspirated before each feeding, measured and returned to the infant. This is done to evaluate how the infant is tolerating the feedings and is further verification that the tube is in the stomach. The amount of the aspirate is subtracted from the total amount of the feeding so that the infant does not receive more volume than he can tolerate. It is not necessary to rinse the tube with water after the feeding; doing so would only increase the volume in the stomach without adding calories. Once the position of the tube has been verified and the stomach contents measured, the feeding can be given. The feeding is allowed to run in slowly by gravity. "Pushing" the feeding with the plunger of the syringe is uncomfortable for the infant and puts him at risk for regurgitation. It is not necessary to restrain the infant's hands to prevent the tube from being removed. If it is dislodged it can be readily replaced. The infant should be observed continually during the feeding, as dislodgment of the tube at that time could easily result in aspiration.

The infant should be held for the feeding. If temperature considerations or the illness of the infant does not allow this, he may be positioned on his abdomen or side, with the head slightly elevated. Tactile contact and a pacifier will help to lessen the deprivation that is experienced by this method of artificial feeding.

Readiness for oral feeding is indicated by the absence of respiratory distress and the neurologic ability to coordinate sucking and swallowing, as well as an adequate gag reflex. These develop at approximately the thirty-fourth week of gestation. When nipple feedings are begun, the nasogastric tube is left in place and its position is assessed before the feeding. The feeding is offered with a soft nipple that does not have an enlarged hole. Gentle rotation of the nipple in the infant's mouth can stimulate sucking. The infant never should be allowed to become fatigued; if he does not take the prescribed amount of formula, the feeding can be finished through the tube. The baby should be observed at each feeding for the presence of appropriate feeding behaviors. These have been described[23] as behavior that indicates hunger, such as crying and sucking on objects, "approach" behavior such as rooting, "attachment" behavior that involves getting the nipple in the mouth and "consummatory" behavior that describes the sucking and swallowing ability of the infant.

The frequency of feeding usually is determined by individual institutions; generally, smaller and younger infants are fed very small amounts at frequent intervals. As the feedings are tolerated, the amount can be increased and also the length of time between feedings.

The young premature infant who is at high risk for necrotizing enterocolitis should be evaluated frequently. The inability to tolerate feedings, as indicated by the presence of repeated aspirates, often is an early sign of the disease and should be regarded with suspicion. Other symptoms include thermal instability, lethargy, abdominal distention and guaiac-positive stools. When the disease is suspected, feeding should be stopped until the infant has been evaluated completely.

HEART RATE AND RESPIRATORY MONITORING

The principles underlying heart rate and respiratory monitoring are discussed in Chapter 7. This section will focus on the common problems associated with monitoring and their solutions.

Common problems include no heart rate or ECG, 60-cycle noise or interference as indicated by a widened baseline, bradycardia and tachycardia false alarms and apnea false alarms.

The majority of problems with monitoring involve electrodes, either because they are not placed correctly or because they have lost their contact with the body. The infant presents some unique problems when electrodes are used; these include the lack of flat areas of skin to which the electrode can adhere, problems with skin irritation because of the adhesive or the electrode paste and the size of the electrodes. When a problem occurs with a monitor, the electrodes should be checked first for looseness or the absence of adequate electrode paste. If the electrodes need to be replaced, the skin should be cleansed with soap and water and dried. The skin of the infant should also be inspected at this time for any areas of irritation or breakdown. The new electrodes should be placed in a different, clean location. Correct electrode placement varies with the parameters that are being monitored and the type of monitor that is being used.

Other sources of malfunctioning are broken lead wires, loss of contact of the lead wire with the cable, broken cables, disconnection of the cable at the monitor and an unplugged monitor. A poor ground may contribute to 60-cycle noise. All these parameters should be checked if changing or repositioning the electrodes does not resolve the problem. Malfunctioning of the monitor itself can be determined by switching the patient's cable to a new monitor; if the problem is resolved, the difficulty is with the monitor.

Although cardiopulmonary monitoring is of great value to the nurse who is caring for the neonate, it does not replace careful observation and assessment of the infant. When a monitor alarm is activated, the nurse must first look at the infant to determine if there is a problem other than at the machine. Her initial observations will determine her course of action; if the infant is pink and crying, the monitoring system can be evaluated. The failure of a monitor to alarm during apnea or bradycardia can be due to the alarm being silenced or not reactivated after an episode. It is essential that the nurse knows how each individual monitor works to avoid this kind of tragedy. The monitor should be checked by the nurse at the beginning of her shift to ensure that the alarm limits are correctly set and the monitor is functioning appropriately.

RESPIRATORY CARE OF THE SICK NEONATE: NURSING RESPONSIBILITIES

The importance of continual assessment of the newborn with respiratory distress has been emphasized in preceding chapters. The

TABLE 8-2.—NURSING ASSESSMENT OF THE INFANT IN RESPIRATORY DISTRESS

ASSESSMENT	FREQUENCY	REASONING	NORMAL RANGE	DEVIATIONS
Color	At least q1h	Can reflect changes in oxygenation and circulation	Pink, pale pink acrocyanosis first 4 hours of life	Cyanosis of mucous membrane, pallor, cyanosis of extremities, jaundice, mottling
Activity	At least q1h	Reflects changes in disease process	Spontaneous activity; responds to stimulation. Changes in state of activity occur throughout 24-hr cycle, i.e., sleep, wake, suck cycles throughout the day	Limp ("floppy"), jittery, seizures, irritable. No changes in state of activity
Position	At least q1h	Prevent pulmonary status, maintain skin integrity, ensure anatomic alignment of airway	Head should be slightly hyperextended; change position q4h or prn	Pressure areas; soft airway obstruction; kinking of endotracheal tube
Temperatures: Axillary	q15′ until stable, then q1h also when blood gas is drawn	Cold stress may produce hypoxia and acidosis	36.3°–36.7° C	Temperature variations when using servo control

O₂ system	As above; check simultaneous with axillary temp. and following addition of water to nebulizer and change of tubing	Contributes to creation of a neutral thermal environment (NTE)	O_2 delivered via hood, nasal prongs or mask should be within 1 degree of the infant's NTE temp. O_2 delivered via endotracheal tube bypasses the upper airway; should be warm (36°–37° C)	Greater than 1° C outside prescribed range
Inner chamber	q15' until stable, then simultaneous with axillary temp.	Hyperthermia and hypothermia increase oxygen consumption	Varies with infant's weight and age. See NTE chart	Outside NTE range
Respiratory effort:				
Rate	At least q1h	Determine changes in disease state	40–60/min. Irregular in premature infant (periodic breathing)	Less than 40 or greater than 60. Any sudden change in rate, labored, apnea
Retractions	At least q1h	Determine changes in disease state as reflected by use of accessory muscles of respiration	Mild retractions may be normal in some premature infants who show no other signs of respiratory distress	Moderate to severe substernal, subcostal, suprasternal or intercostal retractions
Nasal flaring	At least q1h	Determine changes in disease state	No flaring	If present
Grunting	At least q1h	Reflects infant's attempts to compensate for his disease process by breathing against a partially closed glottis, trapping air in alveoli	May be present transiently in the first hour after birth	Often due to cold stress; check temperatures. If grunting is noted, record frequency. Example: grunting audible 50% of the time
Breath sounds	At least q1h before and after suctioning. Following intubation or any acute change in condition	Assess adequacy of ventilation; reflects changes such as pneumothorax, pulmonary edema, malpositioned or blocked endotracheal tube	Equal bilaterally and clear	Decreased, moist, unequal

(continued)

TABLE 8–2.—NURSING ASSESSMENT OF THE INFANT IN RESPIRATORY DISTRESS *(Cont.)*

ASSESSMENT	FREQUENCY	REASONING	NORMAL RANGE	DEVIATIONS
Cardiac status	q1h	Increase metabolic demands; hypoxia and apnea often are reflected in heart rate	120–160/min Regular	Rate less than 120, greater than 160, murmur, change in location of apical impulse
Blood gases	Check 20–30 min after change in FIO_2 and following changes in mechanical ventilation such as CPAP, PEEP, pressure, rate or volume. Obtain blood gases following any major change in infant's condition, or at least q4h during period of acute disease	Assess pH, oxygenation, ventilation. Evaluate response to therapy, protect infant from damage due to oxygen toxicity	Arterial blood gas: PO_2 60–80 pH 7.35–7.45 PCO_2 35–40 $NaHCO_3$ 22–26 O_2 sat. 95–100% BE −3 to +3	PO_2 levels of arterialized capillary samples may be slightly lower. After repeated heel sticks (infants with chronic disease), capillary perfusion may be poor and not reflect arterial values. PCO_2 values may be slightly higher in infants with chronic respiratory disease. Other deviations require immediate attention
Environmental oxygen and delivery system	Measure FIO_2 either continuously or q1h unless condition changes. CPAP and respirator setting should be checked and recorded at least q1h	Damage can occur from excess FIO_2 pressures, rates. Improvement in infant's condition depends on accurately delivered therapy	Stable readings	May be due to poorly calibrated oxygen analyzer problem within system

nurse is in a key position to monitor the infant on a continual basis. Priorities for nursing care of the infant with respiratory distress are:
1. Anticipation of problems.
2. Assessment and evaluation of response to therapy.
3. Awareness of the effect of the total environment on the infant.
4. Provision of opportunities for parent-infant interaction.

Table 8–2 outlines the parameters that the nurse must assess in an infant with respiratory distress. As the infant's condition stabilizes, the frequency of assessments can be decreased. Any deterioration in the infant's status demands a total re-evaluation until the source of distress is identified.

The following sections will examine nursing care of the newborn in respiratory distress. Problems related to the care of an infant receiving oxygen by hood, nasal CPAP and mechanical ventilation will be discussed, as well as special considerations regarding suctioning, stimulation and care of the parents.

Care of the Neonate Receiving Oxygen by Hood

Hoods are utilized to provide a controlled oxygen environment around the infant's head. Generally, oxygen concentrations of 30% or greater cannot be reliably controlled in the incubator due to the large air space within the incubator and the loss of oxygen concentration through portholes when they are opened to provide necessary care. As with other methods of oxygen administration, oxygen delivered through a hood should be warm and humidified.

Special nursing considerations.—*Position.*—Although, traditionally, infants with severe respiratory distress have been positioned supine, recent evidence suggests that oxygenation may be improved in the prone position.[24] Whatever position is used, airway obstruction must be avoided. In the supine position, a small towel roll should be placed under the infant's shoulders to stabilize the position of his head. This roll can be easily changed to ensure that the infant is lying on a dry surface and is protected from evaporative heat loss by this route.

Airway.—Postural drainage and gentle nasal and oral suctioning may be needed to remove secretions. The nares should be kept clear and unrestricted, as the neonate is an obligate nose breather. Nasogastric tubes and phototherapy eye pads should be positioned so that they are not restricting air exchange. Oral care with sterile water or lemon-glycerin swabs should be given at least 3 times a day.

Mechanical considerations.—The water level within the nebulizer should be checked frequently and maintained. Accumulation of water in the tubing from condensation should be drained regularly to promote a free flow of gas into the hood. The flow rate of the oxygen-air mixture should be at least 7 liters to prevent build-up of carbon dioxide.

The oxygen concentration should be measured every hour once the infant has stabilized. Hood temperature may be measured using an indwelling temperature probe and telethermometer. This device is also useful for monitoring temperatures in CPAP.

Environmental Stimulation and Bonding

The oxygen hood, by its physical presence, can interfere with certain goals of nursing care. One problem associated with the high humidity within the hood is difficulty in clear visualization of the infant's face. This can hinder direct observation of the infant and may also interfere with parent-infant attachment. We have observed mothers who have had to delay naming their child due to their obstructed view of his facial characteristics. The process of identification, claiming and attachment on the part of the parents may be prolonged as a result of this therapy. It is our belief that hoods, eye pads or other obstructive

Fig. 8–4. – A large hood provides the infant with opportunities for visual stimulation and spontaneous motor activity.

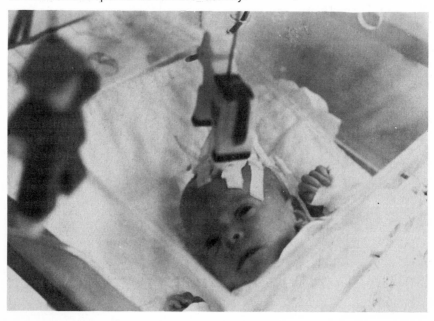

therapies that restrict the parents' and infant's visual contact be briefly removed to give parents an opportunity to see and touch their "whole infant." This also provides an opportunity for eye-to-eye contact between infant and parents, which is so important to the attachment process.[25]

A similar problem of visual deprivation occurs from the infant's perspective. Recent studies have documented the ability of newborns to make visual preferences at an early age.[26, 27] The infant who requires continuous oxygen therapy over a long hospital course should not be deprived of a visually stimulating environment as well as auditory and tactile stimulation.

Infants who receive oxygen via hood for extended periods, such as infants with bronchopulmonary dysplasia, need large hoods that provide room for spontaneous head movement and hand-mouth contact (Fig. 8–4). The nursing staff and parents must create an environment in which growth and development may proceed despite the infant's hospitalization and the restricting nature of the hood. Visual stimulation with mobiles, pictures and frequent personal contact is important. A face mask can be used at various periods throughout the day so that the infant may sit up and change his visual fields. The use of a mask

Fig. 8–5. – Infants who require oxygen for prolonged periods will benefit from the use of an oxygen mask. By inverting the mask, the infant can be bottle fed and held frequently during the day.

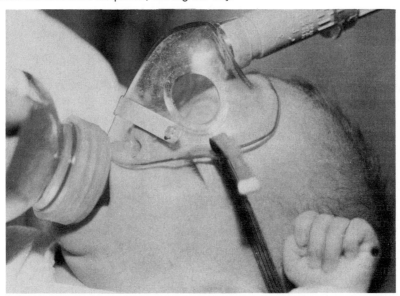

allows for feeding, cuddling, weight bearing and visual stimulation, which would not normally occur when lying flat (Fig. 8–5). Older infants may enjoy the experience of tub baths as long as the oxygen supply remains in place. At this time, various stimulation programs for neonates requiring intensive care are being examined. The effect of such stimulation on long-term growth and development is in active debate.

Care of the Infant Receiving Oxygen Therapy with CPAP

Continuous positive airway pressure (CPAP) is utilized for neonates who are breathing spontaneously but cannot maintain adequate PO_2/PCO_2 levels in relatively high environmental oxygen concentrations. In our institution, an infant with decreased lung compliance resulting in PO_2 levels below 60 in greater than 70% FIO_2 is a candidate for CPAP therapy. Very low CPAP levels (2–4 cm) are also useful in the treatment of apnea. Although there are a number of CPAP delivery systems that are used in neonatal intensive care, CPAP delivered by nasal prongs is most frequently used at Rainbow Babies & Childrens Hospital, as we have seen positive results from this system for a number of years.[28]

SPECIAL NURSING CONSIDERATIONS.—*Position.*—The positions of the neonate's head and the system's nosepiece are of critical importance in the effective delivery of nasal CPAP. If the nasal prongs are not securely placed in the infant's nares, it will be difficult to obtain more than minimal pressure levels. If the nasal prongs are improperly angled, anatomic changes can occur from pressure on the nasal septum or the nares. Figure 8–6 illustrates the proper position of the infant's head and the correct articulation of the nares and nasal prongs, which are supported by the Angel Frame.

To ensure proper positioning, the following steps should be taken when the system is initiated:

1. Select appropriately sized nasal prongs. At present, nasal prongs are manufactured in two sizes, the smaller of which generally is adequate for infants weighing less than 1500 gm.
2. Prepare a "head sling," which will be used to stabilize the position of the nosepiece (Fig. 8–7).
   a) Measure the occipital area of the infant's head, from ear to ear. Add 2 cm to this measurement.
   b) Cut a 3"-wide piece of adhesive tape using your measurement (occiput + 2 cm).
   c) Tape over the top and bottom of the adhesive, leaving only a

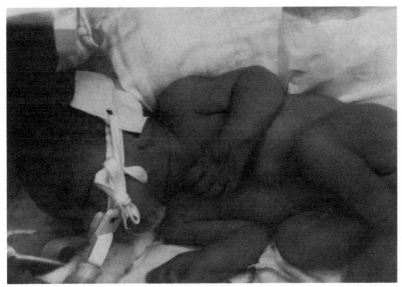

Fig. 8–6.—CPAP nosepiece in place. The headpiece is placed correctly over the occiput. Note the proper positioning of the CPAP mechanism. The headpiece is placed over the occiput and the ties form a straight line with the nosepiece. The prongs are positioned so that there is no pressure on the nose. Note the orogastric tube for gastric decompression. The use of nasal CPAP does not restrict repositioning of the infant.

Fig. 8–7.—Silastic nasal prongs are used in the administration of nasal CPAP. The head sling is made from tape and tied to the nosepiece to stabilize the prongs.

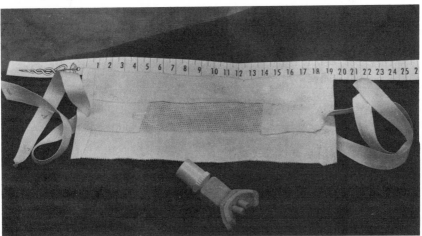

    narrow strip of adhering adhesive in the middle, along the length of the tape.

    d) Insert twill tape in each slit. Later, this will be tied to the nosepiece.

3. The Angel Frame may be used to stabilize the anesthesia bag and tubing of the CPAP mechanism. The infant is placed inside the Frame, with blanket or diaper rolls on each side of the head to minimize head movement. Oxygen is given by mask during this time. A lamb's wool pad is placed under the infant's shoulders and head to prevent irritation from the base of the Angel Frame. When the infant is in the supine position, slight extension of his head should be accomplished using a shoulder roll.

4. Place the head sling under the infant's head at the occipital level. Insert the nasal prongs gently, noting the position that exerts the least amount of pressure on the nasal septum. Using the twill tape, tie the nasal prongs in place. If the sling is too high or too low, the nosepiece will not be held at the correct angle.

5. Adjust the Angel Frame so that the nasal prongs will be stabilized in proper alignment.

6. After the nosepiece is in place, wrinkling or blanching of the nose indicates excessive pressure or improper alignment.

7. Adjust the pressure valve to the prescribed level.

8. Observe the infant's nose from several different angles to ensure that it is not rotated and causing pressure on one side.

9. The infant's position may be changed without disrupting therapy, although realignment of the nosepiece is needed.

Distention of the stomach. — A size 5 or 8 F orogastric tube is inserted and left open to air, to decompress the stomach.

Facial care. — Check for irritation of the face and neck from malposition of the head sling. The twill tape should be placed so that it will not produce facial pressure. The nasal prong nosepiece should be changed every 48 hours or as needed. A hydrocortisone cream may also be used to decrease nasal irritation. Oral and nasal suctioning may be needed frequently. Oral care with sterile water or lemon-glycerin swabs should be done as needed.

Complications. — A variety of air leaks may occur spontaneously or as a result of high-pressure mechanical ventilation. Air leaks generally begin at the alveolar level and extend to a number of other areas from the interstitial space. The most common air leak problem is pneumothorax. Pneumothorax usually produces a fairly rapid deterioration in the infant's condition, including cyanosis, tachypnea, bradycardia, decreased or absent breath sounds and possible shift in apical impulse. A descended liver and decreased blood pressure are also noted frequently. A pneumothorax can be confirmed by transillumination or chest x-ray. Immediate relief from a tension pneumothorax can be accomplished by withdrawal of air by needle and syringe, followed by insertion of a chest tube. Air leaks that extend subcutaneously are identified clinically by crepitus.

Another complication of CPAP is diminished cardiac output. There are different theories regarding why this occurs. It is generally believed that as the infant's condition and lung compliance improve, the continuous pressure can be transmitted through the lungs, causing pulmonary venous compression and reduced blood flow to the heart.[29] Therefore, circulatory status (e.g., warmth of limbs, quality of peripheral pulses) and blood pressure should be evaluated as part of nursing care of these infants.

Infants on CPAP for treatment of respiratory distress syndrome may tire and experience atelectasis and periods of hypercapnia, requiring intermittent bagging. This usually is performed for 5–10 minutes every half hour. The F_{IO_2} during bagging is not increased and the bagging pressure generally is kept between 25 and 30 cm when using nasal CPAP. The infant's mouth must be closed during this time or pressures will not reach the lung. Infants who require frequent bagging require one-to-one nursing care. This procedure often can obviate intubation and the need for constant mechanical ventilation, both of which carry significant risks. The infant should be observed following bagging to ensure that he assumes a normal ventilatory pattern and does not become apneic. The need for frequent assessment of infants receiving nasal CPAP cannot be overemphasized, not only to detect "tiring" and deterioration of condition but also to note improvement that will indicate opportunities for the pressure or F_{IO_2} to be decreased.

Mechanical considerations.—Several aspects of the CPAP mechanism must be routinely checked. These include:

1. The pressure manometer. The manometer must be easily visible at all times. Check to see that it zeros when off the pressure mechanism. Read the pressure every hour. If the pressure has decreased, check for leaks in the system. Leaks can occur anywhere, from the oxygen source to the infant's nose. If no leaks are found, adjust the valve or clamp to attain desired pressure.

2. Pop-off valve. There are two pop-off mechanisms: the underwa-

ter seal and the infant's mouth. Make sure that the water seal is intact and repositioned after bagging and that the infant's mouth and lips are free to open.

3. Humidity. Poor humidification of the system may result in thick pulmonary secretions. High humidity that condenses in the tubing can be dangerous if it empties into the infant's nasopharynx, causing aspiration. High humidity may also lead to water intoxication.

4. Oxygen concentration and temperature. Oxygen concentration should be measured every hour. The neonate's oxygen-air mixture temperature, body temperature and environmental temperature should be measured simultaneously.

Care of the Neonate on a Respirator

Neonates who require mechanical ventilation for their respiratory disease need close surveillance during the critical stages of their disease. Good management demands anticipation of problems and recognition of an improving condition so that the therapy can be quickly tailored to the infant's needs.

The infant on a respirator is intubated via a nasotracheal tube, orotracheal tube or tracheostomy. The airway is attached by an adapter to the respirator tubing. An Angel Frame or other suitable supportive mechanism may be used to stabilize the respirator tubing.

SPECIAL NURSING CONSIDERATIONS. —*Position.* —The intubated infant does not need to be restricted in any position and the older infant with an endotracheal tube or tracheostomy may be cared for in an open crib to provide additional stimulation.

The most important consideration in position is to protect the endotracheal tube from being dislodged. The length of the tube from the mouth, or nose, to the respirator adapter should be measured and recorded on the infant's flow sheet or on a note attached to the incubator wall. This will provide a reference point if the tube appears to slip out of place or is retaped. Originally, the measurement should be made when the tube's proper position has been confirmed by x-ray. The tube alignment should be checked so that it will not pull on the mouth or cause pressure on the naris.

Maintaining a patent airway. — Extubation is a problem that can be prevented by careful tube securement and gentle handling of the infant. Should the tube dislodge and the infant only partially extubate, the length of the tube visible outside the naris or mouth will be increased. This can be determined by comparing the length against that recorded at initial intubation. Do not reintroduce an endotracheal tube blindly, hoping that it will advance down the trachea back to its original location. Chances are that it will not and may traumatize the area, making reintubation more difficult. Extubation can also be noted clinically. Increased respiratory difficulty, crying or audible vocalization, breathing that is out of phase with the respirator and diminished breath sounds are signs of tube displacement. The tube should be completely removed and the infant ventilated with bag and mask until he can be reintubated.

The tube may also dislodge and advance in the opposite direction, into the right mainstream bronchus. If this occurs, it will produce a clinical deterioration due to hyperinflation of the right lung and atelectasis of the left. This situation often is easily detectable, as the visible tube length has shortened and breath sounds on the right are louder than on the left. The tube should be pulled back to its original position until breath sounds are equal. The tube should be taped and an x-ray of its position obtained.

A blocked endotracheal tube may produce a variety of symptoms. Severe distress, including increased retractions, tachypnea, breathing out of phase with the respirator, cyanosis, irritability and decreased breath sounds may be present. The cause usually is a mucous plug that can be loosened using normal saline to irrigate the tube and then removed by suctioning. If the plug cannot be removed, the physician should be notified. A decision to pull the tube, institute bag breathing, suction and then reintubate is made. Endotracheal tubes should not become plugged if the oxygen is well humidified and the endotracheal tube is being suctioned adequately. The use of normal saline routinely with suctioning may help to prevent the formation of mucous plugs.

Suctioning (described in detail later in this chapter) should be done as needed. At this point, it is important to note that suctioning through an artificial airway may cause trauma and produce blood-tinged tracheal aspirate. If this occurs, decrease the suction pressure. Do not apply suction when the catheter is at the carina; rather, withdraw it slightly and then apply the suction.

Blood-tinged aspirate can also be a sign of pulmonary hemorrhage. If the infant's condition shows any other signs of deterioration, the physician should be notified of this finding.

Because suctioning procedures and respirator therapy may introduce pathogens directly into the infant's trachea and lungs, tracheal aspirates should be obtained frequently. The tracheal aspirate is obtained through the use of a sterile specimen trap during suctioning.

Rapid changes in body chemistry.—The infant on a respirator for treatment of respiratory distress syndrome should demonstrate an improvement in lung compliance with time that results in increased PO_2 levels. Other infants may tire and become hypercapneic, necessitating increased respirator cycling rates or pressures. The infant's disease state, his compensatory mechanism and the mechanical control over certain physiologic parameters all contribute to his clinical condition. Close assessment of the infant's clinical condition and laboratory data provide the major evaluation of the therapy and directions for future management.

Complications.—Air-leak complications discussed under nasal CPAP are applicable to respirator therapy. Infants who require intubation for extended periods may require a tracheostomy to prevent tracheal stenosis. Use of high oxygen concentrations, endotracheal intubation and respirator therapy over a "prolonged period" is believed to contribute to the development of bronchopulmonary dysplasia.

Mechanical considerations.—In addition to measuring oxygen concentration and oxygen temperature, the rate, high pressure, low pressure, volume and positive end expiratory pressure all need to be recorded routinely during daily care of the infant. Connections must also be checked systematically from the infant to the wall oxygen source to rule out leaks in the system, loose connections or kinked tubing. Critical changes in the neonate's condition may occur from minor changes in mechanical adjustments. Any deterioration in the infant's status demands that the respirator be evaluated to rule out malfunction. The infant should be bag breathed while the respirator is being checked. Common sources of mechanical variation are:

1. *Fluctuation of the pressure.* Fluctuations may be caused by water in the tubing.

2. *Activation of respirator alarm.* The alarm signals a change in pressure. Activation of the low-pressure alarm may be due to a leak in the system, most commonly due to the infant being disconnected from the respirator. It also is activated when the infant is taken off the respirator for suctioning. If all the respirators alarm at once, the nursery's oxygen pressures or electrical system may be malfunctioning and infants on ventilators will require bag breathing. Activation of the alarm may also be due to high pressure within the system. Increased levels of pressure used for ventilation may be due to kinking of a respirator tube or endotracheal tube or having mucus in the endotracheal tube. Increased or fluctuating positive end expiratory pressure

often is due to water condensation, which should be emptied from the tubing.

3. *Increased humidity in the system.* High humidity may cause water intoxication.

4. *Decreased humidity in the system.* Low humidity may promote plugs in the endotracheal tube.

Because of the variety of mechanical difficulties that may occur, every infant on a respirator needs an anesthesia bag and mask, connected to an oxygen source, at his incubator at all times.

Suctioning

The technique of suctioning carries possible complications for the ill neonate. It is important that the nurse or therapist performing this procedure understand the principles and potential hazards involved. The goal of suctioning is to clear the airway of secretions that can potentially interfere with ventilation. A sterile technique is utilized when suctioning an infant with an endotracheal tube or a tracheostomy to prevent introduction of pathogens into the lower respiratory tract. Use of a sterile technique for suctioning the nasopharynx will reduce the number of organisms mechanically introduced into the infant's upper airway.

NASOPHARYNGEAL AND OROPHARYNGEAL SUCTIONING. — Suctioning can be performed with a bulb syringe or a suction catheter that is either attached to a DeLee suction trap or to mechanical suction. The bulb syringe can be used to suction just the mouth and the external nares; attempts to insert it farther can cause tissue trauma. The use of a suction catheter carries with it the risk of apnea, cardiac irregularities[30] and tissue trauma. To prevent these complications, the catheter should be inserted gently and suction applied only as the catheter is withdrawn. The catheter never should be repeatedly thrust blindly into the oropharynx or swept around the back of the oral cavity. Once the catheter is withdrawn, the infant should be observed and allowed to rest for a few moments; the suctioning then can be repeated as needed. Oxygen can be given if there is a color change, apnea or bradycardia.

SUCTIONING THROUGH A TUBE. — Suctioning carries with it the potential for depriving the infant of oxygen, primarily through the mechanical obstruction that the suction catheter produces. This is particularly true of the smaller uncuffed tubes that are used for infants. For this reason, it is essential that the infant be hyperoxygenated briefly before and after each introduction and removal of the suction catheter.

Care must be taken to insert the catheter only 1–2 cm beyond the carina; insertion "as far as the catheter will go" has been reported as being responsible for perforation and resultant pneumothoraces.[31]

The frequency of suctioning generally is determined by the infant's need and the amount of his secretions. Endotracheal tubes should be suctioned at least every 1 or 2 hours, even if there are minimal secretions, to ensure their patency and to prevent the formation of mucous plugs that would require reintubation. Tracheostomy tubes may require suctioning every 15 minutes initially and then every 2 hours or when necessary.

In order to maintain sterility, two people are required; one person performs the suctioning and the other bag breathes the patient. Small amounts (0.25–0.5 ml) of sterile normal saline can be instilled to help loosen secretions. After the infant is ventilated, the saline is instilled and the bag breathing is repeated to help disperse the saline. The infant then is suctioned. The suction catheter should not be in the airway for longer than 5–10 seconds or bradycardia and hypoxia may occur.

Stimulation

A recent study has demonstrated that the very small and ill neonate can have dramatic changes in PO_2 resulting from what we would consider routine stimulation associated with nursing care.[32] With the advent of the transcutaneous oxygen electrode, one now can visibly observe certain dramatic changes that are produced as a result of tactile stimulation, position and ventilatory changes. Speidel,[32] in a study of neonates receiving intensive care, demonstrated that maneuvers such as changing linen, starting an IV or placing the infant on an x-ray plate produced transient hypoxia in some infants.

Because of our recent experiences with these unstable neonates, we now manage some infants on a "minimal touch" precaution. In practice, the care given to the infant is organized as tightly as possible to minimize the amount of disturbance that we create.

A further consideration for nursing care is the provision of periods during the day when the infant can sleep undisturbed. It must be remembered that the sensory overload in a premature nursery can be tremendous and can place a strain on an infant's physiologic capacities. It has been shown that sleep deprivation in adults causes confusion, disorientation and, in some cases, psychotic reactions.[33] It is possible that sleep deprivation in the infant may similarly disrupt his well-being.

CARE OF THE PARENTS

Care of the parents of the critically ill neonate is discussed in detail in Chapter 12. We would like to add some of our thoughts on this extremely important topic.

When an infant's respiratory problems necessitate rather sophisticated mechanical support, it is important that the parents receive an explanation of what is being done for the infant in terms that they can understand. This explanation is given, in many nurseries, to either parent on the first visit to the nursery. Although the parent should be prepared for what he will see on this visit, we do not believe that a "routine" detailed explanation is indicated the first time a parent visits an extremely ill infant. It is much more important to help the emotionally unprepared parents adjust to the shock of having produced such a small or sick infant. Many parents will not be ready to focus on physiologic or "mechanical" needs of their infant for quite a few days. It is our belief that parents of infants who require therapy, such as CPAP, should be helped to "tune in" to their infant, his behavior and physical characteristics rather than his FI_{O_2}, CPAP level and bilirubin values.

Many neonatal intensive care units utilize "primary care nursing" to provide continuity of care for these families. The primary care nurse helps the parents understand and attach to their infant, work through their feelings during this period and plans with them toward discharge.

REFERENCES

1. Scopes, J. W.: Thermoregulation in the Newborn, in Avery, G. (ed.), *Neonatology* (Philadelphia: J. B. Lippincott Company, 1975), pp. 99–108.
2. Graven, S.: Heat and Body Temperature, in Zachman, R. D. (ed.), *Nursing Manual for the Intensive Care of the Newborn* (Wisconsin Perinatal Center, South Central Region, Madison, Wisconsin (unpublished manual), 1969), pp. 27–35.
3. Klaus, M., and Fanaroff, A.: The Physical Environment, in Klaus, M., and Fanaroff, A. (eds.), *Care of the High-risk Neonate* (Philadelphia: W. B. Saunders Company, 1973), p. 67.
4. Scopes, J. W.: Thermoregulation in the Newborn, in Avery, G. (ed.), *Neonatology* (Philadelphia: J. B. Lippincott Company, 1975), p. 103.
5. Klaus, M., and Fanaroff, A.: The Physical Environment, in Klaus, M., and Fanaroff, A. (eds.), *Care of the High-risk Neonate* (Philadelphia: W. B. Saunders Company, 1973), p. 68.
6. Hey, E., and Monnt, L.: Heat losses from babies in incubators, Arch. Dis. Child. 42:75, 1967.

7. Bruck, K.: Temperature regulation in the newborn infant, Biol. Neonat. 3: 65, 1961.

8. Scopes, J. W.: Thermoregulation in the Newborn, in Avery, G. (ed.), *Neonatology* (Philadelphia: J. B. Lippincott Company, 1975), p. 104.

9. Klaus, M., and Fanaroff, A.: The Physical Environment, in Klaus, M., and Fanaroff, A. (eds.), *Care of the High-risk Neonate* (Philadelphia: W. B. Saunders Company, 1973), p. 66.

10. Du, J., and Oliver, T.: The baby in the delivery room, JAMA 207:1502, 1969.

11. Lutz, L., and Perlstein, P.: Temperature control in newborn babies, Nursing Clin. North Am. 6:113, 1971.

12. Bruck, K.: Temperature regulation in the newborn infant, Biol. Neonate 3:65, 1961.

13. Klaus, M., and Fanaroff, A.: The Physical Environment, in Klaus, M., and Fanaroff, A. (eds.), *Care of the High-risk Neonate* (Philadelphia: W. B. Saunders Company, 1973), p. 67.

14. Battaglia, F. C., and Lubchenco, L. O.: A practical classification of newborn infants by weight and gestational age, J. Pediatr. 71:159, 1967.

15. Dubowitz, L. M. S., Dubowitz, V., and Goldberg, C.: Clinical assessment of gestational age in the newborn infant, J. Pediatr. 77:1, 1970.

16. Amiel-Tison, C.: Neurological evaluation of the maturity of newborn infants, Arch. Dis. Child. 43:89, 1968.

17. Cornblatch, M., Forkes, A., Pildes, R., et al.: A controlled study of early fluid administration in survival of low birthweight infants, Pediatrics 38: 547, 1966.

18. Dreszer, M.: Fluid and electrolyte requirements in the newborn infant, Pediatr Clin. North Am. 24:544, 1977.

19. Gunn, T., Reamon, G., Outerbridge, E. W., and Colle, E.: Peripheral total parenteral nutrition for premature infants with the respiratory distress syndrome: A controlled study, J. Pediatr. 92:612, 1978.

20. Barness, L.: Nutrition in the tiny baby: Update and problems, Clin. Perinatol. 4:377, 1977.

21. Sun, S., Samuels, S., Lee, J., and Marquis, J.: Duodenal perforation: A rare complication of neonatal nasojejunal tube feeding, Pediatrics 55:371, 1975.

22. Royce, S., Tepper, C., et al.: Indwelling polyethylene nasogastric tube for feeding premature infants, Pediatrics 8:79, 1951.

23. O'Grady, R.: Feeding behavior in infants, Am. J. Nursing 71:737, 1971.

24. Wagaman, M. J., et al.: The effects of different body positions on pulmonary function in neonates recovering from respiratory disease, Pediatr. Res. 12:571, 1978.

25. Klaus, M., and Kennell, J.: *Maternal-Infant Bonding* (St. Louis: The C. V. Mosby Company, 1976), p. 77.

26. Miranda, S. B.: Visual abilities and pattern preferences of premature infants and full-term neonates, J. Exp. Child Psychol. 10:189, 1970.

27. Hack, M., Mostow, A., and Miranda, S. B.: Development of attention in pre-term infants, Pediatrics 58:669, 1976.

28. Kattwinkel, J., Fleming, D., Cha, C. C., et al.: A device for administration of continuous positive airway pressure by the nasal route, Pediatrics 52: 131, 1973.

29. Affonso, D., and Harris, T.: Continuous positive airway pressure, Am. J. Nursing 76:570, 1976.
30. Cordero, L., Jr., and Hon, E.: Neonatal bradycardia following naso-pharyngeal stimulation, J. Pediatr. 78:441, 1971.
31. Vaughan, R., Menke, J., and Giacoia, G.: Pneumothorax: A complication of endotracheal tube suctioning, J. Pediatr. 92:633, 1978.
32. Speidel, B. D.: Adverse effects of routine procedures on pre-term infants, Lancet 1:864, 1978.
33. Kornfeld, D., Maxwell, T., and Momrow, D.: Psychologic hazards of the intensive care unit, Nursing Clin. North Am. 3:41, 1968.

9 / Continuous Positive Airway Pressure

THOMAS J. WILLIAMS, B.S., R.R.T.

THEORY AND BASIC TERMINOLOGY

CONTINUOUS POSITIVE AIRWAY PRESSURE (CPAP) now is being used considerably to diminish the morbidity and mortality of hyaline membrane disease. Generally, CPAP is a mode of therapy used after oxygen hood therapy but prior to mechanical ventilation. It is particularly useful for premature infants who lack surfactant, a substance that normally lines the alveoli and keeps them from becoming atelectatic or collapsing at the end of each breath. "Continuous positive pressure to the airway counteracts this tendency to collapse and constitutes a major breakthrough in assisting those babies to make the necessary transition to lung breathing."[1]

Basic Concepts

Continuous positive airway pressure was described by Gregory et al.[2] in 1971. Since then, it has been published that continuous positive airway pressure was clinically used first and the term coined in 1935 by Dr. Alvan Barach, who described the phenomenon as continuous positive-pressure breathing (CPPB).[3] For the past several years, other authors have similarly described CPAP and CPPB as continuous distending pressure (CDP),[4] continuous inflating pressure (CIP),[5] continuous distending airway pressure (CDAP),[6] continuous raised airway pressure (CRAP),[7] continuous positive transpulmonary pressure (CPTPP),[8] continuous positive airway pressure breathing (CPAPB),[9] positive airway pressure (PAP),[10] continuous airway distending pressure (CADP),[11] end expiratory pressure (EEP),[12] continuous elevated airway pressure (CEAP)[13] and nasal end expiratory pressure (NEEP).[14]

Which term is used is really immaterial and insignificant as long as the terms do not get in the way of the ideas. The important point to emphasize is that treatment with CPAP involves connecting a sponta-

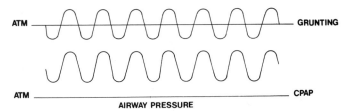

Fig. 9–1.—Pressure versus time diagram illustrates spontaneous breathing with a continuous positive pressure during both inspiration and expiration.

neously breathing infant to a system that applies a constant positive pressure to the airway during both inspiration and expiration. The resultant pressure versus time diagram is shown in Figure 9–1.

Physiologic Effects

CPAP is beneficial in the treatment of the newborn with hyaline membrane disease (HMD) because it is thought to:

1. Re-expand collapsed alveoli, increase surface area and reduce right-to-left intrapulmonary shunting.

2. Increase the functional residual capacity (FRC).

3. Reduce the work of breathing.

"The major defect in HMD is the instability of the alveoli at the end of expiration."[15] This results in a tidal volume and a functional residual capacity that are greatly reduced. "When alveoli which are atelectatic, due to surfactant deficiency or other causes, are opened up or held opened by pressure, a dramatic improvement in oxygenation results. Not only does reexpansion of previously collapsed alveoli greatly increase the surface area for gas exchange in the lungs but it reduces intrapulmonary right-to-left shunting, Such shunting occurs when blood is pumped from the right side of the heart through the lungs which contain no oxygen since they are collapsed. This poorly oxygenated blood returns through the heart back out to the body as if it has been by-passed or shunted around the lungs. Once the air sacs are reopened by CPAP, the blood picks up oxygen on its way through the lungs and delivers it to the body tissues."[1] An increased FRC allows a continuous diffusion of oxygen into the blood at the end of a breath or during periods of nonbreathing. This is important because Kattwinkel *et al.*[16] have shown that premature infants who have periodic breathing or a prolonged time between breaths are not likely to become hypoxemic, bradycardic or apneic if their FRC is increased.

CPAP may also reduce the work of breathing in an infant with respiratory distress syndrome (RDS). Once an elevated FRC is maintained, it is much easier for the infant to increase lung volume slightly than at a greatly reduced volume.

Indications for CPAP

Continuous positive airway pressure has been used most effectively in the treatment of RDS. Through careful and titrated use of CPAP levels, morbidity and mortality due to RDS have decreased markedly. Some newborn intensive care centers have even reported a survival rate approaching 90% in RDS babies.[17] CPAP is not limited, however, to infants suffering from RDS. It has also been used successfully in infants suffering from neonatal milk aspiration[18] or phrenic nerve palsy,[19] in the postoperative management of cardiac and noncardiac thoracic emergencies,[20-23] for pulmonary edema due to a persistent ductus arteriosus[24] and for respiratory failure due to meconium aspiration.[25] In addition, CPAP has also been used to resuscitate newborns at birth and to treat intractable apnea in premature infants.[2]

The CPAP Apparatus

Figure 9–2 shows a typical system for applying continuous positive airway pressure to the newborn through an endotracheal tube. The gas flow into the system is an air/O_2 mixture provided via an air and oxygen flowmeter or oxygen blender to a heated humidifier. The gas flow then passes through an elbow that is attached to an endotracheal tube and to the patient. As the patient exhales, gas exits through a T-piece, a corrugated anesthesia tube and through a reservoir bag (capacity 500 ml). "The screw clamp on the reservoir bag is used to control the outflow of gas and to maintain a constant positive pressure within the system which is indicated on the pressure gauge."[26] The side arm extends below a column of H_2O and acts as a safety valve. Should inadvertent kinking of the exhalation tubing occur, the total pressure in the system cannot exceed the level that the safety valve is set to prevent. In this type of system, the side arm tubing usually is placed approximately 12 inches below the water level. This would allow the safety valve to pop off when 30 cm H_2O is reached. It is important to realize, however, that this safety valve will prevent excessive pressures but will not eliminate sustained pressures. Should the exhalation tubing become kinked, the total system pressure may increase beyond 30 cm H_2O. At this point, the safety valve will prevent pressures from exceeding 30 cm H_2O but the infant still will have to exhale against 30 cm H_2O for as long as the kinked tubing goes unnoticed. The safety valve, although important and necessary, is simply a visual alarm. It is not audible and does not warn the clinician of a problem.

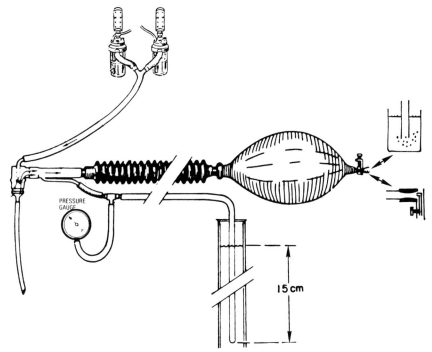

Fig. 9–2.—System for applying continuous positive airway pressure (CPAP) through an endotracheal tube during spontaneous breathing.

Regulation of CPAP

The level of continuous positive airway pressure is regulated by varying the total number of gas molecules flowing into the system while keeping the outflow or leak constant, or by controlling the inflow of gas molecules while varying the amount of obstruction to outflow.

Gas inflow to the system generally is regulated by a single oxygen flowmeter connected to an oxygen blender or a combination of an air and oxygen flowmeter. It may, however, also be regulated by a demand valve. The latter is a valve that opens and provides gas flow to the patient in response to an inspiratory effort by the patient. "Once flow into the system is established its subsequent movement through the circuit is governed by the resistance to flow. The latter is determined by the diameter and length of tubing. The wider and shorter the tubing, the less the resistance and the more the flow."[1]

There are three methods of regulating the number of gas molecules leaving a CPAP system. One is by adjusting a screw clamp on the distal end of the exhalation tubing or over the tail of an anesthesia bag; another is by placing the exhalation tubing under a column of water and the last is via an inverse Venturi.

ADMINISTRATION OF CPAP

CPAP was first provided therapeutically in newborn infants via an endotracheal tube. Subsequently, numerous investigators have described the use of nasal prongs, a face mask or a head hood to administer CPAP in an attempt to avoid the untoward complications of tracheal intubation. Each of these systems is an effective method for increasing arterial blood oxygen (Pa_{O_2}), reducing the inspired oxygen concentration (FI_{O_2}) and providing end expiratory pressure.

Nasal Prongs

Figure 9–3 shows the classic nasal prong device. The nasal piece consists of an endotracheal tube connector for attachment to the CPAP apparatus, an angled flange to allow the unit to be strapped to the infant's head and two short, narrow tubes for insertion into the nares. At present, there are two sizes of the Silastic nasal prongs available. The large size is for infants greater than 1500 gm and the smaller size is for infants less than 1500 gm.

Fig. 9–3. — Silastic prongs for administration of nasal CPAP.

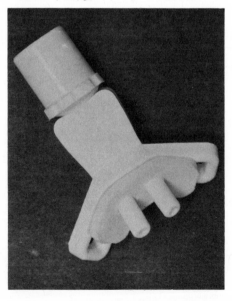

TABLE 9–1.–ADVANTAGES AND DISADVANTAGES OF METHODS OF CPAP THERAPY

NASAL PRONGS	FACE MASK	HEAD HOOD	ENDOTRACHEAL TUBE
Advantages			
1. Ease of application	1. Prevents the complications of endotracheal intubation	1. Ease of application	1. Most efficient method of delivering CPAP
2. Prevents the complications of endotracheal intubation	2. Good accessibility to the patient	2. Quickness	2. Low gas flows can be used
3. Good accessibility to the patient	3. Do not have to wonder where the tube is positioned	3. Closed system requiring low gas flow rates	3. High CPAP pressures can be attained
4. Do not have to wonder where the tube is positioned		4. Do not have to wonder where the tube is positioned	4. Can easily switch to mechanical ventilation
			5. Access to the infant is greatest
			6. No problems with leaks
Disadvantages			
1. Invasive	1. Suctioning causes a loss of CPAP pressure	1. Delays access to the head and face	1. Invasive
2. Prongs should be removed every 2 hr to clean the prongs and external nares and reduce the incidence of nasal irritation and erosion	2. Air insufflation and aspiration	2. Inconvenient when providing nursing care to the head and face	2. Endotracheal tube fixation is difficult and traumatic
3. Is difficult to obtain a good fit	3. Is difficult to obtain a good fit	3. High noise level	3. Endotracheal tube may become kinked, malpositioned or blocked during or following insertion
4. With pressures of 12 cm H_2O an air leak is present through the mouth	4. Head molding and pressure necrosis	4. Loss of pressure when hood is opened	4. Infection, scarring and irritation are possible
5. During periods of crying, the infant loses pressure and inhales room air	5. Delayed access to the face and mouth	5. Neck ulceration	
6. Does not allow mechanical ventilation to be instituted without removing the prongs	6. Does not allow mechanical ventilation to be instituted without removing the mask	6. Vomiting and irritation	
7. Requires high gas flows to obtain high CPAP pressures. High flows may cause cooling and drying effects		7. Gastric distention	

The advantages of nasal prong therapy (Table 9–1) are: the infant does not require intubation, thus eliminating the untoward effects of the latter; they are inserted very quickly and easily into the external nares and accessibility to the patient is excellent.

The disadvantages of nasal prong CPAP (Table 9–1) are: high gas flows are required to provide an end expiratory pressure above 8–10 cm H_2O and this increases the incidence of potential complications of cooling and drying of the upper respiratory tract. It is an invasive method and hard to obtain a good fit.

It is difficult to maintain high levels of CPAP, since the newborn can open his mouth while sucking or crying. During periods of crying, the infant loses pressure and inhales room air. Nasal irritation and erosion are frequent complications during nasal prong CPAP because of the two small tubes that are inserted into the nares. For this reason, the nasal prongs should be removed every 2 hours so that they and the external nares can be cleaned. The most important disadvantage to this type of therapy, however, is that it cannot be used to convert to mechanical ventilation should the infant's clinical condition deteriorate.

Face Mask

Numerous methods are available for affixing a face mask to an infant. One such example is shown in Figure 9–4. "CPAP is applied by positioning a mask over the infant's nose and mouth. The mask is then

Fig. 9–4. – CPAP therapy being administered to an infant via a face mask.

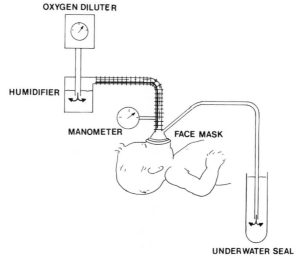

held tightly in position by placing two ties over the hook ring of the mask and around the infant's occiput. A surgical mask is first placed over the occiput to distribute the pressure of the ties more widely."[8]

Although mask therapy has proved to be an efficient and safe method of CPAP delivery in some centers, it has several possible untoward effects (see Table 9–1). Access to the infant's face and mouth is delayed with the use of a mask. The mask must be removed and CPAP pressure is lost during a routine suctioning procedure. Air insufflation and aspiration is possible. With the use of a mask, it is difficult to obtain a good fit and keep the pressure constant. If the mask is too tightly affixed, head molding and pressure necrosis of the face may result. As in nasal prong therapy, another disadvantage is that it cannot be used to convert to mechanical ventilation should the infant's clinical condition deteriorate. The main advantages of mask therapy are that it avoids the complication of tracheal intubation, the clinician does not have to wonder where the tube is positioned and access to the infant is good.

Head Hood

This method of CPAP delivery involves enclosing the infant's head in a chamber with a loosely fitting collar around the neck (Fig. 9–5). "Warmed, moisturized gas, 10 to 20 liters per minute, flows into the chamber and escapes mainly through an outlet tube and to a lesser degree under the neck seal. Pressure in the chamber can be varied by adjustment of the screw clamp on the outlet tube. A length of plastic tubing, its tip 30 cm under water, acts as a safety valve. An anesthesia reservoir bag, connected to a length of corrugated tubing, allows intermittent sighing of the infant. The pressure in the chamber is continuously displayed on an aneroid manometer."[2]

The main advantages of using a head hood for CPAP (see Table 9–1) administration are ease of application, quickness and the elimination of tracheal intubation. The disadvantages of head hood CPAP are numerous (see Table 9–1). It is inconvenient when providing nursing care to the face and head, since access to the infant is delayed. When the hood is opened, CPAP pressure is lost. Too tight a seal around the infant's neck may result in neck ulceration. Gastric distention, vomiting and irritation are also possible sequelae.

Endotracheal Tube

This was the first method used to administer CPAP to newborn infants and it remains the most common today (see Fig. 9–2). The advantages of CPAP by this method (see Table 9–1) are:

1. It is the most efficient method of delivering CPAP.

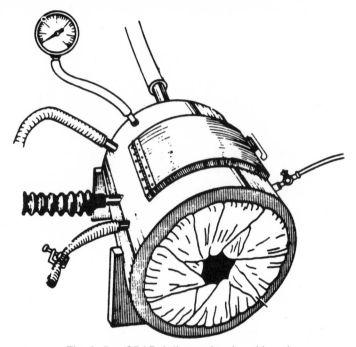

Fig. 9–5.—CPAP delivery via a head hood.

2. Very low gas flow rates may be used because there are few leaks in the system.

3. High CPAP pressures (12–14 cm H_2O) can be attained.

4. If the infant's condition deteriorates, the clinician can easily switch to mechanical ventilation.

5. The clinician has easy access to the entire infant.

6. There are no problems with leaks.

There are disadvantages, however, in the use of this system for CPAP administration (see Table 9–1):

1. The procedure is invasive.

2. Endotracheal tube fixation is difficult and often traumatic.

3. The endotracheal tube may become kinked, malpositioned or blocked during or following insertion.

4. Infection, scarring and irritation are possible sequelae even with good nursing care.

THERAPEUTIC USE OF CPAP

Once it has been clinically determined that CPAP therapy should be implemented, the method of administration must be established.

In general, if CPAP is indicated in an infant under 1000 gm, endotracheal intubation should be implemented. If the infant is larger than 1000 gm, nasal prong therapy should be instituted.

After the method of CPAP administration has been established, the F_{IO_2} must be determined. At the outset of CPAP therapy, the F_{IO_2} that failed to oxygenate the baby in a head hood (usually 0.40–0.60) should be instituted. If the infant is receiving CPAP via nasal prongs and hypoxemia persists at an F_{IO_2} of 0.9, endotracheal intubation should be considered.

Following selection of the method of administration and F_{IO_2}, the pressure setting should be ascertained. Usually the level of end expiratory pressure is begun somewhere between 6 and 7 cm H_2O. If endotracheal tube CPAP is to be administered, start at 4 cm H_2O. If CPAP is to be delivered via nasal prongs, head hood or mask, begin at 6 cm H_2O. A typical rule of thumb is that the maximal pressure level set should not be greater than one-third of the infant's mean arterial blood pressure (Table 9–2).

Once these preliminary steps have been started, the procedure and considerations for utilization of CPAP therapy resemble the following:

1. If CPAP is being administered by any method except endotracheal intubation, a gastric tube should be inserted.

2. During CPAP administration, chest physiotherapy (percussion, vibration and positional changes) should be done hourly. Suctioning should also be performed as an adjunct to this procedure.

3. Following initiation of CPAP, a change in F_{IO_2} or a change in the level of CPAP pressure, an arterial blood gas should be obtained.

4. The Pa_{O_2} of the infant should be maintained between 50 and 70 mm Hg and the pH above 7.20.

5. After discontinuation or removal of CPAP, a chest roentgenogram should be obtained.

When to decrease CPAP therapy: If the infant is not experiencing apneic episodes and his chest roentgenogram, vital signs and blood

TABLE 9–2.—MAXIMAL PRESSURE LEVELS FOR CPAP ADMINISTRATION

WEIGHT (gm)	MAXIMAL CPAP (cm H_2O)
<1000	8
1500	10
2000	12
2500	12
>2500	12

gas results are improving, the following procedure may be utilized:

1. Decrease the oxygen carefully and slowly (2–5%) until an FI_{O_2} of 0.50–0.60 is reached.

2. Once an FI_{O_2} of 0.50–0.60 is reached, begin to decrease the CPAP level 1–2 cm H_2O until a maximal level of 6 cm H_2O is reached.

3. Then decrease the FI_{O_2} until a level of about 0.40 is obtained.

4. Now the CPAP level should be gradually reduced to 2 cm H_2O. Never lower the level of CPAP below 2 cm H_2O while the endotracheal tube still is in place. This results in a lower Pa_{O_2} and FRC for the baby.

5. Maintain the infant at an FI_{O_2} of 0.40 and a CPAP of 2 cm H_2O for at least 4 hours before introducing any further changes.

6. Before CPAP therapy is eliminated, the infant should be thoroughly suctioned, auscultation performed and the FI_{O_2} increased 10%.

7. Immediately following extubation or discontinuation of CPAP, a chest roentgenogram should be obtained.

When to increase CPAP therapy: FI_{O_2} and pressure levels are increased whenever hypoxemia persists.

1. Once the FI_{O_2} reaches 0.70, increase the level of CPAP pressure in increments of 2 cm H_2O until the Pa_{O_2} reaches 50–70 mm Hg. Be sure to monitor blood pressure carefully. Too high a CPAP pressure may cause impedance of venous return and a decrease in cardiac output. It may also precipitate shallow breathing and apnea.

2. If hypoxemia persists at an FI_{O_2} of 0.90 and a CPAP pressure of 8–10 cm H_2O, or apnea occurs concomitantly with bradycardia, or the Pa_{CO_2} is above 60 mm Hg with a pH of 7.25 or below, mechanical ventilation should be implemented.

Weaning from CPAP

Whenever CPAP is applied via nasal prongs, a head hood or a face mask, guidelines for weaning the patient are required. If CPAP is being applied via an endotracheal tube, a specific protocol for weaning and extubation is required. This latter point is especially important, because Harrison et al.[27] have shown that some RDS patients at zero end expiratory pressure had lower Pa_{O_2} values prior to tracheal extubation than following extubation.

The criteria for discontinuation of CPAP by all methods vary with the infant's disease, maturity and arterial blood gas results. In general, the Pa_{O_2} should be at least 50 mm Hg at an FI_{O_2} of 0.5; the Pa_{CO_2} should be less than 50 mm Hg with no apneic episodes and the chest roentgenogram should be clear or nearly so. If the infant satisfies these criteria and is receiving CPAP at a level of 1–2 cm H_2O via nasal prongs, head hood or face mask, the CPAP level should be reduced to a zero end expiratory pressure (ZEEP) level and the infant immediately placed in a head hood with an F_{IO_2} equal to the concentration received during CPAP therapy. If, however, the infant is receiving CPAP via an endotracheal tube at an end expiratory pressure of 2 cm

Fig. 9–6.–A, mean FRC at 2 cm H_2O CPAP, at ZEEP and after extubation. **B,** mean Pa_{O_2} values at 2 cm H_2O CPAP, at ZEEP and after extubation. (From Berman, L. S., Fox, W. W., Raphaely, R. C., and Downes, J. J., Jr.: J. Pediatr. 89:109–112, 1976. Reprinted by permission.)

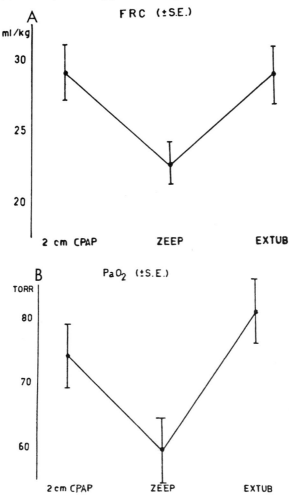

H_2O, extubation should be performed as long as the infant can maintain a Pa_{O_2} greater than 50 mm Hg. Under no circumstances should the level of end expiratory pressure be reduced to zero with the infant still intubated. In these patients at ZEEP, it has been shown that they exhibit a lower FRC (Fig. 9–6, A) and Pa_{O_2} (Fig. 9–6, B) than when 2 cm H_2O is applied or after extubation. This phenomenon probably is best described by stating that the presence or absence of an endotracheal tube seems to make a significant difference in the FRC.[28]

Maintenance of CPAP Therapy

In order to effectively provide and maintain CPAP therapy, four factors should be monitored diligently. They are pressure, temperature, humidity and FI_{O_2}.

PRESSURE. – This is the most important factor governing success or failure of CPAP therapy. CPAP pressure should be increased or decreased according to set guidelines such as color, blood gas analysis, vital signs and chest x-ray. The purpose of CPAP therapy is to apply just enough pressure to keep all the alveoli patent.

TEMPERATURE. – The air/O_2 mixture should be delivered to the infant at approximately body temperature. Inspired gas that is either "too warm" or "too cold" may increase oxygen consumption. In addition, it has been shown that hyperthermia increases the number of apneic spells in the premature infant whereas hypothermia leads to acidosis.

HUMIDITY. – The air/O_2 mixture must be properly humidified to avoid drying of the upper respiratory tract, with subsequent inspissation of secretions. Excessive humidification, however, must also be avoided. This may cause water retention and edema in an infant already severely compromised. Near drowning is also a distinct possibility if H_2O is allowed to pool in the inspiratory portion of the CPAP circuit. More than once a tube filled with water has been picked up and drained in the wrong direction.

OXYGEN CONCENTRATION. – The concentration of inspired oxygen should be titrated in accordance with the arterial blood gas results. The Pa_{O_2} should be kept between 50 and 70 mm Hg.

Complications of CPAP Therapy

All methods of applying continuous positive airway pressure have undesirable side effects. The most frequent complications are pulmonary air leak, inspissated secretions, pressure necrosis and reduction in cardiac output.

PULMONARY AIR LEAK. — This condition may present as interstitial emphysema, pneumothorax or pneumomediastinum. Interstitial emphysema "results from rupture of overdistended alveoli with dissection of air into the perivascular interstitium producing radiolucent areas on the roentgenogram. A pneumomediastinum may develop after a difficult intubation, due to direct trauma to the trachea, bronchus, esophagus or pharyngeal structures, or may be due to overdistention of alveoli with rupture and dissection of air along the perivascular sheaths."[29] A pneumothorax apparently develops when overdistended alveoli rupture and air dissects along the perivascular spaces in a retrograde manner to the root of the lung and breaks into the pleural space. A pneumothorax may occur without clinical warning or without an antecedent change in roentgenographic appearance. The presence of an air leak such as pulmonary interstitial emphysema or a pneumomediastinum, however, should warn the physician that a pneumothorax may occur.

INSPISSATED SECRETIONS. — This problem is a direct result of inadequate humidification of the inspired gas. Either the type of humidifier or nebulizer or the method of using it is insufficient to prevent thickening of secretions and subsequent drying of the mucosa.

PRESSURE NECROSIS. — This condition may present anytime a portion of the CPAP delivery system comes into immediate contact with the infant. Pressure necrosis of the face may occur during mask therapy, of the nares during nasal therapy, of the neck during hood therapy and of the trachea during endotracheal tube therapy. Under some unusual conditions, the pressure necrosis may lead to further sequelae, such as infection or ulceration.[30]

REDUCTION IN CARDIAC OUTPUT. — This is a very unusual complication of CPAP administration during the acute phase of therapy when lung compliance is poor. It is a realistic problem, however, as the infant's condition improves. A reduction in cardiac output occurs when part of the CPAP pressure is transmitted to the mediastinum and great vessels (superior and inferior vena cava). This causes the great vessels to partially collapse, resulting in less blood flow returning to the heart and a subsequent fall in cardiac output. For this reason, it is imperative to lower CPAP levels carefully as the infant's lung compliance and Pa_{O_2} levels improve.

SPECIAL CONSIDERATIONS WHEN USING CPAP

Because the administration of CPAP usually follows oxygen hood therapy and precedes mechanical ventilation, it is a lifesaving process. To ensure safe administration of CPAP, several factors bear special emphasis:

1. *Always observe the baby.* The infant's over-all status can change quickly, so close observation is mandatory. As was mentioned earlier, in most CPAP systems there is no audible or visual low-pressure alarm to warn the clinician of an accidental disconnection of the infant from CPAP therapy. In addition, it is important to monitor the infant's skin color (for the presence or absence of cyanosis or hyperoxia), respiratory rate (for tachypnea or bradypnea), patterns of breathing (grunting, retractions or apnea) and heart rate (tachycardia or bradycardia).

2. *CPAP pressure should be checked frequently.* Too low a pressure will result in atelectasis, a failure to increase FRC and a failure to reduce the right-to-left intrapulmonary shunt. The three causes of sudden and low CPAP pressures are leaks, disconnections and water accumulation in the tubing. Too high a CPAP pressure is also dangerous. Untoward high sustained levels of CPAP pressure can cause pulmonary air leak (pneumothorax, pneumomediastinum or interstitial emphysema) or tension pneumothorax. Usually, too high a pressure is the direct result of overzealous CPAP therapy. Occasionally, however, it is the direct result of an accidentally kinked tube in the expiratory limb of the CPAP circuit.

3. *Arterial blood gases should be monitored frequently.* This is mandatory in order to evaluate the effectiveness of CPAP therapy. The precise measurement of pH, Pa_{O_2} and Pa_{CO_2} is a prerequisite for increases or reductions in F_{IO_2} and end expiratory pressure levels.

4. *Suction the airway when necessary.* "Suctioning, or, as it is often termed, aspiration of secretions, is an extremely beneficial but potentially hazardous procedure which should be performed only when necessary. It is not a routine procedure done on a predetermined basis of once per hour or four times per shift. Suctioning is indicated when there is an accumulation of secretions or presence of obstructive material. It is generally discernible by auscultation of the chest or listening for gurgling sounds in the throat."[31]

5. *Protect the nares, oral cavity and skin from irritation.* "Crust formation can occur due to irritation and tissue breakdown around the nares in nasal CPAP, and in the trachea, mouth, or nose when an ET tube is used. Antibiotic ointments around the outside of the nares may minimize the hazard of infection. Use of hydrocortisone creams to lubricate the ET tube before insertion helps decrease the inflammatory reaction from a foreign body in the trachea. Good oral hygiene is

needed and the mouth should be cleansed with lemon-glycerin swabs or normal saline to prevent drying and cracking."[1]

6. *Watch for distention of the stomach due to insufflation of air.* This problem occurs most often during mask, hood or nasal CPAP. It can be obviated by placement of an orogastric tube.

7. *Construct the CPAP apparatus carefully.* Most CPAP systems are designed as in Figure 9–2. Although this system is adequate for therapy, it is not optimal by modern standards. In addition to the components shown in Figure 9–2, every CPAP apparatus should incorporate an oxygen analyzer, overtemperature electrical shutoff alarm and low-pressure alarm.

COMMERCIAL SYSTEMS AVAILABLE

At present, numerous systems are available to administer CPAP to the infant in respiratory distress. Each of these systems is explained in the following discussion.

Citadel CPAP Administration Set (CAS)—Sherwood Medical Industries

The Citadel CPAP Administration Set (CAS) is designed for use with the Citadel Neonate Respiratory Support System (Fig. 9–7). The

Fig. 9–7.—A Citadel CPAP system.

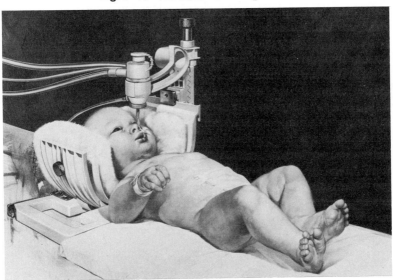

CAS requires a supply of gas, a pressure monitor, a self-purging reservoir bag and a nasal cannula. The CAS appears like a twisted "H." One end is provided with a 22-mm inlet post for connection to an appropriate source of humidified air/oxygen supply. The opposite end of this limb is an outlet to a self-purging reservoir bag. Proximal to this outlet is located a pop-off valve that bleeds off gas if the pressure should exceed 15 cm H_2O (range 14–17 cm H_2O at 15 l/min flow). This valve is provided with an override capability to facilitate bagging the patient.

Face Chamber (FC) 100 – Siemens-Elema AB

The FC 100 consists of a face chamber, an air-oxygen unit and a swivel cradle (Fig. 9–8). The face chamber is a tightly fitting cylindrical piece of aluminum. At one end is an easily removable lid and at the other end a sealing diaphragm is present. The latter is a thin, pliable latex cuff that is filled with small styrene beads. The seal molds against the face of the infant.

The air-oxygen unit consists of an air-oxygen blender, a back pressure compensated flowmeter and a vacuum unit. The oxygen blender allows accurate delivery of FI_{O_2} from 0.21. The flowmeter regulates the total amount of gas flow through the system. Humidity at body

Fig. 9–8.—The Siemens-Elema face chamber (FC 100) is a commercially available CPAP device. (Courtesy of Siemens Corporation, Union, N.J.)

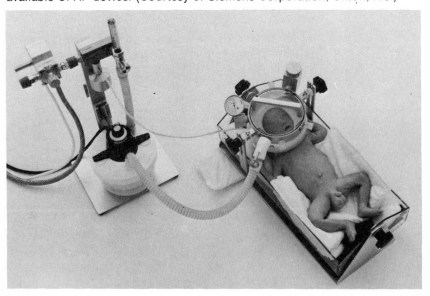

temperature is achieved by using a heated Bennett cascade humidifier. A probe thermometer located just outside the face chamber displays the temperature of the inspired gas. The vacuum device is used to suction the gas from the inside of the latex ring to seal it against the infant's face without exerting pressure.

The swivel crib is an intensive care unit bed. The crib can be used easily in numerous planes to allow multiple positioning of the infant. The crib also has adjustable levels for support of the face chamber.

Use of the FC 100 is simple. The infant is placed into the swivel bed and the face chamber minus the lid is attached to the adjustable levels on the side of the bed. The appropriate size latex ring then is placed over the infant's face and the air evacuated by vacuum. The clinically prescribed FI_{O_2}, flow and temperature are regulated via the air-oxygen blender, flowmeter, heated humidifier and thermometer. A flow rate of at least 12–15 lpm is necessary to eliminate any dead space. End expiratory pressure, monitored and displayed via an aneroid manometer, is adjusted via a pressure regulator attached to a part of the face chamber. Should pressure increase accidentally, a safety pop-off is present, which activates when 20 cm H_2O is reached.

Fig. 9–9. – Carden Valve. Part *A* is a Venturi, which connects to the endotracheal tube. Part *B* is connected to the gas supply.

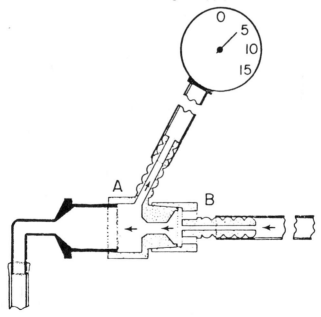

Carden Valve

The Carden Valve is a Venturi tube that creates positive pressure in the airway. It is a lightweight device made of plexiglass that consists of two parts (Fig. 9–9). Part A is a Venturi tube that connects to a pressure gauge, terminating in a 15-mm female adapter for connection to a tracheal tube. Part B consists of a jet that is connected to a fresh gas flow and has eight radially arranged holes for the escape of excess and exhaled gases. Parts A and B are joined together by a 12 mm/2-degree tapered connector.

The Carden Valve is used by attaching it to the endotracheal tube connector of the infant and adjusting the gas flow to deliver the re-

Fig. 9–10.—Front view of Bourns LS150 infant CPAP system. (Courtesy of Bourns Medical Systems, Inc., Riverside, Cal.)

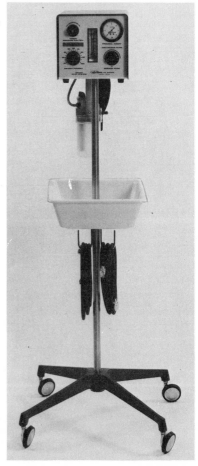

quired amount of end expiratory pressure. When pressures of 5 l/min are used, end expiratory pressures of 5 cm H_2O are attained. When flow is increased to 8 l/min, pressures of 10 cm H_2O are available.

LS150 Infant CPAP System—Bourns Inc.

The Bourns LS150 infant CPAP system is a pneumatically operated device that consists of the CPAP unit itself, a heated humidifier, an external bag and a pedestal/pole assembly (Fig. 9–10). The CPAP unit has controls for flow (continuous or demand), oxygen and end expiratory pressure. The unit is designed to allow the clinician to use conventional CPAP or continuous positive pressure without continu-

Fig. 9–11.—Rear view of Bourns LS150 infant CPAP system connected to an infant. (Courtesy of Bourns Medical Systems, Inc., Riverside, Cal.)

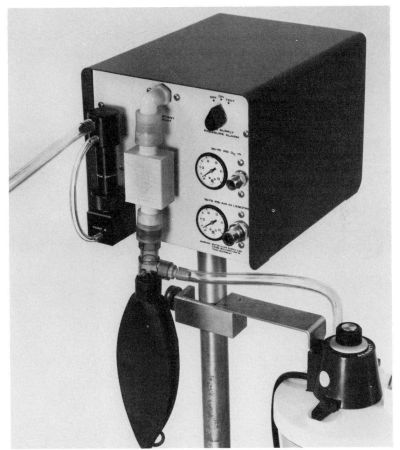

ous flow. The latter, which is termed demand flow, holds the CPAP level in the patient circuit without a continuous flow of gas. During inspiration, the demand valve opens and supplies the required flow of the oxygen-enriched gas to the patient. The required pressure level then is maintained by adjusting the airway pressure control and observing the pressure gauge.

The demand valve also functions to automatically supply an adequate flow to sustain elevated baseline pressure when minimal leaks are encountered.

Because the CPAP unit has an integral air/oxygen blender, the clinician selects FI_{O_2} by turning the O_2 per cent control. Heated humidification is incorporated through use of the modified $Misto_2Gen$ heated humidifier. An external bag allows manual or deep breaths to be provided to the patient. The entire system is provided on a pedestal/pole assembly for ease of use and mobility.

To use the Bourns CPAP system, the clinician attaches the humidifier and patient circuit as shown in Figure 9–11. Then the appropriate flow rate (if demand flow is not being used), oxygen per cent and end expiratory pressure are selected.

Fig. 9–12.—Close-up view of Bird Neonatal CPAP Generator. (Courtesy of Bird Corporation, Palm Springs, Cal., 1975.)

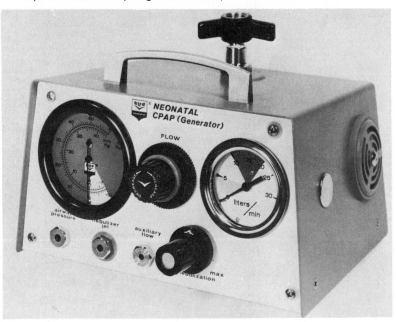

Neonatal CPAP Generator — Bird Corporation

The Bird Neonatal CPAP Generator is a pneumatically operated device that consists of the CPAP unit itself, an oxygen blender, humidifier, manual resuscitator and pedestal/pole assembly (Fig. 9–12). The CPAP unit consists of two controls and two gauges. The controls

Fig. 9–13. — Patient circuit connections for Bird Neonatal CPAP Generator. (Courtesy of Bird Corporation, Palm Springs, Cal.)

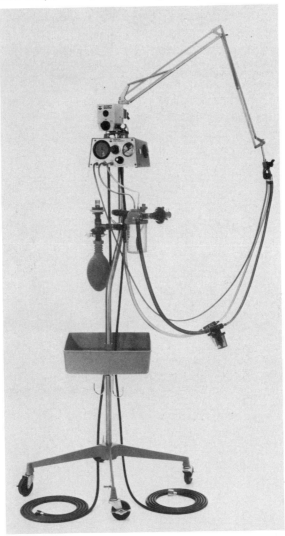

are for flow rate and nebulization whereas the gauges are for displaying the proximal airway pressure and flow rate set. An external air/oxygen blender allows accurate regulation of the FI_{O_2}. Humidification is provided via the Bird 500 ml micronebulizer and nebulization via a small therapy micronebulizer. An external manual resuscitation device allows manual or deep breaths to be provided to the patient. The entire system is provided on a pedestal/pole assembly for ease of use and mobility.

To use the Bird Neonatal CPAP Generator, the clinician attaches the system as shown in Figure 9–13. Then the appropriate flow rate and oxygen concentration are selected. The nebulizer control is adjusted for proper aerosol production. End expiratory pressure is selected by rotating the red control lever located on the bottom of the Bird outflow housing and reading the pressure on the appropriate gauge.

REFERENCES

1. Affonso, D., and Harris, T.: Continuous positive airway pressure, Am. J. Nursing 76:570, 1976.
2. Gregory, G., et al.: Treatment of the idiopathic respiratory distress syndrome with continuous positive airway pressure, N. Engl. J. Med. 284: 1333, 1971.
3. Gregory, G., et al.: Continuous PPB therapy for neonatal respiratory distress, Hosp. Practice 7:100, 1972.
4. Chernick, V., and Vidyasagar, D.: Continuous negative chest wall pressure in hyaline membrane disease, Pediatrics 49:753, 1972.
5. Robertson, N. R.: CPAP or not CPAP?, Arch. Dis. Child. 51:161, 1976.
6. Wolfsdorf, J.: The acute case of respiratory problem in the neonate, infant and child, Int. Anesthesiol. Clin. 13:92, 1975.
7. Williams, T. J.: Unpublished data.
8. Ackerman, B. D., et al.: Continuous positive airway pressure applied by means of a tight-fitting facemask, J. Pediatr. 85:408, 1974.
9. Haller, J. A., et al.: Use of continuous positive airway pressure in the improved postoperative management of neonatal respiratory emergencies, Ann. Thorac. Surg. 15:607, 1973.
10. Gupta, J. M., VanVliet, P. K. J., Vonwiller, J. B., Abrahams, N., and Fisk, G. C.: Positive airway pressure in respiratory distress syndrome, Med. J. Aust. 3:91, 1974.
11. Boros, S. J., and Reynolds, J. W.: Prolonged apnea of prematurity: Treatment with continuous airway distending pressure delivered by nasopharyngeal tube, Clin. Pediatr. 15:123, 1976.
12. Fox, W. W., Berman, L. S., Downes, J. J., and Peckham, G. J.: The therapeutic application of end-expiratory pressure in the meconium aspiration syndrome, Pediatrics 56:214, 1975.
13. Williams, T. J., and Syrentsen, W. A.: The many descriptions of CPAP, Respir. Care 22:1282, 1977.
14. Boros, S. J., and Reynolds, J. W.: Hyaline membrane disease treated with

early nasal end expiratory pressure: One year's experience, Pediatrics 56: 218, 1975.

15. Vidyasagar, D.: Physiological Basis and Clinical Implications of Continuous Negative Chestwall Pressure in Hyaline Membrane Disease, in Keuskamp, D. H. G., *Neonatal and Pediatric Ventilation* (Boston: Little, Brown and Company, 1974).

16. Kattwinkel, J., *et al.*: Apnea of prematurity: Effects of continuous positive airway pressure (CPAP), cutaneous stimulation, and levels of urinary biogenic amines. Abstract of paper presented at joint meeting of the American Pediatric Society and The Society in Pediatric Research held at the Sheraton Park Hotel, Washington, D. C., May 1–3, 1974, Pediatr. Res. 8: 468/194, 1974.

17. Gluck, L.: Special problems of the newborn, Hosp. Practice 13:84, 1978.

18. Newth, C. J. L., *et al.*: Neonatal milk aspiration pneumonia—a possible additional use for continuous positive airway pressure, Crit. Care Med. 1: 145, 1973.

19. Bucci, G., *et al.*: Phrenic nerve palsy treated by continuous positive pressure breathing by nasal cannula, Arch. Dis. Child. 49:230, 1974.

20. Stewart, S., *et al.*: Spontaneous breathing with continuous positive airway pressure after open intracardiac operations in infants, J. Thorac. Cardiovasc. Surg. 65:37, 1973.

21. Hatch, D. J., *et al.*: Continuous positive airway pressure after open heart operations in infancy, Lancet 2:469, 1973.

22. Crew, A. D., *et al.*: Continuous positive airway pressure breathing in the postoperative management of the cardiac infant, Thorax 29:437, 1974.

23. Gregory, G. A., *et al.*: Continuous positive airway pressure and pulmonary and circulatory function after cardiac surgery in infants less than three months of age, Anesthesiology 43:426, 1975.

24. Robertson, N. R.: Prolonged continuous positive airways pressure for pulmonary edema due to persistent ductus arteriosus in the newborn, Arch. Dis. Child. 49:585, 1974.

25. Fox, W. W., *et al.*: The therapeutic application of end-expiratory pressure in the meconium aspiration syndrome, Pediatrics 56:214, 1975.

26. Lough, M. D., Doershuk, C. F., and Stern, R. C. (eds.): *Pediatric Respiratory Therapy* (Chicago: Year Book Medical Publishers, Inc., 1974).

27. Harrison, V. C., Heese, H. de V., and Klein, M.: The significance of grunting in hyaline membrane disease, Pediatrics 42:549, 1968.

28. Berman, L. S., *et al.*: Optimum levels of CPAP for tracheal extubation of newborn infants, J. Pediatr. 89:109, 1976.

29. Kirkpatrick, B. V., Felman, A. H., and Eitzman, D. V.: Complications of ventilator therapy in respiratory distress syndrome, Am. J. Dis. Child. 128:496, 1976.

30. Krauss, D. R., and Marshall, R. E.: Severe neck ulceration from CPAP head box, J. Pediatr. 86:286, 1975.

31. Williams, T. J., and Hill, J. W.: *Handbook of Neonatal Respiratory Care* (Riverside, Cal.: Bourns Life Systems, 1975).

10 / Mechanical Ventilators

THOMAS J. WILLIAMS, B.S., R.R.T.

WITHIN THE PAST 3 DECADES, a plethora of mechanical ventilators have been designed to treat the newborn suffering from acute respiratory failure. With the advent of each new mechanical ventilator has come an array of features and a wide variety of new controls designed to be more physiologic, simpler to operate, more versatile and safer than its competitors and predecessors.

What has remained elusive, however, is the basic fact that each of these machines performs the mechanical process of ventilation by substituting for the bellows action of the thoracic cage and diaphragm. Some machines simply perform this substitution differently or better than others.

A mechanical ventilator should do what the patient cannot do or cannot do well enough, whether it has to do with the work of breathing or another problem. The primary purpose of a mechanical ventilator is to perform alveolar minute ventilation and arterial oxygenation with minimal circulatory impairment and minimal trauma to the lung. Every mechanical ventilator available today performs this function to varying degrees.

It must be understood, however, that artificial ventilation via a mechanical ventilator is only a means of gaining time for self-recovery. For this reason, it is imperative that each member of the critical care team master the physical characteristics and limitations of the type of mechanical ventilator to be used. This is imperative because some research centers report excellent therapeutic results with one type of mechanical ventilator, whereas other centers obtain equally good results with another type of ventilator. On the basis of this, we can underline the importance of becoming familiar with the properties of the ventilator used. We cannot, however, objectively testify to the superiority of one mechanical ventilator over others. Among mechanical ventilators for the newborn there exist great differences in their principles of operation and over-all functional characteristics.

DEFINITION OF TERMS

Before we discuss the performance of mechanical ventilators, it is necessary to define the various terms commonly used. Because there is no international standard in this respect, most of the terms as they are used in this chapter are consistent with those proposed by the American National Standards Institute.*

Airway Pressure (P_{aw}). — The pressure at a *specific* point in the patient's airway. For most newborn mechanical ventilators this point is at the machine end of the endotracheal tube (proximal airway) and is termed proximal airway pressure (measured in cm H_2O).

Peak Inspiratory Pressure (PIP). — The peak pressure attained during the inspiratory phase. This pressure can be obtained by directly observing the pressure gauge (measured in cm H_2O).

End Inspiratory Pressure (P_{Iend}). — The airway pressure at the end of the inspiratory phase. This pressure can be obtained by directly observing the pressure gauge (measured in cm H_2O).

Alveolar Pressure (P_A). — The pressure in the alveoli (measured in cm H_2O).

Pressure Drop. — The difference between proximal airway pressure and alveolar pressure (measured in cm H_2O).

Ventilator Pressure (P_{vent}). — Pressure at a specified point in the ventilator or patient circuit. This may be measured at the outlet port of the ventilator, at the humidifier, at the manifold, or at the proximal airway. The measured pressure is displayed on the ventilator pressure gauge. Most newborn mechanical ventilators measure pressure at the proximal airway. For these ventilators, ventilator pressure equals airway pressure (measured in cm H_2O).

Maximum Safety Pressure ($P_{s}max$). — The highest gauge pressure that can be attained in the patient system during malfunction of the ventilator but with functioning safety mechanisms (measured in cm H_2O).

Maximum Working Pressure ($P_{w}max$). — The highest gauge pressure that can be attained in the patient system during the inspiratory phase when the ventilator is functioning normally. This may be limited by a ventilator control to less than $P_{s}max$ (measured in cm H_2O).

Inspiratory Flow ($\dot{V}_I$). — The volume of gas per unit time passing through the machine end of the endotracheal tube during inspiration. This flow will usually be constant during the inspiratory phase for controlled mechanical ventilation (CMV) and continuous during

---

*American National Standard for Breathing Machines for Medical Use Z79.7 – 1976.

the inspiratory phase for intermittent mandatory ventilation (IMV) (measured in l/min).

Expiratory Flow ($\dot{V}_E$).—The volume of gas per unit time passing through the machine end of the endotracheal tube during expiration. This flow will usually be constant during the expiratory phase for controlled mechanical ventilation (CMV) and continuous during the inspiratory phase for intermittent mandatory ventilation (IMV) (measured in l/min).

Resistance (R).—Resistance equals the pressure gradient divided by the flow $\left(R = \dfrac{cm\ H_2O}{l/sec} \right)$.

Airway Resistance (R_{AW}).—The pressure difference per unit of flow across the airway. This may be measured during either inspiration or expiration $\left(R_{AW} = \dfrac{cm\ H_2O}{l/sec} \right)$.

Compliance $\left(\dfrac{\Delta V}{\Delta P} \right)$.—The relationship between the volume delivered into a closed system and the corresponding pressure increase within that closed system (measured in ml/cm H_2O).

Lung Compliance $\left(C_L = \dfrac{\Delta V}{\Delta P} \right)$.—The elasticity of the respiratory system is expressed as its compliance. The measurement is normally made under static conditions and is defined by the change in volume produced by a unit of pressure change. The respiratory system compliance is composed of the lung and chest wall compliance (measured in ml/cm H_2O).

Ventilator System Compliance (C_{vent}).—The sum of all the portions of the internal machine, plus those parts external to it (patient tubing, humidifier, bacteria filter, etc.), which are pressurized during the inspiratory phase.

Ventilatory Expiratory Resistance ($R_{vent\ exp}$).—The total resistance to gas flow from the patient connection port through the expiratory port of the patient system to the atmosphere $\left(\dfrac{cm\ H_2O}{l/sec} \right)$.

Frequency (patient) (f_{pat}).—The number of patient-initiated spontaneous breaths per minute ($\times$/min) or (min^{-1}) $\left(\dfrac{1}{T_I + T_E} \times 60 \right)$.

Frequency (ventilatory) (f_{vent}).—The number of ventilator delivered breaths per minute ($\times$/min) or (min^{-1}).

Frequency (f).—The *total* number of patient and ventilator delivered breaths per minute ($\times$/min) or (min^{-1}).

Tidal Volume (V_T). — The volume of gas entering or leaving the patient during inspiration or expiration (measured in ml).

Minute Volume ($\dot{V}_E$). — Volume of gas exhaled per minute. During IMV this is the sum total of all spontaneous and ventilator delivered tidal volumes (measured in liters [1]).

Volumetric Displacement. — The volume of gas passed per breath during the inspiratory phase through the patient connection port of the ventilator when the pressures at the intake to the ventilator and at the outlet from the patient connection port are equal to atmospheric pressure. May also be called the preset tidal volume (measured in ml).

Preset Ventilator Minute Volume (V_{min} preset). — The sum of all the preset ventilator tidal volumes (volumetric displacement) occurring within a period of 1 minute (measured in l/min).

Inspiratory Pause Time (T_{IP}). — The interval from the end of inspiratory flow to the beginning of expiratory flow (plateau period). Also called inspiratory hold. In theory, introducing an inspiratory pause improves gas distribution in the lung by prolonging inspiration for a set period of time (measured in seconds).

Inspiratory Phase Time (T_I). — The interval from the initiation of inspiratory flow to the beginning of expiratory flow (measured in seconds).

Expiratory Pause Time (T_{EP}). — The interval from the end of expiratory flow to the initiation of inspiratory flow (measured in seconds).

Expiratory Phase Time (T_E). — The interval from the initiation of expiratory flow to the beginning of inspiratory flow (measured in seconds).

Inspiratory-Expiratory Phase Time Ratio (T_I/T_E). — The ratio of the inspiratory phase time to the expiratory phase time. Also commonly called I : E Ratio.

Ventilator Cycle Time $= T_I + T_E$. — The sum of inspiratory time and expiratory time (measured in seconds).

Patient Circuit (C_{pat}). — That portion of the ventilator external gas system through which gas passes to the patient.

Fail Safe Mechanism – Ventilator. — A safety mechanism that permits the patient to breathe ambient air during a malfunction of the ventilator.

Flow Pattern. — The characteristic shape of the flow curve being emitted from the ventilator and going to the patient. This may be constant flow, nonconstant flow, constant pressure or nonconstant pressure.

Power. — The type of energy used to drive the ventilator system. This may be compressed gas, electricity or both.

UNDERSTANDING VENTILATOR/LUNG INTERACTION
THROUGH WAVEFORM ANALYSIS

In order to discuss the performance of a mechanical ventilator, the clinician must consider the mechanical function of the ventilator as well as the physical effect it creates in the lung. Ventilators operate by creating variations with time to volume, flow and pressure. These variations can be analyzed by viewing the subsequent waveforms they create. These waveforms are easily obtained by testing any ventilator according to International Standards Organization (ISO) speci-

Fig. 10–1.—Schematic of testing device for characterizing mechanical ventilators according to International Standards Organization. (This material is reproduced with permission from the American National Standard for Breathing Machines for Medical Use 79.7, copyright 1976 by the American National Standards Institute, copies of which may be purchased from the American National Standards Institute at 1430 Broadway, New York, N.Y. 10018.)

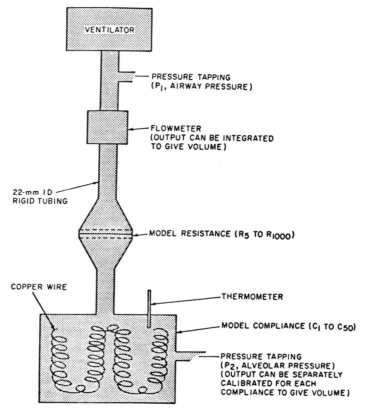

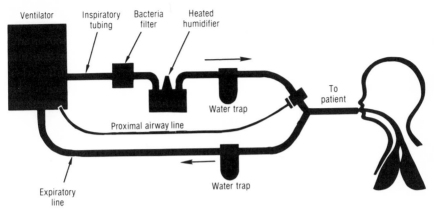

Fig. 10–2. – Gas flow pattern from ventilator to patient.

fications. This is important because every mechanical ventilator must deliver a certain volume of gas into a patient's lung, under a certain amount of pressure, with a particular type of flow pattern. On some mechanical ventilators, these variables can be altered by lung characteristics (airway resistance and lung compliance), while on others they may be regulated by the clinician's astute turning of the ventilator "controls." Essentially the ISO has standardized test procedures for all mechanical ventilators (Fig. 10–1). This then allows the clinician to compare mechanical ventilators as well as to predict what changes in pressure, flow or volume will occur in the face of increasing or decreasing airway resistance and/or lung compliance.

In the following descriptions the clinician will be introduced to several types of waveforms as well as the interrelationships with the terminology discussed previously.

In each of the waveforms shown, it should be understood that gas must flow under pressure and volume simultaneously from the ventilator through the various components in the ventilator patient circuit to the airway and then into the patient's lungs (Fig. 10–2). Once the gas reaches the patient's lungs, it must then be terminated and the patient allowed to exhale.

Pressure vs. Time Waveforms

From Figure 10–2 it can be seen that the ventilator has an internal compliance as well as an external compliance (patient circuit). Added together, this gives a total ventilator system compliance. After the beginning of inspiration a certain volume of gas at a prescribed FI_{O_2} is delivered into the patient circuit. This volume of gas causes an increase of pressure in the patient circuit and in a flow of gas through the proximal airway to the patient. During the inspiratory phase, proximal airway pressure and alveolar pressure increase gradually, with the proximal airway pressure always being higher than the alveolar pressure. The pressure difference across the proximal airway (pressure drop), which is largely determined by the size of the endotracheal tube and connector, determines the flow of gas through the proximal airway to the patient.

Inspiration is terminated when the flow of gas into the patient circuit (not necessarily the patient) is stopped and when the exhalation valve of the ventilator or patient circuit is opened. The expiratory flow from the patient is exhaled through the expiratory portion of the patient circuit and then through the exhalation valve. During exhalation, the patient can exhale either to the atmosphere (zero end expiratory pressure – ZEEP) or to some value above the atmosphere (positive end expiratory pressure – PEEP).

Figure 10–3 shows a typical pressure vs. time waveform that results if ventilation occurs in this manner. The diagram illustrates the following information:

1. There is a pressure vs. time waveform for gas at the proximal airway as well as gas in the lung (alveoli).

2. In order for gas to flow from the ventilator through the patient circuit into the lungs, pressure must gradually decrease. Therefore, pressure at the proximal airway must always be lower than at the ventilator.

3. The difference between the proximal airway pressure and the alveolar pressure (P_A) is the pressure drop across the airway. The latter pressure is determined by the flow, the size of the endotracheal tube and connector and the airway resistance.

Fig. 10–3. — Pressure vs. time waveform without an inspiratory pause.

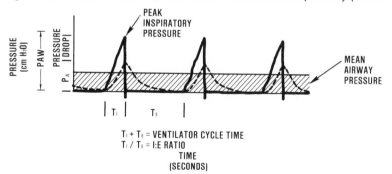

$T_I + T_E$ = VENTILATOR CYCLE TIME
T_I / T_E = I:E RATIO
TIME
(SECONDS)

4. In order for gas to flow from the patient through the expiratory portion of the patient system, alveolar pressure must be higher than proximal airway pressure. This is the period of expiratory flow.

5. When airway pressure and alveolar pressure are equal, there is zero flow because there is no pressure gradient.

6. When airway pressure and alveolar pressure become equal, it cannot be ascertained by the ventilator pressure gauge, since there is no time lag during the period of zero flow. The only exception to this is when an inspiratory pause is used, as shown in Figure 10−4.

7. The inspiratory phase time is the period from the start of inspiration to the start of exhalation.

8. The expiratory phase time is the period from the start of exhalation to the start of inspiration.

9. The sum of the inspiratory phase time and the expiratory phase time is the ventilator cycle time. The inverse of this times 60 is the frequency.

10. An integral taken over one breath (one cycle) produces the mean airway pressure.

Figure 10−4 shows a typical pressure vs. time waveform that results if ventilation occurs with an inspiratory pause. The latter is obtained by not allowing the exhalation valve of the ventilator to open at the same instant gas flow into the system is stopped. The net result of this effect is that for a certain period of time (usually 0.2−2.0 seconds) the pressures in the patient circuit and the alveoli are allowed to equalize. This causes an additional volume of gas to be delivered from the patient circuit into the alveoli initially, and then at the point of pressure equalization there exists a period of no flow because there is no pressure gradient. This period from the end of in-

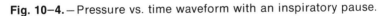

Fig. 10−4.−Pressure vs. time waveform with an inspiratory pause.

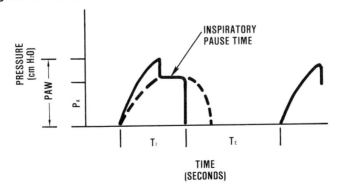

spiratory flow to the beginning of expiratory flow is called the inspiratory pause time.

Following the inspiratory pause time, the exhalation valve is allowed to open and the patient exhales to the atmosphere (zero end expiratory pressure – ZEEP), or to some level above atmosphere (positive end expiratory pressure – PEEP).

Figure 10–4 shows a typical pressure vs. time waveform for an inspiratory pause. Statements 1 through 5 and 7 through 10 above for Figure 10–3 are also true for Figure 10–4.

11. When airway pressure and alveolar pressure become equal, it *can* be ascertained by the ventilator pressure gauge, since there is a time lag during the period of zero flow.

12. The point at which pressures equalize during the inspiratory pause period is the alveolar pressure of the patient.

Clinically, these relationships shown on the ventilator pressure gauge are very important because they illustrate the changes in airway resistance and lung compliance that can occur during mechanical ventilation.

Flow vs. Time Waveforms

Figures 10–5 and 10–6 show a typical flow vs. time waveform without an inspiratory pause period and with an inspiratory pause period for a nonconstant flow generator (described in the Classification Section below). Regardless of the type of flow pattern elicited by the ventilator, the following statements are true:

1. Any flow above the resting level is termed an inspiratory flow.
2. A flow below the resting level is termed an expiratory flow.

Fig. 10–5. – Flow vs. time waveform without an inspiratory pause.

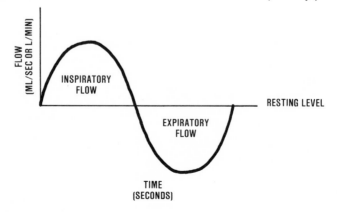

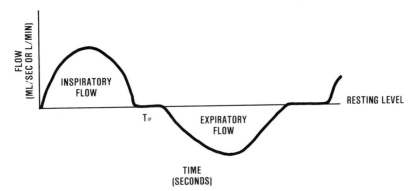

Fig. 10–6.—Flow vs. time waveform with an inspiratory pause.

3. The total area under the inspiratory flow curve is the inspiratory tidal volume.

4. The total area under the expiratory flow curve is the expiratory tidal volume.

5. If the total area under the inspiratory flow curve equals the total area under the expiratory flow curve, then the inspired tidal volume equals the expired tidal volume.

Volume vs. Time Waveforms

Figures 10–7 and 10–8 show the typical volume vs. time waveforms that result if ventilation occurs without an inspiratory pause period and with an inspiratory pause period.

Figure 10–9 shows the combination of pressure, flow and volume waveforms both with an inspiratory pause period and without an inspiratory pause period.

Fig. 10–7.—Volume vs. time waveform without an inspiratory pause.

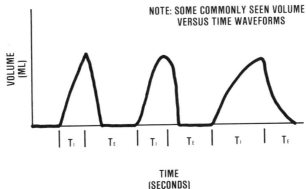

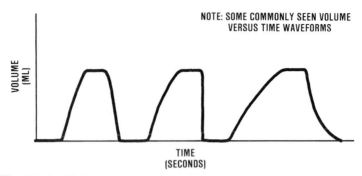

Fig. 10–8. — Volume vs. time waveform with an inspiratory pause.

CLASSIFICATION OF POSITIVE-PRESSURE VENTILATORS (TABLE 10–1)

Few aspects of intermittent positive-pressure ventilation (IPPV) are more intimidating or cause more confusion than the classification of ventilators. This is unfortunate, since the major purpose of classification is to enable the ventilator and its behavior to be understood

Fig. 10–9. — Pressure, flow and volume vs. time waveform without and with an inspiratory pause.

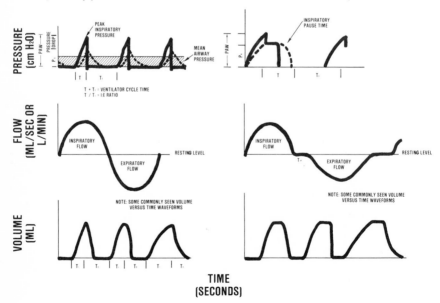

TABLE 10–1.—VENTILATOR CLASSIFICATION

	Beginning of Inspiration				Inspiration				End of Inspiration			Expiration			Power Source			Safety Device			
	Assister	Assister-controller	Controller	IMV	Constant flow	Nonconstant flow	Constant pressure	Nonconstant pressure	Volume	Pressure	Time	Passive	Subambient	PEEP	Pneumatic	Electrical	Both	Pressure limited	Volume limited	Time limited	Fail safe valve
Bourns BP200		X	1	X	X						X	X		X			X			X	X
Bourns LS 104–150	X	X	X	X	X				X			X	X	X			X	X	X	X	X
BABYbird			1	X	X					1	X	X	X	X	X			X	X		
Biomed MVP–10			1	X	X						X	X		X	X			X		X	X

X = primary function.
1 = Alternative method of adjustment.

more readily. Classification is a method of allowing the clinician to look at any ventilator and obtain a rudimentary idea of its capabilities. From there the clinician can predict what the ventilator will do in several given situations. Before we can start to discuss and compare the different infant mechanical ventilators available today, we will have to set up some standard classifications.

There are four basic phases of ventilation:
1. Beginning of inspiration (or end of expiration).
2. Inspiration.
3. End of Inspiration.
4. Expiration.

Ventilators are classified by the way they change from phase to phase and also by the way they operate in any one of the four phases.

Beginning of Inspiration

In this phase of ventilation, the classification depends on how the patient or ventilator initiates the inspiratory phase. This can be accomplished by the patient (assister), the ventilator (controller), through a combination of both (assister-controller) or with intermittent mandatory ventilation (IMV).

A ventilator is an assister if it allows the patient to "trigger" or start the ventilator in response to the patient's inspiratory effort. In order for the patient to trigger the ventilator, the latter must possess a minimum triggering pressure, flow and volume and rapid response time. When the patient is on an assister, he determines his own frequency of ventilation (e.g., Bourns LS104 – 150).

A ventilator is classified as a controller if the machine itself initiates inspiration due to the ventilator settings and not in response to the patient's inspiratory efforts. These settings may be an actual respiratory rate control (e.g., Bourns BP200) or a combination of inspiratory and expiratory timers (e.g., BABYbird and Biomed MVP-10) to initiate inspiration. In order for a ventilator to be called a controller, it must be able to maintain a preset frequency independent of the patient's spontaneous rate.

The next classification for this phase is a combination of the first two. A ventilator is classified as an assister-controller if it allows the patient to initiate inspiration as an assister but also allows a predetermined frequency to be used as a "back-up" in case of bradypnea or apnea (e.g., Bourns LS104 – 150).

An example would be a patient who is assisting the ventilator at 40 respirations/minute. The ventilator rate control is set at 30 respirations/minute. If the patient's respiratory rate starts to slow or he becomes apneic, the ventilator "guarantees" a minimum rate of 30 respirations/minute.

Intermittent mandatory ventilation allows the patient to breathe spontaneously from an independent or integral gas supply and to receive periodic machine-controlled breaths at a preselected respiratory rate and tidal volume. Adequate minute ventilation is obtained through careful combination of spontaneous and machine-controlled breaths.

Inspiration

The manner in which a ventilator delivers the volume of gas during the second phase of ventilation determines the inspiratory flow pattern classification. A ventilator is classified into one of four inspiratory flow patterns — constant flow, nonconstant flow, constant pressure or nonconstant pressure.

A constant-flow generator is one that holds the flow during inspiration at a constant rate and is unaffected by changes in lung characteristics. Sometimes it is called a straight-line flow pattern because the flow, when plotted on a graph, goes almost instantaneously to a predetermined point and remains constant until the beginning of expiration (Fig. 10–10). A true constant-flow generator will not decrease its

Fig. 10–10. — Characteristics of a constant-flow generator.

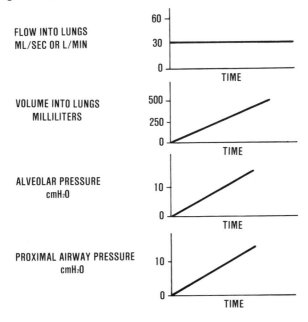

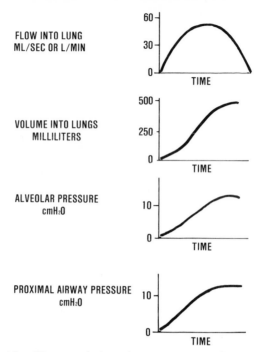

FLOW INTO LUNG
ML/SEC OR L/MIN

VOLUME INTO LUNGS
MILLILITERS

ALVEOLAR PRESSURE
cmH₂O

PROXIMAL AIRWAY PRESSURE
cmH₂O

Fig. 10–11. — Characteristics of a nonconstant-flow generator.

flow in the face of increased resistance. Most of the constant-flow type of ventilators available today will show a slight decrease in flow with high resistance even though we classify them as constant-flow generators.

The nonconstant flow pattern is the flow speculated to be most physiologic to normal respiration. The flow is low at the beginning of inspiration, speeds up to a peak at midinspiration and then decreases to zero at the end of inspiration (Fig. 10–11). This type of flow pattern is found on all piston-driven ventilators that utilize a wheel (none of the currently U.S.-manufactured infant mechanical ventilators is piston driven via a wheel). The wheel moves at a constant speed, but the piston, which is attached to the wheel's outside diameter, moves slowly at the beginning of inspiration, fastest toward the midpoint and slows again at the end of inspiration.

A constant-pressure generator is one that will maintain a constant pressure in the patient circuit but which decreases its flow in the face of high resistance. As the pressure in the lungs increases, the flow decreases (Fig. 10–12). This characteristic is found in almost all

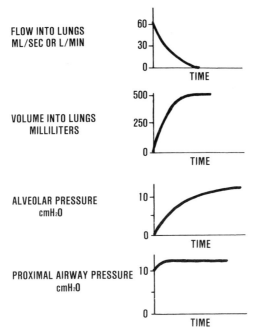

Fig. 10–12. – Characteristics of a constant-pressure generator.

pressure-cycled ventilators. Sometimes it is called a constant-pressure generator because it maintains a constant pressure between the ventilator and the airway. The flow rate will remain variable, changing with the resistance or compliance of the patient.

A nonconstant-pressure generator is similar to a constant-pressure generator except that pressure varies during inspiration instead of being constant. The variation in pressure is constant; the pressure waveform is constant and independent of changes in lung characteristics (Fig. 10–13).

End of Inspiration

The way in which the inspiratory cycle is terminated determines the method of cycling. Under this classification, there are three basic types of ventilators — volume cycled, pressure cycled and time cycled. A ventilator is placed into one of these three categories by the way in which inspiration is normally ended. A volume-cycled ventilator begins the expiratory phase of ventilation when a preset tidal volume has been delivered into the breathing circuit. A volume-cycled ventilator will show an increase in the pressure reading when the compli-

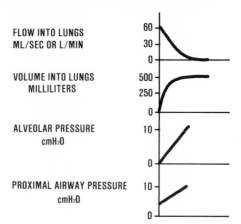

FLOW INTO LUNGS
ML/SEC OR L/MIN

VOLUME INTO LUNGS
MILLILITERS

ALVEOLAR PRESSURE
cmH₂O

PROXIMAL AIRWAY PRESSURE
cmH₂O

Fig. 10–13.—Characteristics of a nonconstant-pressure generator.

ance of the lungs is decreased or the resistance in the patient's airway is increased. It will still deliver a constant tidal volume if there are no leaks in the patient circuit or at the proximal airway.

Much confusion has arisen about the classification of some primary volume ventilators. Most volume ventilators contain a safety device that relieves pressure and consequently a volume at a predetermined point. When this device is used, it is possible to set a pressure at which the ventilator will release pressure to the atmosphere. This may appear to simulate a pressure-cycled ventilator because the ventilator is still in the inspiratory phase until the predetermined volume has been delivered to the atmosphere, not the patient. Instead, it is said to be pressure limited. Some ventilators incorporate both of these features while others possess one or the other.

Pressure-cycled ventilators begin the expiratory phase of ventilation when the preset pressure has been reached in the ventilator as long as an inspiratory plateau is not used. Since the pressure remains constant, an increase in airway resistance and a decrease in lung compliance or a leak will lower the tidal volume.

Time-cycled ventilators end the inspiratory phase of the respiratory cycle when a preset inspiratory time has passed. Following inspiration, the exhalation valve opens and the patient exhales the delivered tidal volume. A respiratory rate control or an expiratory time control does not qualify a ventilator to become time cycled because neither of these terminates inspiration.

Expiration

The manner in which a ventilator allows exhalation to occur determines this type of classification. Exhalation may be broken down as follows:

1. Passive (positive-atmosphere) exhalation.
2. Subambient (positive-negative) exhalation.
3. Positive end (positive-positive) expiratory pressure (PEEP).
4. Retarded (positive-expiratory resistance).

POSITIVE-ATMOSPHERE (Fig. 10–14,A).—This type of exhalation allows the patient to exhale his tidal volume without delay at the beginning of exhalation. In this type of classification, the ventilator produces a positive pressure in the patient's lungs during inspiration whereas during exhalation pressure returns to atmosphere (zero level).

POSITIVE-NEGATIVE (Fig. 10–14,B).—In this type of classification, the ventilator produces a positive pressure in the patient's lungs during inspiration whereas during exhalation pressure drops to below atmosphere in the patient's lungs and patient circuit.

POSITIVE-POSITIVE (Fig. 10–14,C).—In this type of classification, the ventilator produces a positive pressure in the patient's lungs during inspiration whereas during exhalation pressure remains above atmosphere.

POSITIVE-EXPIRATORY RESISTANCE (Fig. 10–14,D).—In this type of classification the ventilator produces a positive pressure in the patient's lungs during inspiration whereas a retard or expiratory flow gradient on the ventilator reduces gas outflow from the patient circuit and thereby the patient. Theoretically reducing expiratory flow rate increases expiratory time while minimizing alveolar collapse.

The four phases of ventilation with their classifications can be summarized as follows:

Phase I — Beginning of Inspiration
a) Assister
b) Controller
c) Assister-controller
d) Intermittent mandatory ventilation
Phase II — Inspiration
a) Constant-flow generator
b) Nonconstant-flow generator
c) Constant-pressure generator
d) Nonconstant-pressure generator

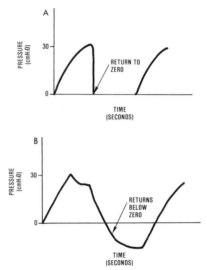

Fig. 10–14.—A, pressure vs. time waveform indicating positive-atmosphere pressure pattern. **B,** pressure vs. time waveform indicating positive-negative pressure pattern. *(Continued.)*

Phase III — End of Inspiration
a) Volume cycled
b) Pressure cycled
c) Time cycled
d) Flow cycled (PR series)
Phase IV — Expiration
a) Passive
b) Subambient
c) PEEP
d) Expiratory resistance

In addition to the above information, it is important to determine where a ventilator gets its power, and what types of safety devices it incorporates. The power source may be:

1. Pneumatic — operated by pressurized gas; e.g., BABYBird, Biomed MVP-10

2. Electrical — operated by electricity; e.g., Bourns LS 104 – 150

3. Pneumatic and electrical — operated by pressurized gas and electronically controlled; e.g., Bourns BP200.

The safety device may be:

1. Pressure limited — the maximal pressure is limited and adjusted by a pop-off valve.

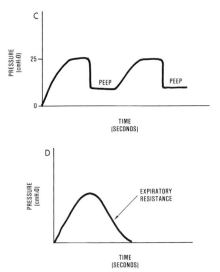

Fig. 10–14. (cont.)—C, pressure vs. time waveform indicating positive-positive pressure pattern. **D,** pressure vs. time waveform indicating positive-expiratory resistance pressure pattern.

2. Volume limited—a maximal volume is set on the ventilator. The machine may deliver less but never more than this volume.

3. Time limited—a maximal time period that may not be exceeded is set on the ventilator. This time period may be fixed (1:1 ratio limit Bennett MA-I) or adjustable (BABYbird and Bourns BP200).

4. Fail safe valve—a one-way valve that opens and allows the patient to inhale room air if the machine fails.

Although all currently manufactured mechanical ventilators possess a fail safe valve, it is important to realize that the patient must breathe through the patient circuit before he can open the one-way valve. In an infant mechanical ventilator, the patient must be able to generate at least −3 cm H_2O to breathe through the patient circuit plus −1 cm H_2O for the one-way valve.

PRINCIPLES OF MECHANICAL VENTILATION

The principle on which all positive-pressure mechanical ventilators work is the achievement of a pressure gradient to produce a flow of gas into the lung. The difference between one ventilator and another lies in their innate capability of meeting this challenge when faced with a wide variety of clinically changing disorders. The crucial difference in mechanical ventilators lies in the number and types of available features offered that allow:

1. Simplicity, versatility, ease of operation and reliability.
2. A wide range of respiratory rates.
3. Accurate delivery of V_T over a wide range of values.
4. Various modes of ventilation such as assist-control, control, inspiratory plateau, PEEP, IMV, CPAP and spontaneous breathing.

TABLE 10-2.—THE IDEAL INFANT VENTILATOR

Operational Characteristics
  Volume or time cycled
  Assist/control, control and IMV modes
  Tidal volume range 5–150 ml
  Respiratory rate 1–80 breaths per minute°
  Variable inspiratory flow rate 0–20 l/min
  Variable I:E ratio 3:1–1:10
  Adjustable peak inspiratory pressure limit 10–80 cm H_2O
  PEEP or CPAP capability to 15 cm H_2O
  Inspiratory plateau 0–2.0 seconds
Alarms (Audible and Visual)
  High and low pressure
  Apnea
  Loss of PEEP/CPAP
  Power failure and power disconnect (electrical)
  Loss of air and/or oxygen inlet pressure (pneumatic)
  Overtemperature
  High and low oxygen concentration
  Failure to cycle
Monitors
  Proximal airway pressure
  Proximal airway temperature
  Inspiratory O_2 concentration
  Exhaled tidal volume
  Respiratory rate (spontaneous and machine)
  Inspiratory time and expiratory time
  I:E ratio
  Mean airway pressure
Ventilator Characteristics
  Small, compact
  Easily detachable, multisterilizable patient circuit
  Servo-control of F_{IO_2}, inspiratory gas temperature and tidal volume
  Output jacks for continuous, periodic or remote recording of pressure, flow and volume waveform
  Output jacks to allow connection of ventilator alarms to a remote alarm at the nurses' station
  Functional with nonflammable anesthetics
  May be used on a transport vehicle

°At this time respirator rates of 80 breaths per minute are more than adequate, although some researchers are advocating rates as high as 120 breaths per minute. This may become a clinical requirement in the future.

---

5. Adequate heated humidification of the inspired gas.
6. Variable or constant flow rates.
7. Adjustable $F_{I_{O_2}}$ concentrations.
8. A wide variety of audible and visual alarms and/or indicators.
9. An adjustable pressure relief valve.
10. Maximal and minimal pressure capabilities.
11. Low cost.
12. Minimal noise.
13. Ease of maintenance or repair.

See Table 10–2 for an example of the ideal ventilator.

Ventilator Controls and Indicators

The controls of a ventilator are important (Table 10–3). In a well-thought-out design, their number is reduced to a minimum, their functions are self-evident and as many as possible are calibrated. The number of controls available will vary from machine to machine, depending on the number of features available. In general, however, the following are the most common controls and indicators found on volume- or time-cycled pressure-limited ventilators:

1. Minute volume.
2. Respiratory rate.
3. Tidal volume
4. Inspiratory time.
5. Expiratory time.
6. I:E ratio.
7. Peak flow.
8. Mode control.
9. Pressure limit.
10. Oxygen.
11. Inspiratory pause.
12. PEEP.
13. Sigh.
14. Sensitivity.
15. Manometer pressure.
16. Alarms.

MINUTE VOLUME. — The minute volume is the product of the respiratory rate (RR) and tidal volume (V_T). Therefore, to set this modality accurately on a ventilator, the clinician must estimate the necessary V_T of the patient needed to produce effective alveolar ventilation as well as a normal respiratory rate. In order to estimate the V_T of the patient, the clinician should do two things:

1. Determine or estimate the patient's body weight. In general, a

TABLE 10-3.—SPECIFICATIONS OF VARIOUS VENTILATORS—
COMPARISON OF CONTROLS

	V_T	T_1	T_E	RR	FLOW	INSP. PLAT	I:E RATIO	PEEP CPAP	PRESS. LIMIT	INSP. TIME LIMIT	SIGH
Bourns LS104–150	X			X	X	X		X	X		X
Bourns BP200				X	X		X	X	X	X	
BABYbird		X	X		X			X	X	X	
Biomed MVP–10		X	X		X			X	X		

newborn requires 3 ml/lb or 7 ml/kg to ventilate adequately. Therefore, a 3-kg infant would need 21 ml of tidal volume to produce effective alveolar ventilation.

2. Compute the ventilator-system compliance. This is the amount of ventilation in milliliters that is lost in the machine, tubing and humidifier each time the ventilator cycles. In other words, it is ventilation that never reaches the patient due to expansion and compressibility of the ventilator tubing system. The amount of ventilator system compliance varies with each mechanical ventilator as well as the type and amount of tubing, humidifier and presence or absence of a bacteria filter. It may be calculated mathematically by using the formula $C = V/P$ where C equals compliance, V equals volume change and P equals pressure. In most circumstances, the compliance will be approximately 0.3 ml/cm H_2O on the ventilator pressure gauge. Therefore, if 25 cm H_2O is required to deliver a V_T of 18 ml, 7.5 ml (25×0.3) is being lost with every breath.

If the clinician wants to ventilate the patient adequately, he must add V_T and compliance loss together. Then, to this number the respiratory rate is multiplied and the product obtained is the minute volume (not minute ventilation). Example: 3-kg infant

f 35

Machine compliance = 0.3 ml/cm H_2O

3 kg × 7 ml = 21 ml (V_T)

If we assume that it will take 25 cm H_2O to put 18 ml into the patient's lungs, then:

25 cm H_2O × 0.3 ml/cm H_2O = 7.5 ml loss/breath

(V_T + loss) × f = MV

(18 + 7.5) × 35 = MV

25.5 × 35 = MV

892.5 = MV

Therefore, the minute volume control on the machine must be set at 0.89 liter to satisfy the patient's ventilatory requirements.

It is apparent from this discussion that two points should be carefully considered:

1. The volume loss due to machine/tubing compliance must be accurately determined to avoid hypoventilating or hyperventilating the patient.

2. Ventilatory requirements depend on the basal metabolic rate, body weight and ventilation/perfusion ratio of the lungs. Few of these points usually are known, which is a good reason for setting a ventilator to provide more than the estimated requirement, since this avoids the danger of hypoventilation. Under all circumstances, the patient must be ventilated.

Respiratory rate. — All ventilators possess some method of regulating the number of breaths per minute. In some machines, the respiratory rate is regulated by a calibrated control whereas in others it is the result of the inspiratory and expiratory time controls. From a practical standpoint, it is much easier to use a ventilator when the clinician merely has to adjust one dial instead of several. Many modern-day mechanical ventilators possess a calibrated control for respiratory rate.

Tidal volume. — Most mechanical ventilators control tidal volume delivery directly by means of a calibrated dial. Others, however, regulate it indirectly through setting of the minute volume and respiratory rate. Several foreign-produced mechanical ventilators work in this latter manner. In the United States, most ventilators possess a tidal volume dial and a respiratory rate control.

With this method of volume delivery, the tidal volume becomes an important modality as a measure of ventilation. In these types of ventilators, the tidal volume set on the machine must be sufficient to provide the patient with effective alveolar ventilation. If the tidal volume is set too low, hypoventilation results. Likewise, if the tidal volume is set too high, hyperventilation ensues. It is important to recognize this relationship and understand it thoroughly. An example will illustrate an interesting point.

$$V_T \times RR = MV$$

30 ml × 40 = 1200 ml	NORMAL
20 ml × 40 = 800 ml	HYPOVENTILATION
40 ml × 40 = 1600 ml	HYPERVENTILATION

In this situation, a change in V_T of 10 ml with a constant RR produces normal or abnormal ventilation.

Another method of controlling tidal volume is to multiply inspiratory time by inspiratory flow rate:

If $T_I = 0.5$ seconds

and $V_I = 20$ ml/sec (1.2 l/min)

then $V_T = 10$ ml

This method of tidal volume computation is utilized with the BABYbird, Bourns BP200 and Biomed MVP-10 infant ventilators.

INSPIRATORY TIME. — The inspiratory time period is the duration of time between initiation of inspiratory flow and the beginning of expiratory flow. It is the phase in which the ventilator produces positive pressure in the chest. On some mechanical ventilators this phase is controlled by the inspiratory time and inspiratory pause controls whereas in others it is governed by the I:E ratio and respiratory rate controls.

EXPIRATORY TIME. — The expiratory time period is the duration of time from the start of expiratory flow to the start of inspiratory flow. On most mechanical ventilators, the process occurs passively; however, on some (BABYbird, Biomed MVP-10), a control labeled Expiratory Time is adjusted. On most ventilators, the expiratory phase may also be controlled by the use of PEEP or expiratory resistance. PEEP, as was mentioned earlier, holds gas in the lung at end exhalation while expiratory resistance lengthens exhalation, thereby theoretically preventing alveolar collapse. This latter point, although postulated, lacks clinical documentation. Should it be clinically proved, virtually any ventilator could be adapted externally to provide this function by placing a variable restriction in the expiratory portion of the patient circuit.

INSPIRATORY/EXPIRATORY(I:E) RATIO. — The I:E ratio is the relationship between the inspiratory time and the expiratory time. During normal ventilation, this value usually is 1:2 (inspiration lasts for one-third and exhalation for two-thirds). In certain situations, such as bronchopulmonary dysplasia, it may be advantageous to reverse this ratio to 4:1. In others, such as high-compliance, low-resistance states, it may be necessary to alter the I:E ratio to 1:4. In most ventilators it is possible to vary the I:E ratio by changing inspiratory time, expiratory time, respiratory rate or flow.

PEAK FLOW. — The peak flow controls the rate at which the positive-pressure breath will be delivered during inspiration. Usually this control is calibrated in ml/sec or liters per minute (l/min). In general, newborn mechanical ventilators have a peak flow rate from 0 to 20 l/min (0–325 ml/sec).

MODE CONTROL.—The mode control allows selection of the method of operation. In some mechanical ventilators this dial allows control, assist-control, IMV and CPAP whereas in others only a given combination is possible.

PRESSURE LIMIT CONTROL.—This control limits the amount of system pressure that may be developed in the inspiratory phase. When the preset pressure limit is reached, inspiration is terminated immediately. Usually this control is adjustable from 0 to 80 cm H_2O in newborn mechanical ventilators.

OXYGEN.—The oxygen control allows adjustable selection of $F_{I_{O_2}}$ from 0.21 to 1.00. To obtain greater than 21% oxygen, the ventilator must be connected to an oxygen source.

INSPIRATORY PAUSE.—This control delays the opening of the exhalation valve until after the positive-pressure breath is delivered and flow has terminated. Usually this control is adjustable from 0 to 2.0 seconds.

PEEP.—Positive end expiratory pressure usually is available from 0 to 20 cm H_2O. In general, the PEEP level is adjusted by turning the PEEP control clockwise or counterclockwise and observing the pressure gauge. In some ventilators, the PEEP circuit is leak compensated to maintain stable PEEP levels even in the presence of minor leaks.

SIGH.—A sigh is a periodic deep breath that all spontaneously breathing patients perform at least 6–8 times per hour. The purpose of a sigh is to hyperexpand the lung, thus preventing areas of microatelectasis that otherwise would develop due to the inflation of the lung with a constant tidal volume. Some mechanical ventilators provide a method of sighing a patient. This may be done manually by depressing a button or it may mean setting a sigh volume (usually 1½ times the V_T), a sigh pressure (1½ times the pressure gauge) and the number of sighs per hour. When IMV is the primary method of ventilatory support, sighs are not necessary since the mandatory or ventilator-delivered breath is delivered at a greater volume than the patient's spontaneous breath. Thus, in effect it is a sigh breath.

SENSITIVITY.—This control is present only in machines that allow the ventilator to assist the patient. The sensitivity control adjusts the amount of negative pressure applied to the ventilator's circuit that the patient must exert to start the ventilator. In some ventilators, the sensitivity control may be called patient-triggering effort. It is important when setting this control to adjust it to meet the patient's demands. If it is set incorrectly, the machine may self cycle or force the patient to exert a larger effort to trigger the machine.

MANOMETER PRESSURE. — This is the amount of pressure that is measured and displayed on the ventilator pressure gauge each time the machine cycles. In some infant ventilators it is an indication of total system pressure (machine + patient circuit + patient) whereas in others it is an indication of proximal airway pressure (patient pressure). A manometer does not reflect lung pressure. The manometer pressure is dependent on three factors:
1. The patient's airway resistance.
2. The V_T of each ventilator breath.
3. The inspiratory flow rate.

In a volume-cycled ventilator, systematic recording of the manometer pressure over several hours or days indicates an improvement or decline in patient lung compliance. As the amount of pressure on the manometer decreases, the lung compliance of the patient increases and vice versa.

ALARMS. — The presence or absence of alarms does not constitute a good ventilator but it does indicate a potentially safe ventilator. The availability of a wide variety of audible and visual alarms ensures prompt recognition of a change in the patient, the machine or a combination of both that otherwise may go undetected. All mechanical ventilators should possess alarms for power failure or power disconnect (if electrically operated), loss of inlet pressure (if pneumatically powered), low pressure, high pressure, failure to cycle and overtemperature. Other alarms such as decrease in oxygen percent, high end expiratory pressure, loss of PEEP pressure and apnea are optional features that are advantageous to possess but not absolutely necessary.

LEARNING A NEW MECHANICAL VENTILATOR

Because of the wide variety of mechanical ventilators available today, something must be said about approaching a new or totally unfamiliar ventilator. All too often, the very appearance of a different machine with tubing, controls and other paraphernalia frightens and baffles would-be users. This phenomenon should never occur, because a ventilator does not have to appear awesome, difficult or confusing simply by its external design.

The easiest method of approaching a new mechanical ventilator is to look at the control panel and then to classify the machine. Follow this step by observing the number and types of alarms available, type of humidification system, visual monitors and meters and assembly of the tubing. This acquaints you in general with what the machine obviously can do. To find out how it does each function, how well it performs it and everything else, read the instruction manual supplied by the manufacturer. Never attempt to operate a mechanical ventilator on a patient without a thorough understanding of its function, controls and capabilities.

After diligent study of the instruction manual, the potential operator should practice assembling the tubing, humidification system, etc., in order to be able to perform the procedure quickly and accurately. The finest ventilator designed is useless if it cannot be assembled when the need arises. The next step to learning a ventilator is setting it up in a mock clinical situation, using a test lung that allows varying lung compliances and airway resistances. This allows the operator to turn the various controls of the ventilator in response to simulated clinical situations and to observe its response. This step is extremely important. The place to find out how a ventilator behaves is in a laboratory environment using a test lung and not in the intensive care unit on a patient.

The last step to learning a mechanical ventilator is to practice setting one up along with a person experienced in its over-all operation. This individual then can check over the machine before it is connected to the patient and point out any minor considerations that should be taken into account.

Advantages of Using a Ventilator

The advantages of mechanical ventilation are:

1. It eliminates the necessity for manually ventilating a patient with a resuscitation device.

2. Better gas distribution and increasing alveolar gas exchange are possible.

3. Alveolar ventilation and diffusion often are increased through the modalities of inspiratory pause and PEEP.

4. Larger and/or fixed volumes and respiratory rates can be given to the patient.

5. The presence of an endotracheal tube allows better control of the airway.

6. The patient is monitored more easily.

Disadvantages of Using a Ventilator

The disadvantages of mechanical ventilation are:

1. There are alarmingly few individuals in every hospital who understand the setup, function and operation of the ventilator.

2. The performance of the ventilator is directly proportional to the knowledge of the operator.

3. A ventilator is subject to mechanical failure.

4. The ventilator induces a false sense of security in the operator and often is not monitored as carefully as necessary.

5. Most mechanical ventilators have incomplete alarm systems.

6. No ventilator at present will indicate changes in the patient as rapidly as a clinician.

7. It often is difficult to wean patients.

8. Infections can be easily induced through the humidification device or patient circuit.

9. Most ventilators are not simple to operate.

10. Most ventilators lack portability for transport of critically ill patients.

Hazards of Using a Ventilator

1. The patient may be hypoventilated or hyperventilated if the ventilator is not adjusted correctly.

2. Leaks occurring from misfitted or improperly fitted rubber or plastic hoses and disconnections may go undetected because of incomplete alarm systems.

3. Many ventilators can self cycle, leading to improper ventilation and abnormal I : E ratios.

4. Many ventilators will continue to cycle even when disconnected from the patient.

5. A dirty air supply system may allow water and other particulate matter to enter the oxygen blender. This will result in inaccurate oxygen concentrations.

6. Inadvertent kinking of the ventilator patient circuit tubing may go undetected due to lack of an audible high-pressure alarm.

7. The humidification system may overheat.

8. Excessive condensation of water in the patient circuit may result in an accidental lavage of the patient.

9. Inappropriate humidifier water levels may result in different levels of tidal volume delivery.

10. Pressure relief valves may fail, with the result usually a pulmonary air leak.

NEWBORN MECHANICAL VENTILATORS
Bourns LS104–150 Infant Ventilator

Description

The Bourns LS104–150 Infant Ventilator (Fig. 10–15) is an electrically operated volume-, time- or pressure-cycled device. It is a constant-flow generator that is capable of functioning as an assister, controller or assister-controller. The ventilator can provide zero end expiratory pressure (ZEEP), a positive end expiratory pressure (PEEP), continuous positive airway pressure (CPAP) or a combination of techniques termed intermittent mandatory ventilation (IMV). During all modes of operation, the clinician can limit the amount of pressure delivered by the ventilator by adjusting the pressure-relief valve or high-pressure alarm. Tidal volume is controlled by adding patient volume (7–10 ml/kg) + volume lost in patient circuit (machine compliance × pressure generated) together and setting the machine volume control to this level.

The Bourns Infant Ventilator system consists of three major mechanical systems: the oxygen blender, infant ventilator and humidification system.

Major Mechanical System (Fig. 10–16)

1. OXYGEN BLENDER. — OXYGEN in the range 30–75 psi (1) and COMPRESSED AIR in the range 15–75 psig (2) are connected to the OXYGEN BLENDER (3) via standard DISS fittings. Inlet pressures are measured and displayed on the appropriate INLET PRESSURE GAUGES (4). If either air or oxygen or both inlet gas pressures are too low for accurate blending, an audible battery-operated ALARM will sound (5). The presence of two PRESSURE REGULATORS (6) balances the pressures before directing the gas to a calibrated differential GAS BLENDING VALVE (7). The latter allows selectable O_2 concentrations between 21% and 100% (± 3% accuracy). Gas flow then is directed through a calibrated ROTAMETER (8) to provide a visual index of flow to the patient. Flow then proceeds to a DEMAND VALVE with adjustable modes (9). In the IPPB mode, gas is supplied to meet the demands of the patient or ventilator. In the CPAP mode, the clinician can select continuous flows up to 20 liters per minute. The flow is directed out of the blender past a SAFETY VALVE (10), which opens in the event of malfunction of the upstream components. This mechanism allows gas supply to the patient or ventilator at all times. A special outlet is pro-

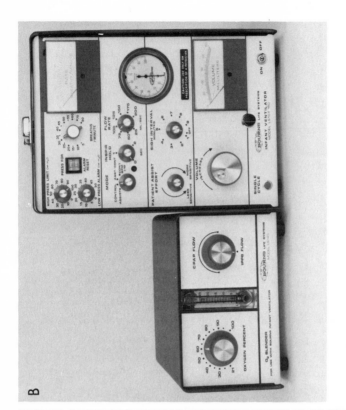

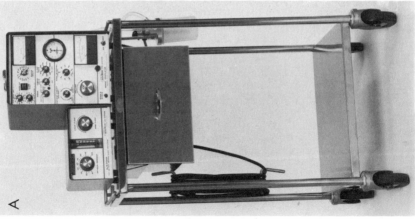

Fig. 10–15.—Bourns LS104–150 Infant Ventilator. **A**, ventilator system with oxygen blender and Mistogen heated humidifier on mobile cart. **B**, front view of oxygen blender and ventilator. (Courtesy of Bourns Medical Systems, Inc., Riverside, Cal.)

vided on the O_2 blender to power the ventilator PEEP VALVE (11).

2. INFANT VENTILATOR.—The Bourns Infant Ventilator is a pneumatic apparatus, electrically powered and electronically controlled. The ventilator supplies gas to the infant by the action of a PISTON-CYLINDER combination (12) that is connected to the MACHINE VOLUME CONTROL (13) on the front of the ventilator. A VOLUME METER (14) will continuously display the setting of the volume control. The piston, on its backstroke, is charged with controlled F_{IO_2} gas from the OXYGEN BLENDER (15). The piston normally rests in the rearward position. When an inspiration signal is received, the piston moves forward, pushing the gas mixture to the patient. The CHECK VALVES (16) in the manifold ensure that the gas will flow in the proper direction. The adjustable PRESSURE RELIEF VALVE (17) is located in the manifold and ensures that the gas delivered to the patient will not exceed the pressure setting of the relief valve. The volume delivered by the piston is preset by a stroke-control mechanism. Gas delivered by the piston is held in the patient circuit during inspiration by the EXHALATION VALVE (18), ensuring delivery to the patient's lungs. The pressure developed by the ventilator is self-compensating for the infant ventilator combination and will rise to a level necessary for preselected volume delivery. The pressure shown on the ventilator PRESSURE GAUGE (19) is measured just inside the machine and is not the same pressure as in the lung.

Because gas is compressible and TUBING WALLS (20) are not rigid, not all the gas delivered by the piston reaches the patient. As the pressure in the tubing increases, an increasing amount of gas remains in the tubing system during inspiration. This gas is "lost" in the compliance of the ventilator system and does not reach the patient. Therefore, it is necessary to calculate the lost volume to determine the volume delivered to the patient. Although this can be done mathematically, it is also easily accomplished with a Bourns Ventilation Calculator.

When the inspiratory stroke of the ventilator is complete, the EXHALATION VALVE (18) opens, allowing the patient to exhale.

Positive end expiratory pressure (PEEP) (21) is generated and maintained by an inverted JET VENTURI (22). When the patient pressure is above the PEEP level, the patient can exhale freely through the Venturi. When the patient pressure drops to the PEEP level, the PEEP level generated by the jet Venturi prevents additional gas from escaping and, therefore, maintains the patient pressure at the PEEP level. If a leak is present in the system, the PEEP level can be maintained

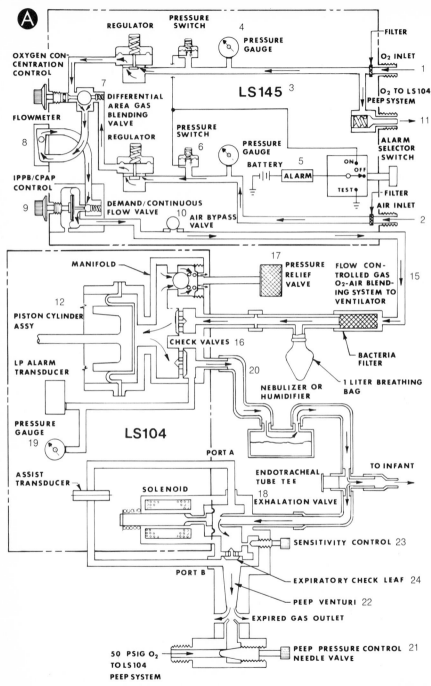

Fig. 10–16.—A, pneumatic flow diagram of Bourns LS104–150 Infant Ventilator and oxygen blender. *(Continued.)*

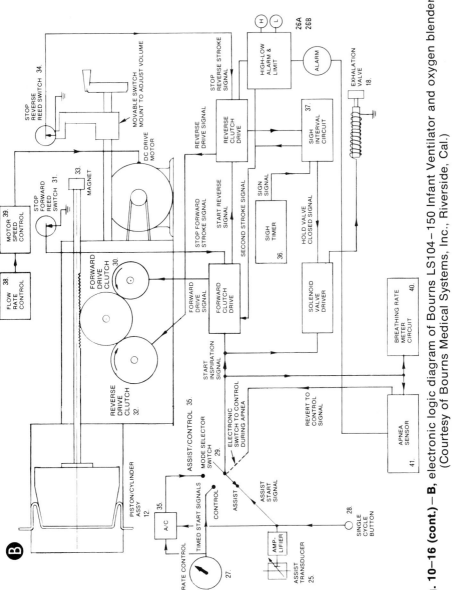

Fig. 10–16 (cont.)–B, electronic logic diagram of Bourns LS104–150 Infant Ventilator and oxygen blender. (Courtesy of Bourns Medical Systems, Inc., Riverside, Cal.)

by opening the SENSITIVITY CONTROL needle valve (23), which will allow gas to flow into the patient circuit and maintain the PEEP level. The PEEP level is controlled by the PEEP needle valve.

When the infant attempts to inhale, the negative pressure generated in the tubing circuit is trapped by the EXPIRATORY CHECK VALVE (24) and is sensed by the ASSIST TRANSDUCER (25). The assist transducer will start the inspiratory stroke of the piston and begin delivering gas to the infant in less than 35 milliseconds after the negative pressure is applied. If PEEP is being applied, the assist transducer still will function, since the back of the transducer is connected to the PEEP system. The transducer now senses a reduction in pressure on the patient side of the expiratory check leaf. It should be noted that in the case of power failure, the infant still can breathe through the ventilator. Gas can be drawn into the ventilator through the PISTON CHECK VALVES (16) when the infant sucks on the ventilator with more than a 1 cm H_2O effort.

A high/low PRESSURE SENSOR (26 A and B) is provided, which will sound an audible alarm and give a visual indication whenever pressures above or below the settings are reached.

The operation of the ventilator is controlled by an electronic logic system. These electronic signal paths are used to operate and control the ventilator. The initiation of a cycle is caused by the RATE CONTROL TIMER (27), the ASSIST TRANSDUCER (25) or the SINGLE-CYCLE BUTTON (28). The source of the start inspiration signal is controlled by the MODE SELECTOR SWITCH (29). The start inspiration signal closes the EXHALATION VALVE (18) and actuates the FORWARD CLUTCH (30). When the piston has reached the full forward position, a magnet on the piston shaft actuates the forward REED SWITCH (31). The forward reed switch signal disengages the forward drive clutch, opens the exhalation valve and engages the REVERSE DRIVE CLUTCH (32). The reverse drive clutch returns the piston to the reset-volume position. When the piston is at the correct back position, the PISTON SHAFT MAGNET (33) actuates the REAR REED SWITCH (34). The rear reed switch signal disengages the REVERSE DRIVE CLUTCH (32). The ventilator now is ready to start a new inspiration but waits in expiration until a new inspiratory start signal is reached. If the rate control timer initiates an inspiration start signal before the piston has returned to the resting position, the start signal will be ignored and the ventilator will wait for the next cycle before starting an inspiration.

The volume delivered by the ventilator is controlled by the position of the reverse reed switch.

In the ASSIST-CONTROL MODE (35), the machine cycles in the same manner as in the control mode except for the added feature of allowing the infant to breathe at his own rate. This is accomplished by letting the ASSIST TRANSDUCER SIGNAL (25) override the RATE CONTROL SIGNAL (27) as long as the infant is trying to breathe on his own. The instant the infant stops breathing on his own, the machine reverts to the control setting.

A sigh is initiated when the SIGH TIMER (36) sends a signal to the SIGH CONTROL (37). The sigh control then will maintain the exhalation valve closed through the piston return stroke and immediately initiate a second cycle. The result is a double-volume breath.

The INSPIRATORY FLOW RATE (38) is controlled by a MOTOR SPEED CONTROL CIRCUIT (39).

An INSPIRATION HOLD (40) may be initiated by activation of the control. This delays the exhalation valve from opening until after the hold period.

The inspiration start signal is also used by the rate meter circuit and the apnea sensor. The RATE METER CIRCUIT (41) integrates the inspiration start pulses and displays the breathing rate of the infant. The APNEA SENSOR (42) is functional in the assist mode and determines if the breathing rate drops to below 60% of the control rate setting for more than 10 seconds. If apnea has occurred by this criteria, the sensor electronically reverts the mode selector to the control setting for a 5-second period and sounds an audible alarm.

3. HUMIDIFICATION SYSTEM.—The gas supplied by the ventilator may be humidified (43) on the way to the infant by the modified Mistogen heated humidifier or modified DeVilbiss Ultrasonic. The heated humidifier gives variable heat control to provide 100% humidity of the inspired gas. Included with the Mistogen heated humidifier is a probe thermometer for monitoring temperature of the inspired gas leaving the humidifier and an audio overtemperature alarm with electrical power shutoff. The modified ultrasonic nebulizer has a reduced water output suitable for infant ventilation (0–30 ml per hour adjustable) and a low compliance nebulizer cup.

Preliminary Operation of the Bourns Infant Ventilator (Figs. 10–15 and 10–17)

1. *Oxygen Blender:*

   a) Connect 50 psi oxygen and 50 psi compressed air to the blender.

   b) Turn the LOW PRESSURE ALARM switch to TEST, then to the ON position. If the alarm fails to sound in the TEST position, replace the battery.

   c) Select the desired oxygen concentration.

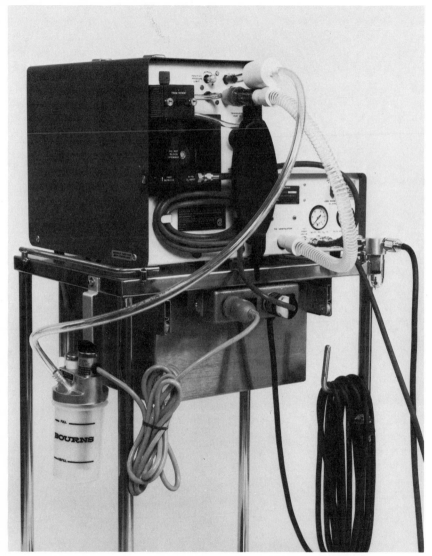

Fig. 10–17. – Rear view of Bourns LS104 – 150 Infant Ventilator. (Courtesy of Bourns Medical Systems, Inc., Riverside, Cal.)

d) Set CPAP FLOW/IPPB FLOW control to the desired level.

2. *Infant Ventilator:*

a) Plug the ventilator into a 117-VAC, 60-Hz grounded electrical source.

b) Turn the PATIENT ASSIST EFFORT control counterclockwise. This controls the effort required to trigger the ventilator in the assist and assist-control modes. The response time is 35 milliseconds.

c) Turn off the SIGH INTERVAL.

d) Set the MODE selector to CONTROL.

e) Set the BREATHING RATE to 30 bpm.

f) Adjust the POSITIVE PRESSURE LIMIT to the maximal pressure (full clockwise).*

g) Set the MACHINE VOLUME control to 30 ml.

h) Set the FLOW RATE to 100 ml/sec.

i) Set the INSPIRATORY HOLD to zero.

j) Occlude the proximal airway connection and read the peak pressure displayed on the PRESSURE GAUGE.

k) Calculate system compliance by dividing the ventilator volume setting by the peak pressure (e.g., volume = 30 ml; pressure = 90 cm H_2O; machine compliance = volume/pressure = 0.33 ml/cm H_2O).†

l) Readjust all controls as desired.

m) Set the alarms to the desired levels.

3. *Humidifier, Overtemperature Alarm and Ultrasonic Nebulizer*

a) Fill the desired unit with sterile water. If the ultrasonic nebulizer is being used, the area around the cup should be filled with tap water and the cup itself filled with sterile distilled water. If the pass-over humidifier is being used, turn the power switch of the Mistogen overtemperature alarm to the ON position. The green indicator must come on. Press the TEST button. The red OVERTEMP indicator and audible alarm must activate. Turn the POWER switch of the overtemperature alarm to the OFF position and then back to the ON position.

---

*On the Bourns Infant Ventilator, the maximal amount of pressure delivered to the patient can be limited by either the HIGH-PRESSURE ALARM or the POSITIVE-PRESSURE LIMIT. The high-pressure alarm stops the piston when the preset pressure is reached. Inspiration thus is terminated due to pressure (pressure cycled). The pressure-relief valve also limits the amount of pressure that can be delivered to the patient, but it holds this pressure until the piston has completed its forward stroke. Inspiration thus is terminated due to time (time cycling) and provides the clinician the capability of using an inspiratory plateau.

†A machine compliance in the range 0.25–0.40 ml/cm H_2O is typical. A higher machine compliance value may indicate that the water level in the humidifier is too low, or that there is excess tubing or leaks within the system. As long as the water level in the humidifier and the tubing length remains constant, the machine compliance should remain the same.

  b) Plug the unit into a 117-VAC, 60-Hz grounded electrical outlet.

  c) Turn the unit on to the desired temperature.

Using the Bourns in a Clinical Situation

  1. *Spontaneous Breathing:*

  a) Select the desired oxygen concentration.

  b) Adjust the CPAP FLOW/IPPB FLOW control to the desired level as indicated on the FLOWMETER.

  2. *CPAP:*

  a) Select the desired oxygen concentration.

  b) Adjust the CPAP FLOW/IPPB FLOW control to the desired level as indicated on the FLOWMETER.

  c) Adjust the PEEP control knob to the level of end expiratory pressure desired (read on ventilator manometer).

  d) Adjust the POSITIVE PRESSURE LIMIT to the desired level.

  3. *IMV:*

  a) Select the desired oxygen concentration.

  b) Adjust the CPAP FLOW/IPPB FLOW control to the desired level as indicated on the FLOWMETER.

  c) Set the BREATHING RATE to the desired level.

  d) Set the FLOW RATE to the desired level. Variations in flow rate affect the I:E ratio. As flow rate increases, inspiratory time decreases and I:E ratio decreases.

  e) Set the MACHINE VOLUME to the desired level. The machine volume = patient's tidal volume + volume lost in patient circuit – e.g., 7 – 10 ml/kg + (machine compliance × pressure generated).

  f) Set the MODE selector to CONTROL.

  g) Adjust the POSITIVE-PRESSURE LIMIT to the desired level.

  h) Turn the ventilator ON. This activates the visual POWER ON light.

  4. *Volume Ventilation:*

  a) Select the desired oxygen concentration.

  b) Adjust the CPAP FLOW/IPPB FLOW control to IPPB FLOW.

  c) Set the BREATHING RATE to the desired level.

  d) Set the FLOW RATE to the desired level. Variations in flow rate affect the I:E ratio. As flow rate increases, inspiratory time decreases and I:E ratio decreases.

  e) Set the MACHINE VOLUME to the desired level. The machine volume = patient's tidal volume + volume lost in patient circuit – e.g., 7 – 10 ml/kg + (machine compliance × pressure generated).

  f) Set the MODE selector.

  g) Adjust the level of PEEP if desired.

  h) Adjust the POSITIVE-PRESSURE LIMIT to the desired level.

i) Set the SIGH INTERVAL if desired. Never use in combination with PEEP.

j) Turn on the ventilator.

k) Adjust the alarm controls.

5. *Inspiratory Plateau:*

a) Select the desired oxygen concentration.

b) Adjust the CPAP FLOW/IPPB FLOW control to IPPB/FLOW.

c) Set the BREATHING RATE to the desired level.

d) Adjust the FLOW RATE to the desired level. Variations in flow rate affect the I:E ratio. As flow rate increases, inspiratory time decreases and I:E ratio decreases.

e) Set the MACHINE VOLUME to the desired level. The machine volume = patient's tidal volume + volume lost in patient circuit−e.g., 7−10 ml/kg + (machine compliance × pressure generated).

f) Set the MODE selector.

g) Set the INSPIRATION HOLD control to the desired level.

h) Turn on the ventilator.

i) Adjust the POSITIVE PRESSURE LIMIT at some value above that occurring in the patient system.

j) Set the alarms to selected values.

Advantages of Bourns LS104−150

1. All modes of ventilation, spontaneous breathing, assist, control or assist-control.

2. Capability to perform ZEEP, PEEP, CPAP, inspiratory plateau or IMV.

3. Can compensate for small leaks during CPAP or PEEP.

4. Accurate selectable control of inspired O_2 concentration 21−100% ± 3%.

5. Audible and visual high-pressure alarm (ventilator).

6. Audible and visual low-pressure alarm (ventilator).

7. Audible apnea alarm (ventilator).

8. Audible alarm for loss of gas inlet pressure (blender).

9. Respiratory rate and volume meter.

10. Precise delivery of V_T.

11. Rapid response time of 35 milliseconds.

12. Minimal internal compliance.

13. Variable control of I:E ratio, including reverse ratio capability.

14. Heated humidification or continuous, controllable nebulization.

15. Simple, easy to connect patient circuit, which includes a heated humidifier and infant bacteria filter.

16. Precise FI_{O_2} concentrations even with varying inlet pressures.

17. Adjustable pressure-limit control.

18. Visual display of air and oxygen inlet pressures.

19. Visual indication of flow to the patient.

20. Audible overtemperature alarm with an electrical power shutoff to the heater.

Disadvantages of Bourns LS104–150

1. Cost.

2. Humidifier awkward to refill.

3. Pressure limited to inspiration not visible from front of unit, nor readily accessible.

4. PEEP or CPAP must be controlled from back of ventilator.

5. Many expensive accessories are necessary to make unit operational.

SPECIFICATIONS FOR BOURNS LS104–150 INFANT VENTILATOR

On/Off control	
Breaths/minute control	5–80 bpm, or 1 breath every 2 minutes to 8 bpm with ÷ 10 switch
Mode control	Assist, control, assist-control or ÷ 10
Inspiration hold control	0–2 sec
Flow rate control	25–200 ml/sec
Patient assist effort	−0.05 cm H_2O to −1.0 cm H_2O
Response time	35 msec
Sigh interval	Every 1–9 minutes, or off
Sigh volume	Double preset tidal volume
Tidal volume	5–150 ml
Oxygen % control	21–100% with LS145 oxygen blender ± 3% accuracy
Flow rates for CPAP and IMV modes	0–20 l/min
Audible and visual alarms	High-pressure limit (ventilator)
	Low pressure (ventilator)
	Apnea (ventilator)—lasts for 5 seconds; unit reverts to control mode for 10 seconds when rate drops to 60% of control setting
	Low pressure (oxygen blender)—indicates low air and/or oxygen pressure
	Overtemperature—indicates that the temperature at the proximal airway is 104° F
Visual indicators	Air inlet pressure gauge
	Oxygen inlet pressure gauge
	Proximal airway pressure gauge
	Flowmeter (oxygen blender)
	Rate meter
	Volume-selected meter

BABYbird Infant Pressure Ventilator

Description

The BABYbird (Fig. 10–18) is a pneumatically operated time-cycled ventilator. It is a constant, or continuous, flow generator that functions as a controller. The ventilator can provide zero end expiratory pressure (ZEEP), positive end expiratory pressure (PEEP), continuous positive airway pressure (CPAP), a combination of techniques termed intermittent mandatory ventilation (IMV) or an inspiratory plateau. During all modes of operation, the clinician can limit the amount of delivered pressure by adjusting the overpressure relief valve. The tidal volume is controlled by adjusting the inspiratory flow rate and inspiratory time control.

Major Mechanical Systems (Figs. 10–19 and 10–20)

The BABYbird consists of three major mechanical systems: supply, patient and ventilator. Four auxiliary mechanical systems are also present. They are for the low-pressure alarm, expiratory flow gradient, inspiratory time limit and BABYbird circle.

1. SUPPLY SYSTEM.—Oxygen and compressed air, each at 50 psi (45–55 psi) pressure, are connected to the OXYGEN INLET (1) and AIR INLET (2) of the OXYGEN BLENDER (3). Pressures are balanced by dual pressure regulators before being directed to a calibrated proportioning valve, which continuously selects O_2 concentrations between 21% and 100% (± 3%). The operating pressure leaving the blender (2 psi lower than the lowest source gas pressure) enters the INLET MANIFOLD (4) after passing through a sintered bronze filter and registers in the green "safe" pressure range (45–55 psi) of the inlet SUPPLY PRESSURE GAUGE (5). All mechanical systems are connected to the inlet manifold; therefore, one operating pressure and selected gas concentration enters all systems.

2. PATIENT SYSTEM.—Gas from the common inlet manifold is directed to the FLOW REGULATOR (6), which is a pressure-reducing valve (regulating pressures with fixed and variable orifices resulting in a calibrated flow system with the FLOW GAUGE [7] indicating liters per minute). Gas flow then is directed to the NEBULIZER control (9), which regulates pressures to the NEBULIZER JET (10) (determining aerosol particle production). When adjusting the nebulizer control to the "minimum" position, the nebulizer control valve internally diverts pressure/flow from the 500-ml in-line nebulizer jet to the nebulizer AUXILIARY PORT (12) (producing fewer particles). Pressure/flow

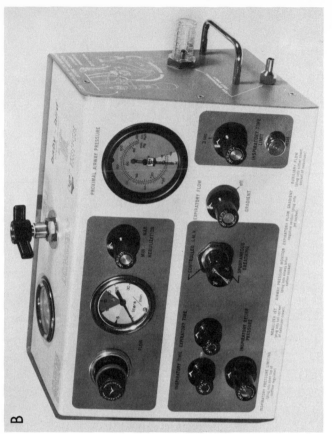

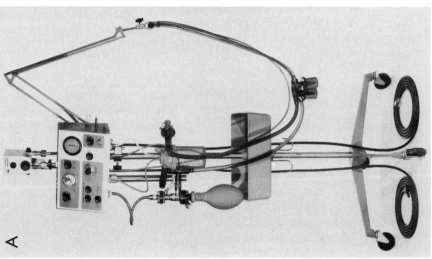

Fig. 10–18.—A, BABYbird ventilator complete. **B,** BABYbird control panel. (Courtesy of Bird Corporation, Palm Springs, Cal.)

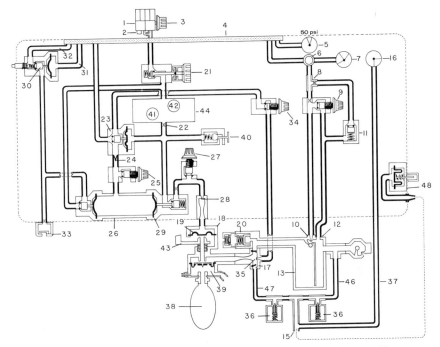

Fig. 10–19. — Pneumatic flow diagram for BABYbird ventilator. (Courtesy of Bird Corporation, Palm Springs, Cal.)

greater than the nebulizer control orifice can accommodate is directed through a CALIBRATED T CONNECTION (8) and spring tension BYPASS VALVE (11) to the in-line nebulizer AUXILIARY PORT (12). The selected total liter per minute gas flow must enter the patient system by way of the 500-ml IN-LINE NEBULIZER (13).

The flow of gas enters the inspiratory tubing of the BABYbird circle due to the closed one-way flapper check valve in the SHUTTLE VALVE (17) and the closed OVERPRESSURE GOVERNOR VALVE (20) (adjusted to relieve at 65 mm Hg). The flow of gas is directed to the PATIENT AIRWAY CONNECTION (15). Pressure changes within the patient and/or the ventilator are monitored at the proximal airway and displayed on the PROXIMAL AIRWAY PRESSURE GAUGE (16). Gas continues its flow through the expiratory limb to the open, lower one-way flapper check valve in the SHUTTLE VALVE (17), to the OUTFLOW VALVE (18), against a DIAPHRAGM (19) under atmospheric pressure. By adjusting the position of the red-colored HANDLE (43) closer to the diaphragm, increases in resistance are encountered by the continuous gas flow. This resis-

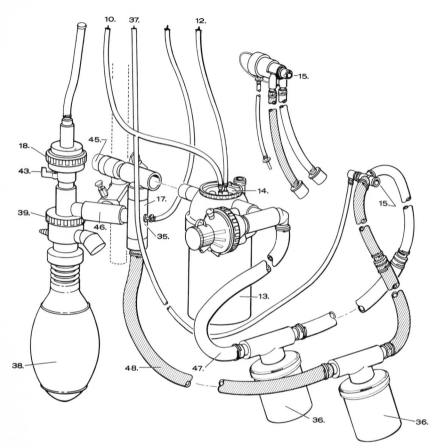

Fig. 10–20.—Close-up of BABYbird patient circuit. (Courtesy of Bird Corporation, Palm Springs, Cal.)

tance manifests itself through the entire BABYbird circle system, resulting in an elevated baseline pressure (CPAP or PEEP).

3. VENTILATOR SYSTEM.—In the "Controlled IMV" mode, manifold pressure is directed through the ROTARY SWITCH (21) to the inlet of the MARK 2 (44) time-cycled servo device. Flow exits through a FIXED-ORIFICE OUTLET (22) (operating pressure between 15 and 18 psi), pressurizing the inspiratory interrupter switch and via the right side of the compound LOCKOUT CARTRIDGE (26) to the INSPIRATORY PRESSURE-RELIEF CONTROL (27) and to the VENTURI JET (28) (pressurizing the top of the DIAPHRAGM [19] in the OUTFLOW VALVE [18] and closing the exit from the patient system).

The MARK 2 INSPIRATORY TIMER CONTROL (41) regulates the time that the diaphragm in the outflow valve interrupts the exiting continuous gas flow, resulting in a pressure build-up in the patient's continuous flow system.

The pressure applied against the DIAPHRAGM (19) in the OUTFLOW VALVE (18) is regulated by the INSPIRATORY PRESSURE-RELIEF CONTROL (27), resulting in the selection of ventilation pressure.

If for any reason the pressure in the patient's continuous flow system increases over the selected inspiratory relief pressure, e.g., a cough, the difference is released to the atmosphere. The increased pressure against the lower side of the outflow valve diaphragm, being higher than the selected pressure on the top side diaphragm, forces the diaphragm from its seat, allowing the excess pressure to be relieved.

Auxiliary Mechanical Systems (see Figs. 10–19 and 10–20)

1. LOW-PRESSURE ALARM (30). — This system ensures reliable operation of the MARK 2 time-cycled servo above its minimal safe operating pressure (45 psi). The system consists of two connections from the COMMON INLET MANIFOLD (4) to the pneumatically activated cartridge. One MANIFOLD CONNECTION (31) directs the proper operating pressure (50 psi) to the diaphragm side of the cartridge, which is pressurized, and, in turn, forces the valve to close against an adjustable selected spring tension (45 psi). This action interrupts continuation of pressure/flow from the other MANIFOLD CONNECTION (32) through the cartridge. When the operating pressure against the diaphragm drops (below 45 psi), the valve opens and gas flow from the distal MANIFOLD CONNECTION (32) is directed to the AUDIBLE ALARM (33).

2. EXPIRATORY FLOW GRADIENT CONTROL (34). — This system selects and maintains a zero or subambient baseline (0 to -10 cm H_2O or 0 to -8 mm Hg). This is accomplished in the following manner: from the INLET MANIFOLD (4) pressure/flow is directed through the normally open INSPIRATORY INTERRUPTER CARTRIDGE (23) to the EXPIRATORY FLOW GRADIENT CONTROL (34). This pressure/flow regulates the amount of pressure or flow to the expiratory (negative) VENTURI JET (35) IN THE SHUTTLE VALVE (17). The accelerated gas flow forces the DIAPHRAGM (19) in the OUTFLOW VALVE (18) off its seat before entering the atmosphere.

The created pressure drop in the shuttle valve negative Venturi lowers resistance to the continuous flow in the patient circuit, so that in case of a high selected liter flow per minute, an undesirable elevated baseline will not result.

The expiratory flow gradient system supplies a continuous flow to the expiratory (negative) jet when the ROTARY SWITCH (21) is in the "Spontaneous" mode, but only during the expiratory phase when in the "Controlled IMV" mode. During the inspiratory phase, the pressure from the MARK 2 outlet orifice pressurizes the INSPIRATORY INTERRUPTER (23) switch, blocking the manifold gas pressure flow.

3. INSPIRATORY TIME LIMIT (25). — This system interrupts (locks out) a prolonged ventilator inspiratory phase when a preset safety inspiratory time limit is reached (time 0 to infinity).

If the inspiratory time of the MARK 2 servo exceeds the selected inspiratory time limit selected, two events will occur. First, the spring tension plunger DIAPHRAGM (29) recoils, interrupting gas flow from the MARK 2 servo fixed ORIFICE OUTLET (22) to the VENTURI JET (28), terminating the inspiratory phase, thus dropping the patient breathing circuit to baseline pressure. Second, gas flow through the now open left side of the cartridge activates an AUDIBLE ALARM (33). Depressing the RESET BUTTON (40) releases the pressure against the INSPIRATORY INTERRUPTER CARTRIDGE (23) diaphragm. The inspiratory interrupter cartridge returns to the normally open position and reopens the gas flow passage from the INLET MANIFOLD (4) to repressurize the COMPOUND LOCKOUT CARTRIDGE (26), preparing the system for the next inspiratory phase.

4. BABYBIRD SAFETY CIRCLE (SEE FIG. 10–20). — This system allows for exchange of the patient circuit.

Assembly:

1. Assemble the patient circuit as shown in Figure 10–20. Fill the humidifier with sterile water to the full level.

2. Attach the air and oxygen hose assembly to the oxygen blender. Fifty psi (5 kg/cm²) pressure is required.

Clinical Operation of the BABYbird Infant Pressure Ventilator (see Figs. 10–18 and 10–20)

Continuous Positive Airway Pressure (CPAP):

1. Connect the infant ventilator system as shown in Figures 10–18 and 10–20.

2. Fill the humidifier with sterile water to the full level.

3. Switch master control to SPONTANEOUS mode.

4. Select desired OXYGEN concentration.

5. Adjust the FLOW RATE control to 10 lpm.

6. Set the EXPIRATORY FLOW GRADIENT to zero.

7. Adjust the OUTFLOW VALVE to the desired level of end expiratory pressure.

8. Turn the NEBULIZER control to maximum or minimum.

9. Set the INSPIRATORY TIME LIMIT control to 3 seconds.

10. Set the OVERPRESSURE RELIEF VALVE. This is done by occluding the proximal airway connection with the ventilator in operation and adjusting the OVERPRESSURE RELIEF VALVE so that the peak pressure indicated on the PROXIMAL AIRWAY PRESSURE GAUGE equals the desired maximal pressure. NOTE: the OVERPRESSURE RELIEF VALVE should be set above the maximal normal pressure.

11. Connect the infant ventilator to the patient.

Intermittent Positive Pressure Ventilation (IPPV):

1. Follow steps 1, 2 and 4 – 10 as outlined in the CPAP section.

2. Switch master control to IMV mode.

3. Adjust the INSPIRATORY TIME CONTROL to the desired interval.

4. Adjust the EXPIRATORY TIME CONTROL to the desired interval. NOTE: When a change in respiratory rate is desired and not a change in tidal volume, only the expiratory time of the BABYbird should be altered.

Intermittent Mandatory Ventilation (IMV):

1. Follow all steps outlined in IPPV operation section.

2. Turn the INSPIRATORY and EXPIRATORY TIME CONTROLS to the IMV interval desired.

Advantages of BABYbird

1. Continuous flow system — minimal internal compliance loss.

2. Controlled mechanical ventilation patterns — IPPV, IMV or inspiratory hold.

3. Controlled end expiratory pressure selection — CPAP, PEEP or ZEEP.

4. Selection of patient ventilation techniques — spontaneous, controlled or IMV.

5. Inspiratory time limit control to back up MARK 2 servo during an inlet pressure decrease.

6. Selection of I : E ratio patterns — variable I : E ratio application.

7. Selectable full range oxygen concentration 21 – 100%, ± 3%.

8. Audible inlet gas supply failure alarm.

9. Audible adjustable overpressure/obstruction alarm.

10. Audible ventilator inspiratory time limit alarm.

11. Inspiratory time limit control to back up inspiratory time function if a low operating pressure source occurs — spontaneous mode results.

12. Continuous, controllable nebulization.

13. Continuous proximal airway pressure monitoring.

14. Two indexed quick exchange patient circuits.

SPECIFICATIONS FOR BABYBIRD INFANT PRESSURE VENTILATOR

Spontaneous breathing/ventilator on control	
Inspiratory time control	0.4–2.5 sec
Expiratory time control	0.4–10.0 sec
Inspiratory flow control	0–30 l/min
Nebulization control	Minimum to maximum
Inspiratory relief pressure control	13–81 cm H_2O
Oxygen concentration	21–100%, ± 3%
PEEP	0–20 cm H_2O
Inspiratory time limit control	0 to infinity, normally set at 3 sec
Expiratory flow gradient	0 to −10 cm H_2O
Reset control	Dumps pressure during inspiratory phase
Proximal airway pressure gauge	−10 to 100 cm H_2O
Audible alarms	Low pressure—when pressure from the oxygen blender is less than 45 psi
	Operating pressures below preset levels
	Inspiratory time limit
Visual indicators	Operating pressure
	Proximal airway pressure gauge
	Flow

15. Self-testing unit—for training and operating unit.

16. Check list on side panel.

17. Schematic circle assembly diagram on side panel.

Disadvantages of BABYbird

1. Complicated circle system, too many components.

2. Expiratory flow gradient control necessary for eliminating flow resistance in circle confusing to many operators.

3. No heated humidification system.

4. Self-test unit not externally accessible for sterilization.

5. No manual ventilator override control.

6. Confusing terminology between "inspiratory time" and "inspiratory time limit."

7. No reducing valve to compensate for fluctuations in line pressure before entering ventilator systems.

Bourns BP200 Infant Pressure Ventilator

Description

The Bourns BP200 Infant Pressure Ventilator (Fig. 10–21) is an electronically controlled and pneumatically operated time-cycled device. It is a constant, or continuous, flow generator that functions as a controller. The ventilator can provide zero end expiratory pressure (ZEEP), positive end expiratory pressure (PEEP), continuous positive airway pressure (CPAP), a combination of techniques termed intermittent mandatory ventilation (IMV) or an inspiratory plateau. During

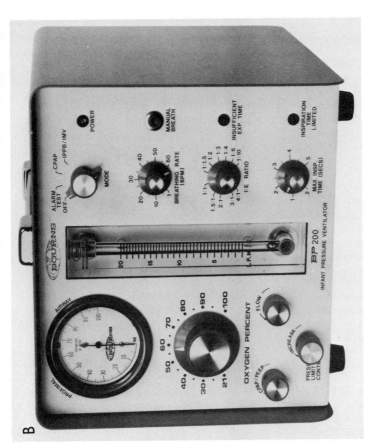

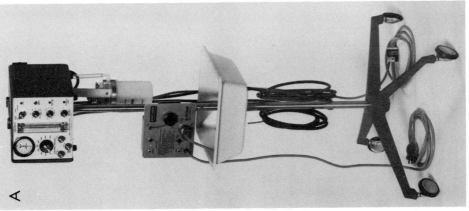

Fig. 10–21.—A, Bourns BP200 infant pressure ventilator complete. **B**, BP200 front panel. (Courtesy of Bourns Medical Systems, Inc., Riverside, Cal.)

all modes of operation, the clinician can limit the amount of delivered pressure by adjusting the pressure-limit control. The tidal volume may be controlled by setting the inspiratory flow rate and regulating I : E ratio or the maximal inspiratory time control.

Major Mechanical System (Fig. 10–22)

Oxygen in the range 30–75 psi (1) and compressed air in the range 15–75 psig (2) are connected to the rear of the ventilator via standard fittings. The incoming gas passes through a sintered bronze FILTER (3)

Fig. 10–22.—BP200 infant pressure ventilator flow diagram. (Courtesy of Bourns Medical Systems, Inc., Riverside, Cal.)

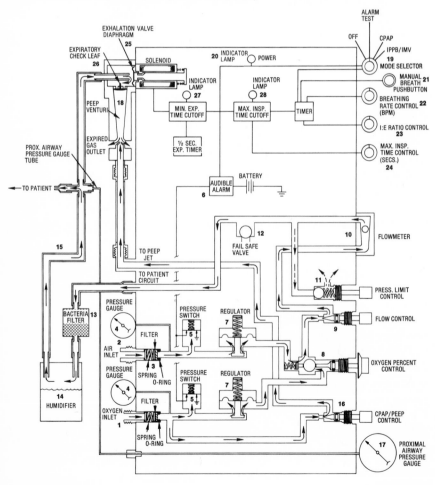

before going to the oxygen and air pressure GAUGES (4) and electronic PRESSURE SWITCHES (5). The pressure gauges display the respective inlet pressures and the electronic pressure switches look for the presence or absence of gas pressure. If either air or oxygen or both inlet gas pressures are too low for accurate blending, an audible battery-operated ALARM (6) will sound. The presence of two PRESSURE REGULATORS (7) balances the pressure to within ± 2 cm H_2O of each other, with the output being approximately 10 psi, before directing the gas to a calibrated differential gas BLENDING VALVE (8). The latter allows selectable O_2 concentrations between 21% and 100% (± 3% accuracy). Blended gas flow then is directed through an adjustable needle valve for precise control of FLOW RATE (9) and through a calibrated ROTAMETER (10) to provide a visual index of the flow going to the patient. Flow then proceeds past the PRESSURE LIMIT CONTROL (11) and SAFETY VALVE (12) to the bacteria filter (13), heated humidifier (14) and the VENTILATOR PATIENT CIRCUIT TUBING (15). The adjustable pressure limit control assures the clinician that the gas delivered to the patient will not exceed the preset pressure level. The safety valve provides a means for the patient to breathe room air if a loss of air and oxygen inlet pressures occurs.

Should an end expiratory pressure be desired in addition to the continuous flow, it is available by adjusting the CPAP/PEEP CONTROL (16) and reading the pressure displayed on the PROXIMAL AIRWAY PRESSURE GAUGE (17). The latter control is powered by gas from the OXYGEN INLET (1). End expiratory pressure is generated and maintained by an INVERTED JET VENTURI (18). When the patient pressure is above the CPAP (PEEP) level, the patient can exhale freely through the Venturi. When the patient pressure drops to the PEEP level, the PEEP level generated by the jet Venturi prevents additional gas from escaping and, therefore, maintains the patient pressure at the PEEP level.

The ventilator may be used as described above to provide continuous flow or to deliver CPAP without activating the MODE SELECTOR (19), if desired. Activation of the mode selector turns on the electronic portion of the ventilator. This is indicated visually by the yellow POWER PILOT LIGHT (20). In the alarm test position, this allows functional checking of the alarm battery and audible alarm buzzer. In the CPAP position, it allows use of the MANUAL BREATH PUSHBUTTON (21). The latter control allows one manual breath on each actuation, with inspiratory time being controlled by the ventilator settings of BREATHING RATE (22), I:E RATIO (23) and MAXIMAL INSPIRATION TIME (24).

To deliver controlled mechanical ventilation (CMV), the MODE SELECTOR (19) is turned to the IPPB/IMV position. BREATHING RATE (22) and I : E RATIO (23) then are adjusted by turning the calibrated controls to the desired levels. During inspiration, gas is held in the patient circuit by the EXHALATION VALVE DIAPHRAGM (25), ensuring delivery to the patient's lungs. The EXPIRATORY CHECKLEAF (26) ensures that gas will flow in the proper direction during inspiration and expiration.

Since the ventilator is a continuous-flow device, two situations may arise during CMV. First, the exhalation phase may be too brief. This could occur if the BREATHING RATE CONTROL (22) was inadvertently set to 60 bpm and the I : E RATIO CONTROL (23) to 4 : 1. In this situation, the patient would have an inspiratory time period of 0.8 second and an expiratory time period of 0.2 second. Should this situation arise, the INSUFFICIENT EXPIRATORY TIME INDICATOR (27) lights and the ventilator overrides the I : E RATIO CONTROL and automatically prolongs the exhalation time period to 0.45 – 0.55 second.

Second, the inspiration time phase may be too long. This could occur if the BREATHING RATE CONTROL (22) was inadvertently set to 1 bpm and the I : E RATIO CONTROL (23) to 1 : 1. In this instance, inspiratory and expiratory time would each be 30 seconds in duration. This situation is alleviated, however, by proper adjustment of the MAXIMAL INSPIRATION TIME CONTROL (24). This control is adjustable from 0.2 to 5.0 seconds. It limits the inspiration time independent of the BREATHING RATE (22) and I : E RATIO CONTROLS (23). It may be used as an override to prevent excessive inspiratory time periods or as a primary control of inspiratory time at lower breathing rates. During the normal IPPV mode of operation, this control should be set at a level above the inspiratory time period the patient actually is receiving. This will prevent the MAXIMAL INSPIRATION TIME CONTROL (24) from overriding the I : E RATIO CONTROL (23). During the IMV mode of operation or when using reverse I : E ratios, this control should be set at whatever length of inspiration the clinician wants the patient to receive. An INSPIRATION TIME-LIMITED INDICATOR (28) provides visual display that the MAXIMAL INSPIRATION TIME CONTROL (24) is overriding the BREATHING RATE (22) and I : E RATIO CONTROLS (23) and terminating inspiration.

Assembly:

1. Assemble the patient circuit as shown in Figure 10–23. Fill the humidifier with sterile water to the full level.

2. Attach the air hose assembly to the rear of the ventilator; 15–75 psi (1–5 kg/cm²) pressures at flow rates of up to 22 lpm are required.

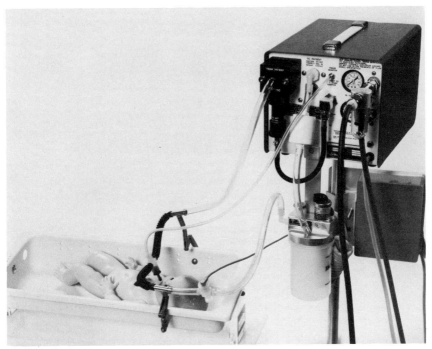

Fig. 10–23.—BP200 infant pressure ventilator. Close-up of patient circuit connected to baby. (Courtesy of Bourns Medical Systems, Inc., Riverside, Cal.)

3. Attach the oxygen hose assembly to the rear of the ventilator; 30–75 psi (2–5 kg/cm²) pressures at flow rates of up to 30 lpm are required.

Clinical Operation of the BP200 Infant Pressure Ventilator

Continuous Positive Airway Pressure (CPAP):

1. Connect the infant ventilator system as shown in Figure 10–23.

2. Fill the heated humidifier with sterile water to the full level. Do not overfill. Select the desired setting of warm, tepid or cold on the heated humidifier.

3. Plug the electrical cord of the ventilator and heated humidifier into a properly grounded 117-VAC, 60-Hz or 220-VAC, 50-Hz source.

4. Attach the air and oxygen hose assemblies to an appropriate gas source.

5. Switch the MODE SELECTOR CONTROL from the OFF position to "Alarm Test," then to CPAP mode.

6. Adjust FLOW control to the desired level as indicated on the

flowmeter. NOTE: The gas flow rate should be adjusted to provide sufficient gas mixture to meet the infant's peak inspiration demands.

7. Adjust for the desired CPAP level by turning the CPAP/PEEP control and observing the PROXIMAL AIRWAY PRESSURE GAUGE.

8. Select the desired OXYGEN concentration.

9. Set the PRESSURE LIMIT CONTROL. This is done by occluding the endotracheal tube tee with the ventilator in operation or while depressing the MANUAL BREATH PUSHBUTTON and adjusting the PRESSURE LIMIT CONTROL so that the peak pressure indicated on the PROXIMAL AIRWAY PRESSURE GAUGE equals the desired maximal pressure. Use an inspiration period long enough to generate the desired pressure. NOTE: The PRESSURE LIMIT CONTROL should be set above the maximal normal pressure.

10. Connect the infant ventilator to the patient. NOTE: The MANUAL BREATH PUSHBUTTON is operational in the CPAP mode only. Inspiratory time is controlled by the ventilator settings of BREATHING RATE, I : E RATIO and MAXIMAL INSPIRATION TIME CONTROLS.

Intermittent Positive Pressure Ventilation (IPPV):

1. Connect the infant ventilator system as shown in Figure 10–23.

2. Fill the heated humidifier with sterile water to the full level. Do not overfill. Select the desired setting of warm, tepid or cold on the heated humidifier.

3. Plug the electrical cord of the ventilator and heated humidifier into a properly grounded 117-VAC, 60-Hz or 220-VAC, 50-Hz source.

4. Attach the air and oxygen hose assemblies to an appropriate gas source.

5. Switch the MODE SELECTOR CONTROL from the OFF position to "Alarm Test," then to IPPB mode.

6. Turn the PRESSURE LIMIT CONTROL to 80 cm H_2O (maximum counterclockwise).

7. Set the BREATHING RATE CONTROL to the desired level (usually 30–40 per minute).

8. Set the I : E RATIO CONTROL to the desired level (usually 1:2). NOTE: Reverse I : E ratio capability is provided.

9. Set the MAXIMAL INSPIRATION TIME CONTROL to the desired level. In the IPPB mode of operation, this is when the INSPIRATION TIME-LIMITED INDICATOR stops blinking.

10. Adjust the FLOW CONTROL so that the desired pressure level, as indicated on the PROXIMAL AIRWAY PRESSURE GAUGE is approximately 5 cm H_2O higher than desired.

Example: If the physician does not want the patient to receive more than 20 cm H_2O pressure, adjust the FLOW CONTROL to a level where

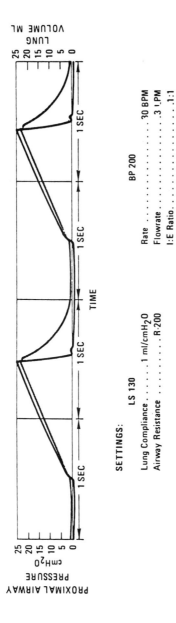

VOLUME ML
LUNG

25 20 15 10 5 0

1 SEC

1 SEC

TIME

1 SEC

1 SEC

SETTINGS:

LS 130

Lung Compliance 1 ml/cmH₂0
Airway Resistance R-200

BP 200

Rate . . . . 30 BPM
Flowrate . . . . .3 LPM
I:E Ratio. 1:1
Prox. Airway Pressure 25cmH₂0
Pressure Limit. . . . . Maximum

25 20 15 10 5 0
cmH₂0
PRESSURE
PROXIMAL AIRWAY

Fig. 10–24.—Pressure-time diagram indicating preliminary ventilator settings.

25 cm H_2O is being reached per breath as indicated on the pressure gauge. This is a preliminary setting only.

11. Use the PRESSURE LIMIT CONTROL to reduce the pressure as indicated on the PROXIMAL AIRWAY PRESSURE GAUGE to the desired level.

Example: Pressure limit is used to reduce pressure from 25 cm H_2O to 20 cm H_2O. This results in a pressure waveform similar to that shown in Figure 10–24. Note the gradual rise of inspiratory flow and the subsequent plateau.

To set the PRESSURE LIMIT CONTROL, occlude the proximal airway connection with the ventilator in operation and adjust the PRESSURE LIMIT CONTROL so that the peak pressure indicated on the front panel PROXIMAL AIRWAY PRESSURE GAUGE equals the desired maximal pressure.

12. Adjust for the desired PEEP level by turning the CPAP/PEEP CONTROL and observing the PROXIMAL AIRWAY PRESSURE GAUGE.

13. Select the desired OXYGEN concentration.

14. Connect the infant ventilator to the patient. NOTE: The PRESSURE LIMIT CONTROL should be set above the maximal normal pressure unless an inspiratory plateau is desired.

Intermittent Mandatory Ventilation (IMV):

1. Follow all steps outlined in IPPV operation section.

2. Turn the BREATHING RATE CONTROL to the desired level.

3. Adjust the MAXIMAL INSPIRATION TIME CONTROL to the level of inspiratory time desired. NOTE: During low breathing rate IMV, the primary control of inspiratory time is the MAXIMAL INSPIRATION TIME CONTROL and not the I:E RATIO CONTROL.

Inspiratory Plateau:

1. Follow all steps outlined in IPPV operation section.

2. Adjust the PRESSURE LIMIT CONTROL to terminate the pressure at the desired level. Plateau duration is affected by inspiratory time (BREATHING RATE and I:E RATIO CONTROLS) and flow rate.

Advantages of Bourns BP200

1. Continuous flow system—minimal internal compliance loss.

2. Controlled mechanical ventilation patterns—time cycled, pressure limited (inspiratory hold) or volume limited.

3. Controlled end expiratory pressure selection—CPAP, PEEP or ZEEP.

4. Selection of patient ventilation techniques—spontaneous, controlled or IMV.

5. Calibrated selection of I : E ratio from 4 : 1 to 1 : 10.

6. Calibrated selection of respiratory rate from 1 to 60 bpm.

7. Integral oxygen blender.

8. Continuous display of proximal airway pressure.

9. Simple, easy to connect patient circuit that includes a heated humidifier and infant bacteria filter.

10. Precise FI_{O_2} concentrations even with varying inlet pressures.

11. Audible alarms for loss of air or oxygen, air and oxygen and power failure.

12. Ventilator controls grouped by logical function — pneumatic versus electronic.

13. Manual breath capability — in CPAP mode only.

14. Adjustable pressure limit control from 10 to 80 cm H_2O.

15. Integral test for functional integrity of alarm battery.

16. Visual indicators for insufficient expiratory time and inspiratory time limited.

17. Integral override to ensure 0.45 – 0.55 second for exhalation.

18. Visual display of air and oxygen inlet pressures.

19. Accurate selectable control of inspired oxygen concentration 21 – 100%, ± 3%.

20. Visual indication of flow to the patient.

Disadvantages of Bourns BP200

1. No schematic patient circuit assembly on side panel.

2. No check list on side panel.

3. No self-testing unit for training and operating unit.

4. Lacks an incorporated emergency manual resuscitator.

5. Does not provide continuous nebulization.

SPECIFICATIONS FOR BOURNS BP200 INFANT PRESSURE VENTILATOR

Mode control	Off, alarm test, CPAP, IPPB/IMV
Breathing rate control	1 – 60 breaths per min
I : E ratio control	4 : 1 – 1 : 10
Maximal inspiration time control	0.2 – 5 sec
Inspiratory flow range	0 – 20 l/min
Minimal expiratory time	Internally preset 0.45 – 0.55
Pressure limit	10 – 80 cm H_2O
PEEP	0 – 20 cm H_2O
Oxygen concentration	21 – 100%
Proximal airway pressure gauge	0 – 100 cm H_2O
Audible alarms	Power failure or power disconnect (electrical)
	Inadequate air and/or oxygen pressure
	Overtemperature electrical shutoff alarm
	(not integral to ventilator)

Visual indicators

Power pilot light — indicates that ventilator is plugged into a properly functioning electrical outlet

Insufficient expiratory time — indicates incompatible settings, which causes internal timer to not allow an exhalation phase of less than 0.5 second

Inspiration time limited — indicates setting on maximal inspiratory time control reached

Air inlet pressure gauge

Oxygen inlet pressure gauge

Proximal airway pressure gauge

Overtemp — indicates that temperature at the proximal airway has reached 104° F (not integral to ventilator)

Biomed MVP-10 Infant Ventilator

Description

The Biomed MVP-10 infant ventilator (Fig. 10 – 25) is a pneumatically operated time-cycled device. It is a constant, or continuous, flow generator that functions as a controller. The ventilator can provide zero end expiratory pressure (ZEEP), positive end expiratory pressure (PEEP), continuous positive airway pressure (CPAP) or a combination of techniques termed intermittent mandatory ventilation (IMV). During all modes of operation, the clinician can limit the amount of delivered pressure by adjusting the MAXIMAL PRESSURE CONTROL. Tidal volume is controlled by adjusting the inspiratory flow rate and inspiratory time controls.

Major Mechanical System (Fig. 10 – 26)

Oxygen and compressed air (50 psi) are connected to the rear of the ventilator via standard fittings and directed to the respective flowmeters. The setting of the air and oxygen flowmeters on the front of the ventilator regulates the amount of flow that is titrated together for both total flow requirements and oxygen concentration delivery. The constant flow of gas at the predetermined oxygen concentration then passes through the patient tubing, humidifier and past the patient wye and out the expiration tubing and valve. During intermittent positive pressure ventilation, the diaphragm of the exhalation valve is pressurized by the servo line and thus closes the exhalation valve. This causes the total pressure to build in the system to increase the volume of gas to be delivered to the path of least resistance (the patient).

Assembly:

To assemble the Biomed MVP-10 infant ventilator system, follow the directions below and refer to Figures 10 – 25 and 10 – 27.

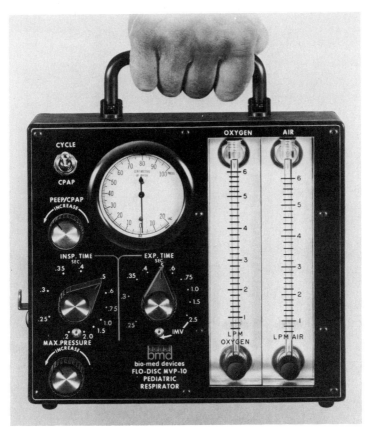

Fig. 10–25.—Biomed MVP–10 infant ventilator. Close-up of front panel. (Courtesy of Bio-med Devices, Inc., Stamford, Conn.)

1. Attach the oxygen hose assembly to the rear of the ventilator; 50 psi (5 kg/cm²) pressure is required.

2. Attach the air hose assembly to the rear of the ventilator; 50 psi (5 kg/cm²) pressure is required.

3. Place exhalation valve on bracket at side of MVP-10. If required, exhalation valve may be positioned closer to the patient and the connecting hose shortened to reduce system compliance.

4. Connect a 12"-long section of ⅛" ID tubing between the expiration valve control connection and the EXPIRATION VALVE fitting on the rear of the MVP-10.

5. Connect 4–6 feet of ⅛" ID tubing from the patient wye to the PRESSURE GAUGE fitting on the rear of the MVP-10.

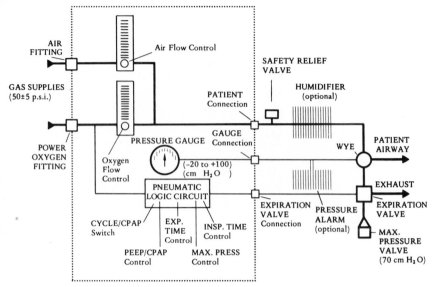

Fig. 10–26. — Pneumatic flow diagram of Biomed MVP–10. (Courtesy of Bio-med Devices, Inc., Stamford, Conn.)

6. Insert a humidifier (Bard-Parker "U-MID/LO" or equivalent) on the downstream side of the SAFETY RELIEF VALVE installed on the PATIENT fitting at the rear of the MVP-10.

7. Connect approximately 3 feet of ¼" ID tubing between the humidifier outlet and the patient wye. Then, connect another 3 feet of ¼" ID tubing from the patient wye to the exhalation valve.

Clinical Operation of the Biomed MVP-10 Infant Ventilator
Continuous Positive Airway Pressure (CPAP):

1. Assemble infant ventilator as described above.

2. Fill the heated humidifier with sterile water to the full level. Do not overfill. Select the desired temperature setting.

3. Set PEEP/CPAP control fully clockwise.

4. Set CYCLE/CPAP switch to CPAP position.

5. Empirically determine total flow required by setting flow so that the pressure gauge reading does not drop during inspiration.

6. Readjust the oxygen and air flowmeters according to Figure 10–28 to provide the desired FI_{O_2}.

7. Occlude the proximal airway wye and set the CPAP level by adjusting the PEEP/CPAP control to the desired level as indicated on the MVP-10 pressure gauge.

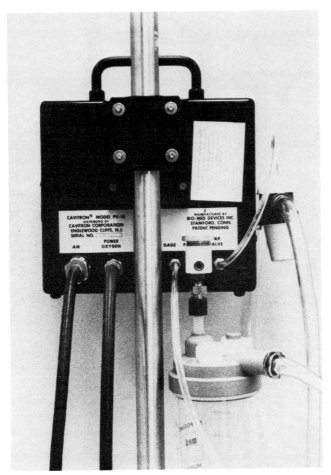

Fig. 10–27.—Rear view of Biomed MVP–10. (Courtesy of Bio-med Devices, Inc., Stamford, Conn.)

8. Connect the infant ventilator to the patient.

Intermittent Positive-Pressure Ventilation (IPPV):

1. Assemble infant ventilator as described above.

2. Fill the heated humidifier with sterile water to the full level. Do not overfill. Select the desired temperature setting.

3. Set the MAX. PRESSURE control fully counterclockwise.

4. Set the PEEP/CPAP control fully clockwise.

5. Set the INSP. TIME and EXP. TIME controls to the required level to obtain the desired respiratory rate and I : E ratio. For example, for a

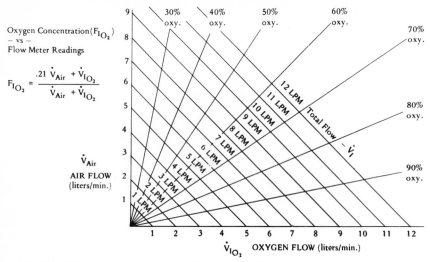

Fig. 10–28. — Oxygen concentration versus flowmeter readings. (Courtesy of Bio-med Devices, Inc., Stamford, Conn.)

respiratory rate of 30 bpm and an I:E ratio of 1:1, the ventilator cycle time will be 2 seconds, with an inspiratory time of 1 second and an expiratory time of 1 second (see Table 10–4). NOTE: When a change in respiratory rate is desired and not a change in tidal volume, only the expiratory time of the MVP-10 should be altered.

6. Determine total flow required by multiplying the required tidal volume by the appropriate multiplication factor (from Table 10–4). Set the air and oxygen flowmeters for this total flow. This is a preliminary setting only.

7. Set CYCLE/CPAP switch in CYCLE position.

8. Set desired oxygen concentration by readjusting the air and oxygen flowmeters (according to Fig. 10–28). Be sure total flow as determined in step 6 is kept constant.

9. Readjust the MAX. PRESSURE control until the desired pressure limit is seen during inspiration.

10. Set the PEEP/CPAP control to the desired level.

11. Connect the infant ventilator to the patient. NOTE: The MAX. PRESSURE control should be set above the maximal normal pressure unless an inspiratory plateau is desired.

Intermittent Mandatory Ventilation (IMV):

1. Follow all steps outlined in IPPV section.

2. Decrease respiratory rate by increasing EXP. TIME control to the desired level.

$$\text{Respiratory Rate} = \frac{60}{\text{Insp. Time} + \text{Exp. Time}}$$

Advantages of Biomed MVP-10

1. Continuous flow system — minimal internal compliance loss.

2. Controlled mechanical ventilation patterns — time cycled, pressure limited (inspiratory hold) or volume limited.

3. Controlled end expiratory pressure selection — CPAP, PEEP or ZEEP.

4. Selection of patient ventilation techniques — spontaneous, controlled or IMV.

5. Continuous display of proximal airway pressure.

6. Simple, easy to connect patient circuit, which includes a heated humidifier.

7. Low gas consumption.

8. Small, compact system ideal for air or land transport.

9. Adjustable pressure limit control from 0 to 80 cm H_2O.

10. Selection of I : E ratio patterns — variable I : E ratio application.

11. May be used in hazardous environments.

Disadvantages of Biomed MVP-10

1. No integral oxygen blender.

2. Humidifier must be passover type and not bubbler or pressure jet. The latter will render the safety relief valve ineffective.

3. Inlet gas pressures must be relatively constant to keep accuracy of settings.

4. No manual breath or external bag capability.

5. When the ventilator is used at altitudes significantly above sea

---

SPECIFICATIONS FOR BIOMED MVP-10 INFANT PRESSURE VENTILATOR

CYCLE/CPAP CONTROL	
Inspiratory time control	0.2 – 2 sec
Expiratory time control	0.2 – 30 sec
Inspiratory flow range	0 – 12 l/min
Maximal pressure control	0 – 80 cm H_2O
Oxygen concentration	21 – 100%
PEEP	0 – 18 cm H_2O
Proximal airway pressure gauge	–20 – 100 cm H_2O
Audible alarms	None
Visual indicators	Proximal airway pressure gauge
	Oxygen flowmeter
	Air flowmeter

TABLE 10-4.—INSPIRATION AND EXPIRATION TIMES AND MULTIPLICATION FACTOR (TO FIND FLOW RATE) FOR VARIOUS RESPIRATORY RATES AND I:E RATIOS

RESP. RATE (breaths/min)	RESP. CYCLE (sec)	I:E RATIO	3:1	2:1	1½:1	1:1	1:1½	1:2	1:3	1:4	1:5	1:6	1:7	1:8
10	6	Insp. Time	4.5	4.0	3.6	3.0	2.4	2.0	1.5	1.2	1.0	.86	.75	.67
		Exp. Time	1.5	2.0	2.4	3.0	3.6	4.0	4.5	4.8	5.0	5.1	5.25	5.33
		Mult. Factor	13.3	15	16.7	20	25	30	40	50	60	70	80	90
15	4	Insp. Time	3.0	2.7	2.4	2.0	1.6	1.33	1.0	0.8	.67	.57	0.5	.44
		Exp. Time	1.0	1.3	1.6	2.0	2.4	2.67	3.0	3.2	3.3	3.4	3.5	3.56
		Mult. Factor	20	22.5	25	30	37.5	45	60	75	90	105	120	135
20	3	Insp. Time	2.25	2.0	1.8	1.5	1.2	1.0	.75	0.6	0.5	.43	.38	.33
		Exp. Time	.75	1.0	1.2	1.5	1.8	2.0	2.25	2.4	2.5	2.57	2.62	2.67
		Mult. Factor	26.7	30	33.3	40	50	60	80	100	120	140	160	180
25	2.4	Insp. Time	1.8	1.6	1.44	1.2	.96	0.8	0.6	.48	0.4	.34	0.3	.27
		Exp. Time	0.6	0.8	.96	1.2	1.44	1.6	1.8	1.92	2.0	2.06	2.1	2.13
		Mult. Factor	33.3	37.5	41.7	50	62.5	75	100	125	150	176	200	225

Rate														
30	2	Insp. Time	1.5	1.33	1.2	1.0	0.8	.67	0.5	0.4	.33	.29	.25	.22
		Exp. Time	0.5	.67	0.8	1.0	1.2	1.33	1.5	1.6	1.67	1.71	1.75	1.78
		Mult. Factor	40	45	50	60	75	90	120	150	180	210	240	270
40	1.5	Insp. Time	1.12	1.0	0.9	.75	0.6	0.5	.38	0.3	.25	.21	.19	.17
		Exp. Time	0.38	0.5	0.6	.75	0.9	1.0	1.12	1.2	1.25	1.29	1.31	1.33
		Mult. Factor	53.3	60	66.7	80	100	120	160	200	240	280	320	360
50	1.2	Insp. Time	0.9	0.8	.72	0.6	.48	0.4	0.3	.24	0.2	.17	.15	.13
		Exp. Time	0.3	0.4	.48	0.6	.72	0.8	0.9	.96	1.0	1.03	1.05	1.07
		Mult. Factor	67	75	83.3	100	125	150	200	250	300	350	400	450
60	1.0	Insp. Time	.75	.67	0.6	0.5	0.4	.33	.25	0.2	.17	.14	.13	.11
		Exp. Time	.25	.33	0.4	0.5	0.6	.67	.75	0.8	.83	.86	.87	.89
		Mult. Factor	80	90	100	120	150	180	240	300	360	420	480	540
70	.86	Insp. Time	.65	.57	.52	.43	.34	.29	.21	.17	.14	.12	.11	.10
		Exp. Time	.21	.29	.34	.43	.52	.57	.65	.69	.72	.74	.75	.76
		Mult. Factor	93.3	105	117	140	175	210	280	350	420	490	560	630

$$\text{Flow Rate Multiplication Factor} = \frac{\text{INSP. TIME (sec)}}{60}.$$

Flow Rate (liters/min) = Tidal Volume (ml) × Mult. Factor.

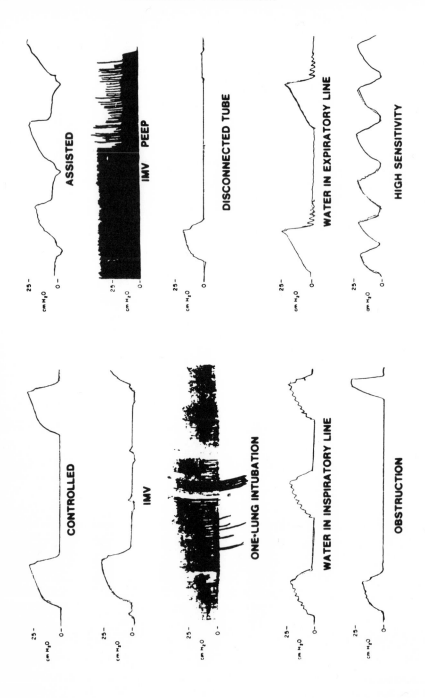

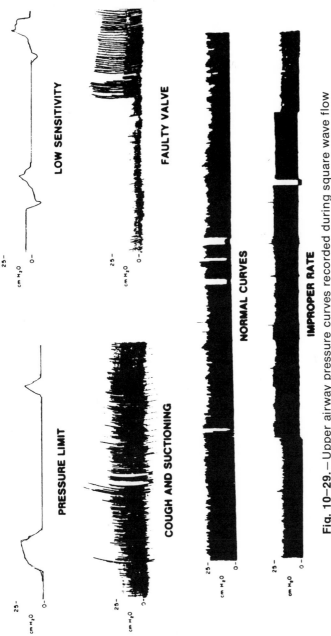

Fig. 10–29.—Upper airway pressure curves recorded during square wave flow mechanical ventilation. (From Rattenborg, C. C., and Mikula, R. J., Crit. Care Med. 5:254, 1977. Reprinted by permission.)

level or in nonpressurized aircraft, the calibration of inspiratory time and expiratory time must be corrected. The actual times will be greater than the panel marking by approximately 2½% for every 1000 feet of altitude.

COMPUTING MACHINE COMPLIANCE AND TIDAL VOLUME IN A TIME-CYCLED CONTINUOUS-FLOW VENTILATOR

Machine Compliance

1. Set respiratory rate at 30 bpm (inspiratory time 1 second, expiratory time 1 second). This will provide an I:E ratio of 1:1.

2. Set flow rate to 3 l/min (3000 ml/min). The ventilator now will deliver 3000 ml/min/30 bpm — 100 ml/breath. Therefore, during each ventilator cycle of 2 seconds (inspiratory time + expiratory time) 100 ml of gas flows through the patient circuit. During inspiration (1.0 sec), 50 ml of this gas is the tidal volume for the patient.

3. Occlude the proximal airway connection and read the peak pressure displayed on the pressure gauge (example: 90 cm H_2O). Machine compliance = volume/pressure = 50 ml/90 cm H_2O = 0.55 ml/cm H_2O.

Tidal Volume

1. Follow steps 1–3 above.

2. Calculate the inspiratory flow rate. This is done by multiplying the desired tidal volume of the patient (7–10 ml/kg) by 60 seconds/inspiratory time. For example, at a respiratory rate of 30 bpm and an I:E ratio of 1:3, the inspiratory time is 0.5 second; 60 seconds/0.5 second = 120. Therefore, for a 3-kg infant whose tidal volume is 30 ml and who will be ventilated at 30 bpm at an I:E ratio of 1:3, the inspiratory flow rate should be 30 ml × 120 = 3600 ml/min (3.6 l/min).

3. Connect the patient to the ventilator patient circuit. The volume of gas delivered to the patient during each ventilator cycle will be less than was calculated in step 2 because of the volume lost in the patient circuit due to compliance. As with the Bourns LS104–150 infant volume ventilator, compensation for this lost volume must be made.

4. With the patient connected to the infant ventilator, read the peak pressure displayed on the pressure gauge (example 30 cm H_2O). Calculate the volume of gas lost in the tubing circuit (peak pressure × compliance) = 30 cm H_2O × 0.55 ml/cm H_2O = 16.5 ml.

5. The 16.5 ml should be added to the patient's desired tidal volume and the total multiplied by 120. For example, patient tidal volume + patient circuit volume = machine volume (30 ml + 16.5 ml ×

120 = 46.5 ml × 120 = 5580 ml (5.58 l/min). Readjust the flow rate to this level.

This method of computing machine compliance and tidal volume may be used with the BABYbird, Bourns BP200 and Biomed MVP-10 infant ventilator.

MONITORING PROXIMAL AIRWAY PRESSURE CURVES

In the past several years, much attention has been directed to the monitoring of proximal airway pressure curves as a guide to correct ventilator function. In breath-by-breath measurements of ventilator function, the upper airway pressure curve serves a purpose similar to that of the electrocardiogram or electroencephalogram. During mechanical ventilation, the following events have characteristic airway pressure patterns: controlled inflation, assisted breathing, intermittent mandatory ventilation and positive end expiratory pressure. Curves with characteristic patterns are also generated by faulty adjustment of sensitivity, respiratory rate or by water accumulation in the patient circuit and by critical complications, such as one-lung intubation, complete airway obstruction or by disconnection of the patient circuit.

Monitoring proximal airway pressure curves will permit a study of short-term and long-term changes reflecting trends of improvement or deterioration, thus preventing catastrophes and alerting personnel when immediate intervention is needed. Figure 10–29 shows proximal airway pressure curves recorded during square wave flow mechanical ventilation, illustrating the various conditions and complications that can be detected by this method.

REFERENCES
1. Lough, M. D., Doershuk, C. F., and Stern, R. C. (eds.): *Pediatric Respiratory Therapy* (2d ed.; Chicago: Year Book Medical Publishers, Inc., 1979).
2. Klaus, M., and Fanaroff, A. (eds.): *Care of the High-risk Neonate* (Philadelphia: W. B. Saunders Company, 1973).
3. Buyer information – BABYbird Ventilator, Bird Corporation, Palm Springs, California.
4. Buyer information – Bourns infant ventilators, Bourns Life Systems, Riverside, California.
5. Buyer information – MVP-10, Bio-med Devices, Stamford, Connecticut.
6. Heironimus, T. W., and Bageant, R. A.: *Mechanical Artificial Ventilation* (Springfield, Ill.: Charles C Thomas, Publisher, 1977).
7. Rattenborg, C. C., and Mikula, R. J.: Ventilator surveillance, Crit. Care Med. 5:252, 1977.

11 / Mechanical Ventilation of Newborn Infants: An Overview

STEPHEN J. BOROS, M.D.

HISTORY

"BEHOLD, the child was dead . . . and he went up and lay upon the child, and put his mouth upon his mouth . . . and the flesh of the child waxed warm . . . and the child opened his eyes." This is the first report of the successful resuscitation and artificial ventilation of a child. It is found in the Bible (2 Kings 4:32–35).

In 1806, Chaussier reported the successful endotracheal intubation and artificial ventilation of an asphyxiated neonate.[1, 2] By the late 1880s, a number of investigators had developed mechanical devices for the artificial ventilation of asphyxiated infants and children. Most of these machines were body chambers that utilized both intermittent positive and negative pressure.[3-5] In 1889, Alexander Graham Bell designed and built such a body-type respirator, specifically for use with premature infants. Although Bell had successfully tested his ventilator with small animals, he was unsuccessful in generating interest within the scientific community for its use with human infants.[6]

In 1950, Bloxsom[7] described his experiences with infant mechanical ventilation using a positive-pressure body chamber, referred to as the "Bloxsom airlock." During a 3-month period in 1950, 55 infants were ventilated with this machine. Forty-four (82%) survived. In 1953, Donald and Lord[8] developed the first servo-controlled, patient-cycled infant ventilator. The machine, a negative-pressure tank-type ventilator, utilized a complex series of lights, mirrors and a photoelectric cell to trigger mechanical inspiration.

In 1959, Smythe and co-workers reported the successful use of intermittent positive-pressure ventilation in the treatment of tetanus neonatorum. Following the introduction of a regimen utilizing both intermittent positive-pressure ventilation and paralytic agents, the mortality from neonatal tetanus fell from greater than 90% to less than 20%.[9-11]

During the early 1960s, pediatricians and anesthesiologists began to experiment with mechanical ventilation in the treatment of infants with severe hyaline membrane disease. Clinical trials of both intermittent positive-pressure ventilation and intermittent negative-pressure ventilation demonstrated significant improvements in survival.[12, 13] The first clinical efforts with intermittent positive-pressure ventilation in the treatment of hyaline membrane disease attempted to mimic the distressed infant's natural respiratory pattern of rapid shallow breathing. The regimen of rapid ventilatory rates and modest tidal volumes proved adequate for the treatment of hypercapnia, but, in most cases, inadequate in the prevention of hypoxia. In 1969, Smith and co-workers[14] meticulously examined the effect of different ventilator variables on oxygenation and ventilation. They observed that arterial oxygenation appeared to vary inversely with respiratory rate and directly with peak inspiratory pressure or tidal volume. Following the publication of these observations and similar observations by Reynolds[15] and others, clinicians involved with neonatal mechanical ventilation gradually converted to a regimen utilizing slow ventilatory rates and relatively high tidal volumes. Again, clinical results were encouraging.

In 1970, Gregory *et al.* applied the principles of continuous positive-pressure breathing, long known to aviation medicine, to the treatment of infants with hyaline membrane disease.[16, 17] Two years following the introduction of continuous positive airway pressure (CPAP), spontaneous breathing against a supra-atmospheric pressure maintained throughout the respiratory cycle and the use of intermittent positive-pressure ventilation in association with positive end expiratory pressure (PEEP), the survival of mechanically ventilated infants increased from less than 25% in 1969 to greater than 70% in 1971.[18] CPAP is discussed in detail in Chapter 10.

POSITIVE END EXPIRATORY PRESSURE

Positive end expiratory pressure (PEEP), a term originally synonymous with CPAP, has come to mean intermittent positive-pressure ventilation in association with a residual supra-atmospheric pressure during expiration. Normally, during intermittent positive-pressure ventilation, exhalation is unobstructed and airway pressures rapidly return to atmospheric levels prior to the next inspiration. PEEP is produced by placing a resistance in the ventilator's expiratory circuit.

When a preset expiratory pressure is reached, further exhalation is stopped by a pressure-sensitive valve. This pressure is held until the beginning of the next inspiration.[19]

The primary clinical effect of PEEP is to improve arterial oxygenation by increasing functional residual capacity (FRC) and decreasing the amount of blood shunted through nonventilated portions of the lung. PEEP increases FRC by trapping gas within the lung. Atelectatic areas are recruited and contact with the inspired gas mixture is reestablished. The amount of gas trapped is determined by both the functional state of the lung and the amount of PEEP used.

Excessive end expiratory pressures may overdistend alveoli and precipitate lung rupture or barotrauma, a fairly common complication. Alveolar overdistention may also, by its effect on the pulmonary capillary bed and great veins, reduce cardiac output.[20]

PEEP is a valuable clinical tool for increasing arterial oxygenation in patients with reduced FRC and increased intrapulmonary shunting. However, it must be used with great care. PEEP obviously is contraindicated in situations in which air trapping or low cardiac output is the primary problem.

NEGATIVE-PRESSURE VENTILATION

The negative-pressure infant ventilator is a body-enclosing tank-type incubator-respirator, tightly sealed at the infant's neck by an iris diaphragm. Negative pressures are generated by a vacuum pump. Up to 60 cm H_2O of negative pressure can be achieved during inspiration and up to -10 cm H_2O can be left as a residual negative pressure during expiration or maintained as a continuous negative pressure.[6] Inspiratory and expiratory times are independently variable and ventilator frequencies of up to 60 breaths per minute can be achieved.[21] The desired air-oxygen mixture is supplied at atmospheric pressure through a clear plastic head box outside the negative pressure compartment (Fig. 11 – 1). The machine produces artificial ventilation by effecting a negative force around the thorax, causing a pressure gradient between the mouth, at atmospheric pressure, and the thorax, at a subatmospheric pressure, resulting in gas flow into the airways. Negative pressure may be applied intermittently, producing intermittent negative-pressure ventilation or continuously producing a continuous transpulmonary pressure similar to CPAP.[22]

The advantages of this system are: (1) infants generally do not require endotracheal tubes, although some infants have required endotracheal intubation because of glottic obstruction secondary to a tight

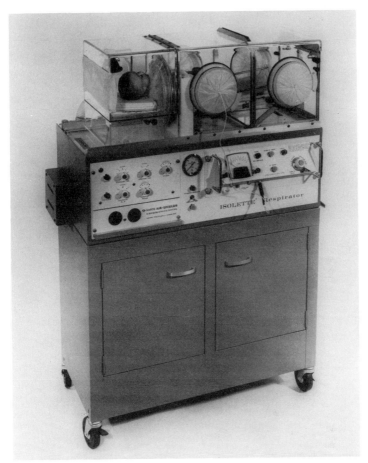

Fig. 11–1.—The Air-Shields Isolette respirator. (Courtesy of NARCO Air-Shields, A Division of Narco Scientific.)

neck cuff;[21] (2) infants are not exposed to positive airway pressures, a key factor, many believe, in the development of bronchopulmonary dysplasia.

The system's disadvantages are its large size and cumbersomeness and the relative isolation of patients within the system. It is difficult to carry out emergency procedures such as chest tube insertions or even routine nursing care while maintaining the vacuum necessary for continued mechanical ventilation or continuous transpulmonary pressure. The tight neck seals necessary to maintain sufficient vacuum have caused skin abrasions and pressure necroses.[23, 25] Despite a powerful servo-controlled heater, the cooling effects of intermittent or continuous vacuum are significant, especially in very small infants. Negative-pressure ventilation is used less frequently today than in years past. Considering all the currently available mechanical ventilators, this system's disadvantages probably outweigh its advantages.

Recently, Bancalari and co-workers[25] developed a more simple system for producing continuous negative pressure, using a smaller chamber that encloses only the chest and abdomen. The authors' preliminary clinical results are encouraging.

INTERMITTENT POSITIVE-PRESSURE VENTILATION

The design and the specific variables of the various positive-pressure infant ventilators are discussed in Chapter 10. Positive-pressure infant ventilators commonly are classified as either pressure preset or volume preset, depending on how they limit tidal volume.

PRESSURE PRESET VENTILATORS

Most pressure preset infant ventilators such as the BABYbird or Bourns BP200 are time-cycled continuous-flow machines. Gas flows through the ventilator circuit throughout the respiratory cycle. Inspiration is terminated on the completion of a preset inspiratory time. These ventilators deliver a volume of gas by generating a constant predetermined inspiratory pressure. The tidal volume delivered is a product of the time over which the inspiratory pressure is applied and the mechanical properties of the system into which the pressure is directed (a low compliant lung accepting less volume per unit pressure than a normal lung).[26] Since inspiratory time is controlled, inspiratory-expiratory (I:E) ratios can be varied at will. Pressure preset ventilators compensate for moderate gas leaks within the ventilator's system but are unable to maintain constant tidal volumes in face of changing resistances and compliances. In general, these ventilators are more compact and less expensive than comparable volume preset machines (see Fig. 10–18).

VOLUME PRESET INFANT VENTILATORS

Volume preset ventilators deliver a preselected volume of gas by means of a piston or bellows and continue to do so in the face of changes in lung compliance and airways resistance. Therefore, when used as strict constant tidal volume machines, they are, theoretically at least, pressure unlimited. Inspiratory gas flow is terminated when the preselected tidal volume is delivered into the patient circuit. The duration of inspiration may be controlled by changing either inspiratory flow rate (the slower the flow the longer the inspiratory time) or by a combination of changes in inspiratory flow rate and using a time-cycling inspiratory hold device.

Although generally referred to as constant tidal volume ventilators, the tidal volume delivered to the patient or the "effective tidal volume" is not truly constant. Some of the tidal volume delivered by the ventilator will be lost within the ventilator and patient circuit. This lost volume is referred to as the compression volume. The ventilator system's compression volume depends on its own internal compliance. The internal compliance values for most infant ventilators range from 0.28 to 0.5 ml/cm H_2O, depending on tubing diameter and length. Assuming that a ventilator's internal compliance is constant, decreases in lung compliance will result in an increase in the gas compressed within the circuit. Since neonatal endotracheal tubes do not have cuffs, an unknown volume of gas will also be lost by leakage between the noncuffed endotracheal tube and the tracheal wall. This volume leak will also increase as lung compliance decreases.

Despite these shortcomings, volume preset infant ventilators are remarkably successful in ventilating infants with severe low-compliance lung disease, often succeeding in clinical situations in which pressure preset ventilators have failed (see Fig. 10 – 15).

INTERMITTENT MANDATORY VENTILATION (IMV)

Prior to the advent of intermittent mandatory ventilation (IMV), mechanical ventilation was considered to be either "assisted" or "controlled." Neither regimen was fully satisfactory. During assisted ventilation, a patient initiated inspiration and set the frequency of breathing. In most clinical situations, assisted ventilation failed because most mechanical ventilators' triggering mechanisms were not sensitive enough to sense the minute changes in airway pressure produced by small infants. Consequently, infants were underventilated. When more sensitive pressure transducers became available, infants then, more often than not, were overventilated. Distressed neonates have very rapid respiratory rates, often in excess of 100 breaths per minute. The tidal volumes of most infant ventilators could not be reduced sufficiently to retain normal minute volumes. Today, assisted ventilation is used little, if at all, in the treatment of neonates.

During controlled mechanical ventilation, respiratory frequency is determined by the ventilator alone, irrespective of the patient's respiratory efforts. Maintaining controlled ventilation often required the use of sedatives or paralytic agents. In addition to their unpredictable effects on blood pressure and cardiac output, these agents, by abolishing all spontaneous muscle activity and muscle tone, often prolonged the time required for weaning from mechanical ventilation.[27, 28]

Prior to IMV, ventilators cycling in either the controlled or assist mode allowed gas flow only during inspiration. If a ventilator failed to cycle at a sufficient rate or if the patient breathed asynchronously or at a rate in excess of the mechanical ventilator, the patient would either receive no gas at all (inspiring against a closed circuit) or would rebreathe previously expired gas. In 1972, Kirby, deLemos and co-workers[28] designed an infant ventilator system that provided a continuous flow of gas throughout the respiratory cycle. When not cycling, this circuit functioned basically as a CPAP or continuous air flow T-tube system. By adding an exhalation valve and a time-cycling device, gas flow was intermittently forced into the patient's lungs.[29] Since gas flow was continuous, the patient was able to breathe spontaneously between machine breaths and the precise level of mechanical ventilatory support necessary could be titrated. Originally designed as a system to wean patients from controlled mechanical ventilation, IMV now is widely used as an intermediate step between CPAP and controlled mechanical ventilation. Clinical experience with the early IMV treatment of borderline respiratory insufficiency of very low birth weight infants and periodic apnea of prematurity has shown significant increases in survival and decreases in morbidity.[30] All infant ventilators currently manufactured in the United States now have IMV capabilities.

SQUARE WAVE VENTILATION

In the late 1960s and early 1970s, E. O. R. Reynolds and co-workers developed a system of infant mechanical ventilation with pressure preset ventilators utilizing low peak inspiratory pressures, prolonged inspiratory times and slow ventilatory rates. Reynolds restricted peak inspiratory pressures to less than 30 cm H_2O because of earlier clinical experiences suggesting that peak inspiratory pressures above this level were critical factors in the later development of chronic postventilator lung disease or bronchopulmonary dysplasia.[31, 32] When peak inspiratory pressures were severely restricted, Reynolds found that significant gains in oxygenation could be achieved by prolonging the time over which peak inspiratory pressures were applied. When inspiratory time was prolonged, plateaued or "squared," proximal airway

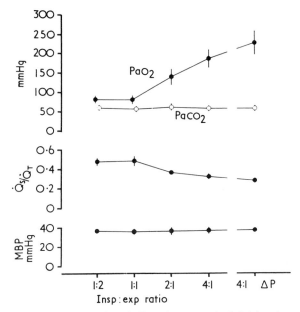

Fig. 11–2.—Effect of altering I:E ratio on arterial blood gas tensions, right-to-left shunt and mean arterial blood pressure. Peak airway pressure constant at 25 cm H_2O in 5 infants and 30 cm H_2O in 1. Respiratory frequency constant at 30/min 4:1; ΔP shows the effect of a 5-cm increment in airway pressure at an I:E ratio of 4:1. (From Reynolds, E. O. R., Arch. Dis. Child. 46:152, 1971. Reprinted by permission.)

pressure waves were produced and significant increases in arterial oxygenation followed[33] (Fig. 11–2). Herman and Reynolds[34] later observed that increased inspiratory times (increased I:E ratios) and modest amounts of PEEP appeared to act synergistically to improve arterial oxygenation. In order to allow enough time during inspiration for optimal gas exchange and enough time in expiration for adequate emptying of the lungs, slower ventilatory frequencies were used. Following the introduction of this ventilator protocol utilizing low peak inspiratory pressures, prolonged inspiratory times and slow ventilatory rates, Reynolds observed an increase in survival among patients with hyaline membrane disease and a significant reduction in the incidence of bronchopulmonary dysplasia.[31]

MEAN AIRWAY PRESSURE

Mean airway pressure is the mean pressure transmitted to the proximal airways throughout the respiratory cycle. It is determined by cal-

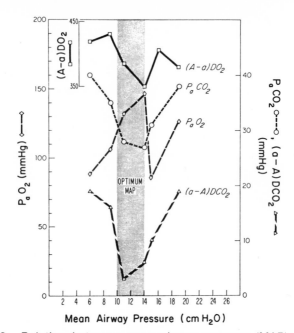

Fig. 11–3.—Relation between mean airway pressure (MAP) and arterial oxygen tension (Pa_{O_2}), arterial carbon dioxide tension (Pa_{CO_2}), alveolar-arterial oxygen difference ($[A-a]DO_2$) and arterial-alveolar carbon dioxide difference ($[a-A]DCO_2$). (From Boros, S., *et al., J. Pediatr.* 91:794, 1977. Reprinted by permission.)

culating the areas beneath the airway pressure waves of both inspiration and expiration, then dividing that area by its appropriate time. Mean airway pressure changes with any change in peak inspiratory pressure, inspiratory time (I:E ratio) or PEEP. It is a composite measure of all pressures transmitted to the airways by a mechanical ventilator and has been shown to be a useful parameter in determining oxygenation and ventilation. Herman and Reynolds,[34] examining the synergistic effect of prolonged inspiratory time and PEEP, observed that gains in oxygenation were directly related to increases in mean airway pressure. A recent clinical study examining the interrelationships between I:E ratios and airway pressure waveforms also suggested that mean airway pressure was a useful ventilator parameter for determining arterial oxygenation.[35] Animal studies have shown that for a given subject at a given time during mechanical ventilation there appears to be an optimal mean airway pressure where gas exchange is best and beyond which alveolar overdistention probably occurs[36] (Fig. 11–3).

Mean airway pressure can be clinically monitored using slightly modified blood pressure monitoring equipment. Several of the newer infant ventilator prototypes now monitor and display mean airway pressures.

ESOPHAGEAL PRESSURE MEASUREMENTS

The measurement of intraesophageal pressures with esophageal balloons or esophageal catheters is simple and often clinically useful in the management of infants receiving positive-pressure ventilation. Pressure changes within the distal third of the esophagus accurately reflect pressure changes within the intrapleural space.[37] The transmission of airway pressures to the intrapleural space and esophagus is extremely variable, the degree of transmission depending on lung distensibility or compliance. Most of the major complications of positive-pressure ventilation result from lung overdistention by excessive airway pressures and characteristically occur at a time when lung compliance is improving. Esophageal pressure measurements can be used to titrate airway pressures in order to prevent lung overdistention. Modanlou and others observed that as hyaline membrane disease improved, more airway pressure was transmitted to the intrapleural space. The transmission of more than 2 cm H_2O of pressure to the intrapleural space was considered to be a harbinger of impending barotrauma and an indication to reduce the levels of therapeutic airway pressure.[38, 39]

Esophageal pressures are measured using water-filled, blind-tipped, side hole feeding tubes attached to standard pressure transducers and recording equipment. The measurement of esophageal pressures is a promising adjunct to neonatal mechanical ventilation.

HIGH-FREQUENCY MECHANICAL VENTILATION

Recently, Bland et al.[40] described a rather unorthodox, but successful, "new" approach to the mechanical ventilation of infants. Returning to the views of earlier investigators, Bland attempted to mimic the distressed infant's natural respiratory pattern of rapid, shallow breathing. Small tidal volumes, modest levels of PEEP and ventilatory rates in excess of 80 breaths per minute were used during mechanical ventilation of 23 infants with hyaline membrane disease. Twenty-one (91%) survived. The remarkable early success of this regimen raises a number of intriguing clinical questions. How does high-frequency ventilation effect the distribution of gas within the lung? Recent work by Stetson and Swyer[41] suggests that the increased air velocities produced by rapid breathing may, by increasing airway turbulence, reduce the stratification of gases within the lung. Does high-frequency ventilation cause air trapping and result in an inadvertent or "silent" PEEP? How does high-frequency ventilation effect mean airway pressure? A mechanical ventilator's cycling frequency is intimately associated with inspiratory flow rate, inspiratory time and ultimately mean airway pressure. Clearly, the early success reported with this mode of mechanical ventilation requires that it be studied thoroughly.

A PRACTICAL APPROACH TO MECHANICAL VENTILATION

Over the years, the staff of the St. Paul (Minn.) Children's Hospital has developed a rather eclectic approach to infant mechanical ventilation. This approach evolved as newer techniques and equipment became available and, it is hoped, will continue to change in response to advances in methodology and technology. The following is not a suggested protocol or a "cookbook" recipe for mechanical ventilation. It is, simply, one institution's approach to infant mechanical ventilation developed through trial and error.

CPAP

Most mechanically ventilated infants have hyaline membrane disease and most have been previously treated with CPAP. CPAP is discussed in detail in Chapter 9. At present, our indications for CPAP are: (1) radiographic evidence of hyaline membrane disease; (2) inability of any infant to maintain a Pa_{O_2} of 60 mm Hg in an FI_{O_2} of 0.5 or a Downes RDS score of 6 or more in an FI_{O_2} of 0.5.[42] CPAP is administered through either nasal prongs or a single nasopharyngeal tube. It is commenced at an FI_{O_2} of 0.5 and an end expiratory pressure of 5 cm H_2O. FI_{O_2} is increased in increments of 0.1, alternated with end expiratory pressure increases of 1 cm H_2O until the level of 7 cm H_2O end expiratory pressure and FI_{O_2} of 0.7 is reached. Arterial blood gases are monitored following each change. If, at these settings, the patient's Pa_{O_2} is less than 60 mm Hg or the Pa_{CO_2} is 60 mm Hg or greater, we proceed to endotracheal intubation and intermittent mandatory ventilation (IMV).

IMV

Intermittent mandatory ventilation is administered through a pressure preset infant ventilator. IMV is started at an FI_{O_2} of 0.7, PEEP of 5 cm H_2O, a peak inspiratory pressure of 25 cm H_2O, a rate of 10 breaths per minute (bpm) and an inspiratory time of 1.0 second. If, at these settings, the patient's Pa_{CO_2} is 60 mm Hg or greater, the ventilator rate is increased in 5-bpm increments to 25 bpm. If the patient's Pa_{O_2} is less than 60 mm Hg, F_{IO_2} is increased in 0.1 increments to 0.8. Inspiratory time then is increased, first to 1.5 seconds, then to 2.0 seconds and the ventilator rate is increased in 5-bpm increments to 25 bpm. If hypoxia persists at these settings, the patient is paralyzed with pancuronium bromide (0.08–0.1 mg/kg) and advanced to the next level of ventilator support, controlled mechanical ventilation.

Controlled Mechanical Ventilation

PRESSURE PRESET VENTILATOR.—Following paralysis, the patient remains on the same pressure preset ventilator. The ventilator is connected via high-pressure tubing to a standard blood pressure transducer and blood pressure processor display module to monitor and display mean airway pressures. The initial ventilator settings are: peak inspiratory pressure 25 cm H_2O; ventilator rate 30 bpm; PEEP 5 cm H_2O; I : E ratio 1 : 1; F_{IO_2} 0.9–1.0.

If the Pa_{CO_2} is 60 mm Hg or greater, the ventilator rate is increased to a maximum of 50 bpm. In our experience, ventilator rates in excess of 50 bpm often are associated with deterioration in arterial oxygenation.

If, at these initial settings, the Pa_{O_2} remains less than 60 mm Hg or attempts to decrease the F_{IO_2} to less than 0.8 are unsuccessful, I : E ratio is increased first to 1.5 : 1, then to 2.0 : 1. If, despite a 2.0 : 1 I : E ratio, hypoxia persists, peak inspiratory pressure is first increased to 30 cm H_2O and PEEP increased to 7–8 cm H_2O. If hypoxia persists, the patient is transferred to a volume preset infant ventilator.

Volume Preset Ventilator

The volume preset ventilator (Bourns LS 104–150) is attached to a pressure transducer and processor display module to monitor mean airway pressure and to a ventilator monitor (Bourns LS 160) to monitor and display I : E ratio. This ventilator has the capability of changing both I : E ratio and proximal airway pressure waveform either by changing inspiratory flow rate or by utilizing an inspiratory time hold device. Decreasing inspiratory flow increases inspiratory time or I : E ratio and produces an elongated triangular pressure wave. The inspiratory time hold increases inspiratory time while keeping inspiratory flow rate constant by producing an inspiratory plateau or "squared" proximal airway pressure wave.

Initially, the ventilator is set to deliver an effective tidal volume (machine tidal volume minus volume lost within the ventilator) of 8–10 ml/kg, a ventilator rate of 25 bpm, PEEP of 5–6 cm H_2O and an inspiratory flow rate that produces an I : E ratio of 1 : 2–1 : 3. The high-pressure limit is set 10 cm H_2O higher than the peak inspiratory pressure generated while ventilating the infant at these settings. The inspiratory time hold is not used at this time.

If the Pa_{O_2} is less than 60 mm Hg or attempts to decrease the FI_{O_2} to less than 0.8 are unsuccessful, PEEP is increased in 1-cm H_2O increments to 8 cm H_2O. If hypoxia persists, I:E ratio is progressively increased using the inspiratory time hold. I:E ratio is first increased to 1:1, then to 1.5:1 while carefully monitoring mean airway pressure and arterial blood pressure.

If Pa_{O_2} remains less than 60 mm Hg or the peak inspiratory pressure generated by the ventilator at these settings is greater than 70 cm H_2O, the inspiratory time hold is discontinued, tidal volume is reduced by 50% and the ventilator rate is doubled.

Once recovery has begun, as witnessed by a consistent decrease in peak inspiratory pressures, patients are weaned from ventilator support in a stepwise fashion, weaning first from the volume preset ventilator to the pressure preset machine, then to IMV and CPAP. Once recovery has started, meticulous attention must be given to airway pressures (peak inspiratory pressures, PEEP and mean airway pressures). As lung compliance improves, more and more airway pressure is transmitted to the intrapleural space. At this point, patients are at significant risk for the adverse effects of elevated airway pressures (hypotension and barotrauma).

REFERENCES

1. Daily, W., Meyer, H., Sunshine, P., and Smith, P.: Mechanical ventilation of newborn infants. III. Historical comments and development of a scoring system for selection of infants, Anesthesiology 34:119, 1971.
2. Faulconer, A., and Keys, T.: *Foundation of Anesthesiology* (Springfield, Ill.: Charles C Thomas, Publisher, 1965) Vol. I, Chaps. 1 and 2.
3. Truehead, W.: Ein Apparat Zur Kunstlichen Respiration bei asphyxia, milth. a.d. sitzprotok, Der Gesselschaft F. Gebertsch, Berlin, 1869–1872, i, 154–156, 2 pl (transactions of the Berlin Obstetrical Society for 1869–1872).
4. O'Dwyer, J.: Fifty cases of croup in private practice treated by intubation of the larynx with a description of the danger incident thereto, Med. Rec. 32:557, 1887.
5. Doe, O.: Apparatus for resuscitating asphyxiated children, Boston Med. Surg. J. 120:9, 1889.
6. Stern, L., Ramos, A., Outerbridge, E., and Beaudry, P.: Negative pressure artificial ventilation. Use in treatment of respiratory failure of the newborn, Can. Med. Assoc. J. 102:595, 1970.
7. Bloxsom, A.: Resuscitation of the newborn infant. Use of the positive pressure oxygen-airlock, J. Pediatr. 37:311, 1950.
8. Donald, I., and Lord, J.: Augmented respiration studies in atelectasis neonatorum, Lancet 1:9, 1953.

9. Smythe, P., and Bull, A.: Treatment of tetanus neonatorum with intermittent positive pressure respiration, Br. Med. J. 2:107, 1959.
10. Smythe, P.: Studies on neonatal tetanus and on pulmonary compliance of the totally relaxed infant, Br. Med. J. 1:565, 1963.
11. Smythe, P.: Treatment of tetanus in neonates, Lancet 1:335, 1967.
12. Stahlman, M., Malan, A., Shepard, F., Blankenship, W., Young, W., and Gray, J.: Negative pressure assisted ventilation in infants with hyaline membrane disease, J. Pediatr. 76:174, 1969.
13. Heese, H. de V., Harrison, V., Klein, M., and Malan, A.: Intermittent positive pressure ventilation in hyaline membrane disease, J. Pediatr. 76:183, 1969.
14. Smith, P., Daily, W., Fletcher, G., Meyer, H., and Taylor, G.: Mechanical ventilation of newborn infants. I. The effect of rate and pressure on arterial oxygenation of infants with respiratory distress syndrome, Pediatr. Res. 3:244, 1969.
15. Reynolds, E. O. R.: Effect of alterations in mechanical ventilator settings on pulmonary gas exchange in hyaline membrane disease, Arch. Dis. Child. 46:152, 1971.
16. Gregory, G., Kitterman, J., Phibbs, R., Tooley, W., and Hamilton, W.: Treatment of the idiopathic respiratory distress syndrome with continuous positive airway pressure, N. Engl. J. Med. 284:1333, 1971.
17. Barach, A., Fenn, W., Ferris, E., and Schmidt, C.: The physiology of pressure breathing. A brief review of its present status, J. Aviation Med. 18:73, 1947.
18. Cumarasamy, N., Nussli, R., Vischer, D., Dangel, P., and Duc, G.: Artificial ventilation in hyaline membrane disease. The use of positive end-expiratory pressure and continuous positive airway pressure, Pediatrics 51:629, 1973.
19. Ashbaugh, D., and Petty, T.: Positive end-expiratory pressure. Physiology, indications and contraindications, J. Thorac. Cardiovasc. Surg. 65:165, 1973.
20. Powers, S., Mannal, R., Neclerio, M., English, M., Marr, C., Leather, R., Veda, H., Williams, G., Custead, W., and Dutton, R.: Physiologic consequences of positive end-expiratory pressure (PEEP) ventilation, Ann. Surg. 178:265, 1973.
21. Llewellyn, M., and Swyer, P.: Mechanical ventilation and continuous distending pressure: The intensive care of the newly born. Physiological principles and practice (P. Swyer, [ed.]), Monogr. Paediatr. 6:90, 1975.
22. Stern, L.: Negative Pressure Ventilation, in Shnider, S., and Moya, F. (eds.), *The Anesthesiologist, Mother and Newborn* (Baltimore: The Williams & Wilkins Company, 1974), p. 252.
23. Fanaroff, A., Cha, C., Sosa, R., Crumrine, R., and Klaus, M.: Controlled trial of continuous negative external pressure in the treatment of severe respiratory distress syndrome, J. Pediatr. 82:921, 1973.
24. Sanyal, S., Mitchell, C., Hughes, W., Feldman, S., and Caces, J.: Continuous negative chest-wall pressure as therapy for severe respiratory distress in older children, Chest 68:143, 1975.
25. Bancalari, E., Gerhardt, T., and Monkus, E.: Simple device for producing continuous negative pressure in infants with IRDS, Pediatrics 52:128, 1973.

26. Lough, M. D., Doershuk, C. F., and Stern, R. C.: *Pediatric Respiratory Therapy* (Chicago: Year Book Medical Publishers, Inc., 1974), p. 123.
27. Noguchi, A., and Boros, S.: The use of pancuronium bromide during the controlled mechanical ventilation of newborn infants, Pediatr. Res. 13:490, 1979.
28. Kirby, R., Robison, E., Schulz, J., and deLemos, R.: Continuous-flow ventilation as an alternative to assisted or controlled ventilation in infants, Anesth. Analg. 51:871, 1972.
29. Downs, J., Klein, E., Desautels, D., Modell, J., and Kirby, R.: Intermittent mandatory ventilation: A new approach to weaning patients from mechanical ventilators, Chest 64:331, 1973.
30. Mannino, F., Feldman, B., Heldt, G., DeLue, N., Wimmer, J., Fletcher, M., and Gluck, L.: Early mechanical ventilation in RDS with a prolonged inspiration, Pediatr. Res. 10:464, 1976.
31. Reynolds, E. O. R., and Taghizadeh, A.: Improved prognosis of infants mechanically ventilated for hyaline membrane disease, Arch. Dis. Child. 49:505, 1974.
32. Taghizadeh, A., and Reynolds, E. O. R.: Pathogenesis of bronchopulmonary dysplasia following hyaline membrane disease, Am. J. Pathol. 82:241, 1976.
33. Reynolds, E. O. R.: Effect of alterations in mechanical ventilator settings on pulmonary gas exchange in hyaline membrane disease, Arch. Dis. Child. 46:152, 1971.
34. Herman, S., and Reynolds, E. O. R.: Methods for improving oxygenation in infants mechanically ventilated for severe hyaline membrane disease, Arch. Dis. Child. 48:612, 1973.
35. Boros, S.: The effect of variations in inspiratory-expiratory ratio and airway pressure wave form during mechanical ventilation: The significance of mean airway pressure, J. Pediatr. 94:114, 1979.
36. Boros, S., Matalon, S., Ewald, R., Leonard, A., and Hunt, C.: The effect of independent variations in inspiratory-expiratory ratio and end expiratory pressure during mechanical ventilation in hyaline membrane disease: The significance of mean airway pressure, J. Pediatr. 91:794, 1977.
37. Hjalmarson, O., Torsten, O., and Riha, M.: Mechanics of breathing in newborn infants with pulmonary disease: Theoretical and methodological aspects, Acta Paediatr. Scand. (supp.) 247:6, 1974.
38. Hinkes, P., Nelson, P., and Modanlou, H.: Esophageal pressure measurements in newborn ventilatory therapy. (In press.)
39. Uauy, R., and Motoyama, E.: Continuous monitoring of esophageal pressure (pes): A simple technique and its potential use, Pediatr. Res. 9:402, 1975.
40. Bland, R., Kim, M., and Woodson, J. L.: High-frequency mechanical ventilation of low birth weight infants with respiratory failure from hyaline membrane disease, Pediatr. Res. 11:531, 1977.
41. Stetson, J., and Swyer, P.: *Neonatal Intensive Care* (St. Louis: Warren H. Green, Inc., 1976), p. 306.
42. Downes, J. J., Vidyasagar, D., Morrow, G. M., and Boggs, T. R.: Respiratory distress syndrome of newborn infants: I. New clinical scoring system (RDS score) with acid-base and blood-gas correlations, Clin. Pediatr. 9:325, 1970.

12 / Care of the Parents

JANE H. DAVIS, A.S.S.S., A.C.S.W.

WITH THE ADVENT OF intensive care units and sophisticated life support systems, a unique stress has been created for the patients' families, who feel both helpless and ineffectual during the crisis. Their forced "wait-and-see position" contradicts natural impulses to mobilize for action during the emergency. Nowhere is the impact greater than on the family of the newborn intensive care unit (NICU) patient that has anticipated a happy event and is suddenly faced with a crisis situation. The parents suffer from a variety of emotional and physical discomforts, including separation from the infant, financial concerns about the usually enormous intensive care unit (ICU) bill, upset of the family routine and distress over the baby's immediate condition and long-term prognosis. Not only do the parents begin to grieve for the normal, healthy infant they did not have but they must accept the possible loss of the sick infant who is theirs. In addition, the fear of a permanently damaged offspring is almost too threatening for them to face immediately.

Because of the ongoing emotional issues experienced by the family in the NICU, it is crucial that the staff have not only sophisticated medical knowledge but an understanding of the variety of emotional responses and needs of the family. They must also be able to apply this understanding in their dealing with the families; the special needs of the families are clearly considered important in offering intensive care to infants.[4]

Although various medical conditions may cause an infant to be brought to the NICU, including prematurity, congenital anomalies, low birth weight, problems around delivery and maternal complications, the staff's goals for the families remain the same: (1) to help families develop appropriate and effective coping mechanisms for dealing with the crisis situation, (2) to assist the necessary grieving process for the expected child and in preparation for the possible loss of the sick infant and (3) to facilitate the bonding process between parents and infant. Integration of the theories of bonding, grieving and crisis is essential in the care of the NICU families; a short description of each of these theories follows.

CRISIS THEORY

This theory incorporates several basic concepts from a variety of philosophies: ego psychology, theories of personality, stress, role, systems and communication. Its concepts have been developed mainly in studies of population groups or communities confronted with states of disaster and then applied to family functioning and breakdown. Of particular relevance to NICU work are the studies by Caplan,[5] Kaplan and Mason,[13] Rapoport[23] and Parad.[20] Parents of NICU patients are suddenly faced with a crisis and experience a psychologically stressful event.

The source of the crisis is external and upsetting to the family's homeostatic, or steady, state. Their customary patterns of coping do not work and a state of tension is created. Erikson[7] identifies crises as two types: (1) developmental crises that occur in the normal psychosocial development of an individual or family and (2) accidental crises that are precipitated by unanticipated, unplanned events usually associated with a loss. Birth of a sick, premature or defective child falls in both categories. It is biologically determined but presents a situation for which neither parent is prepared. (It is suggested by some that the birth of a mentally defective child is a third type of crisis; there is no time for working through the loss of the fantasized normal baby; the unexpectedly abnormal child requires immediate attention.[25])

Crisis therapy is not just short-term psychotherapy but a unique intervention adapted to a specific situation; the occurrence of an acute disorder during the event does not depend on the prior existence of disturbance but rather results from an individual's attempt to cope with a threatening event for which he/she is not sufficiently psychologically prepared.[13] Basically, crisis intervention is brief, ego-supportive and based on the here and now. During the crisis, customary defense mechanisms have become weakened and the ego is more open to outside influence and challenge. A minimal force can produce a maximal effect.[10] The family's motivation for receiving help is increased because they are in great distress.

"The state of active crisis is usually characterized by a series of reactions: first a state of shock, of psychological and physical turmoil that includes aimless activity or immobilization and disturbance in physical, emotional, and intellectual functioning. Then comes a painful preoccupation with the past, during which the events leading up to the state of the crisis are 'reworked.' Finally, there is a period of remobilization and renewed activity and readjustment."[10] During this reorganization, new styles of coping may emerge to help the individual or family deal more effectively with the situation. On the other hand, maladaptive patterns may also develop that can result in a weakened ability to cope in the future.[10] The resulting condition may be the same as, worse than or better than that before the crisis; factors influencing the outcome include: current adaptive capacities, environmental factors, personality structure, prior family functioning and the accomplishment of certain specific psychologic tasks during the crisis.[23] These tasks, for NICU families, are more effectively completed with appropriate staff intervention.

The initial hazardous event that precipitates the crisis requires a solution that is novel to the individual in relation to his previous life experiences and problem-solving activities. This initial stress can be experienced in one of three ways, each accompanied by specific emotional responses: (1) as a threat, exhibited by high anxiety; (2) as a loss, exhibited by depression and mourning; or (3) as a challenge, accompanied by some anxiety but with hope and a release of energy for problem solving.[23] And, as Caplan states in his paper, "Patterns of Parental Response to the Crisis of Premature Birth," the responses to the stress "have, therefore, more enduring significance for mental health than merely the immediate relief from frustration or escape from danger. The discontinuity and imbalance of the customary patterns of behavior and feeling during the crisis period are associated with an increased susceptibility to change, which may be in the direction either of improved mental health or mental illness."[5] Healthy crisis resolution by families in the NICU can be effected by the staff's assistance in three areas: (1) aiding families in the correct, realistic perception of the situation, (2) helping with appropriate verbalization of feelings and management of affect and (3) the development of patterns of seeking and using help.[5, 23] Goals for staff in their help with the crisis should include: relief from symptoms, a return to the previous level of functioning of the family, an understanding by the family members of the factors involved in the crisis and identification of remedial measures that are available to the family through hospital, community and family resources.[23]

THEORIES OF GRIEVING

Grief is a natural, healing process resulting from a loss and occurring over a period of time. The parents of the sick, premature or defective infant experience the loss of the normal, healthy child they did not have and, as a result, grieve for that imagined child. When a dying or dead infant is born, "whether the baby lives one hour or two weeks, whether the baby is a nonviable 500 g or weighs 4000 g, whether or not the mother had had physical contact with her baby, clearly identifiable mourning will be present."[15]

In dealing with the grieving parents, it is essential to understand and identify the symptoms of the normal grieving process: (1) somatic distress, such as tightness in the throat, shortness of breath, sighing, an empty feeling in the abdomen, weakness, intense subjective distress described as tension or mental pain; (2) preoccupation with the image of the deceased; (3) feelings of guilt; (4) loss of warmth and feelings of irritability and anger toward others; (5) loss of normal patterns of conduct. These symptoms may appear immediately after the loss and may be delayed or exaggerated. The duration of the reaction appears to depend on the success with which the person or family accomplishes its tasks of separation from the deceased, readjustment to a new situation in which the deceased is missing and the formation of new relationships.[19]

Two other syndromes — morbid grief reaction and postponed reaction — indicate a distortion of normal grief. Lindemann's[19] classic study of the survivors of the Cocoanut Grove fire in Boston in 1942 indicates that there are several manifestations of these pathologic responses: overactivity without a sense of loss; acquisition of the symptoms belonging to the last illness of the deceased; psychosomatic conditions, such as ulcerative colitis, asthma, an alteration in relationships with friends and relatives, furious hostility or formal wooden affect, lasting loss of patterns of social interaction, with a lack of decision and initiative, self-punitive behavior, such as unwise economic dealings, agitated depression with tension, insomnia and feelings of worthlessness. (Caplan's study suggests that the absence of grief after the birth of a premature child rather than extreme grief may be a sign of pending family disorganization.)[5]

Normal, acute grief, then, is of relatively short duration, usually achieving some degree of resolution within a period of several weeks to several months.[6] However, since the death of a child is a unique event, with parents feeling the loss as if they have lost a part of themselves, their mourning process may last years, and without appropriate intervention, indefinitely.[9] The uniqueness of the grief response to a perinatal death and illness appears to relate to the quality of attachment the survivors have had with the infant who existed as a parental fantasy. Their relationship with the infant has been of high intensity, short duration and with little physical contact. NICU parents are faced with the enormous task of grieving for the actual loss of the expected child and the anticipated loss of the actual child. The task is more difficult for the parents who have had ambivalent feelings about the pregnancy and subsequent[15] conflicts and guilt during the hospitalization.

The stages of grieving have been well described by Kubler-Ross[16] in *On Death and Dying;* they represent emotional changes of the bereaved experience: (1) denial, (2) anger, (3) bargaining, (4) depression, (5) acceptance and lead toward a process of integrating the finality of the loss with reality. The various affective components of the stages (to be discussed more fully later in the chapter) may occur alone or together and it is necessary in NICU work to have an understanding of the variety of emotional responses that accompany a loss. Kubler-Ross's important work focuses on the dying patient; however, she emphasizes that we cannot help the terminally ill patient in a really meaningful way if we do not include his/her family.[16] Observations in our unit indicate that not only do parents of sick infants experience extreme isolation but they are also unprepared for the intensity of their feelings. Friends and relatives are unsure of what to say or how to help. In an attempt to be supportive, they usually offer statements of unrealistic optimism: "I know she'll get better; just wait and see." In many hospitals, grieving parents leave with little or no intervention; nursery and maternity staff are accustomed to dealing with happy, healthy patients. Parents quickly realize that there is no place for grief in the nursery or maternity floor. They become innocent victims of the "conspiracy of silence."[16]

Other factors compound the parents' sorrow: deaths of other children, miscarriages, previously unsuccessful attempts at parenthood, absence of a supportive extended family, lack of other social supports, inability to share sadness with others and marital problems. In a recent study by Benfield, Leib and Reuter,[3] it was found that most parents of critically ill infants who were transferred to a regional center experienced grief reactions similar to those of parents of infants who did not survive. Interestingly, their anticipatory grief did not appear to be associated with the severity of the baby's illness. The degree of maternal grief was found to be related positively to the degree of pleasure at being pregnant and negatively with her age and her confidence in her ability to care for the baby after discharge. The father's anticipatory grief was significantly related to delivery by cesarean section and negatively to mother's age. In another study, Kennell, Slyter and

Klaus[14] found that there was a higher degree of mourning in mothers who had touched their baby before death and who had not talked to their husbands about their loss.

The birth of a defective child who eventually goes home with the family elicits not only an initial acute grief reaction but an enduring chronic sorrow: "unlike acute grief, which is intense and limited in time, chronic grief is prolonged and recurrent. But it follows the same stages as acute grief, except that it is unresolved."[12] However, because the parents experience this chronic sorrow, they are not necessarily immobilized or prevented from receiving some satisfaction from their child. Effective intervention can mean the difference between an adaptive resolution and a maladaptive resolution that can impair family functioning. Staff's involvement with the family of a permanently handicapped infant can make that difference.

THEORIES OF BONDING AND ATTACHMENT

There is accumulating evidence that disturbances in the attachment process between mother and infant are associated with serious disorders in infancy and childhood. Probably the most dramatic of these is in the battered child and failure-to-thrive syndromes; in one study, 25–41% of the reported failure-to-thrive infants were premature.[1] Prematurity or serious illness in the newborn period resulting in maternal-infant separation was a feature in 23–31% of the battered infants.[29] Others have found that the incidence of prematurity, with prolonged separation of mother and infant, is 3 times as high among children who subsequently have been battered than among the general low birth weight incidence.[15] In light of these statistics, early and prolonged separation is believed to be one of the primary factors.

There have been mammalian studies of maternal behavior suggesting that the animal's earliest contact with her young is crucial in determining her later behavior toward her infant. In studies with goats, sheep and cattle, when a mother is separated from her young in the first few hours after delivery and the two then are reunited, the mother will fail to care for her own infant. And, as Klaus notes, "despite the reluctance of many investigators to accept the concept that these patterns may apply to humans, the possibility of their extension to the human should not be neglected when they are found in a large number of species."[15]

Results to date of several long-term studies reveal identifiable differences in mothering performance as late as 6 months after birth. These studies indicate that mothers who had earlier and more contact with their infants showed greater soothing behavior, engaged in significantly more eye-to-eye contact and fondling during feeding, had more reluctance to leave their infants with someone else and usually stood and watched during a physical examination.[15] There is also evidence to suggest that early contact affects aspects of mothering behavior that may have significance for the child's later development; increased maternal attentiveness facilitates later exploratory behavior in infants.[15] Mothers who had earlier contact with their infants were observed to exhibit distinctive linguistic behaviors with their children, such as use of fewer commands, asking more questions, use of fewer adjectives and fewer content words. In another follow-up study with prematures, when tested at 42 months, the children in the early contact group attained significantly higher Stanford-Binet scores, according to Kennell in a 1975 conference on maternal attachment and mothering disorders.[21] Although high mourning is also related to increased contact, the advantages of early contact do seem to outweigh the disadvantages.

Early contact between family and infant is the most natural and desirable condition, and results suggest that separations should be avoided whenever possible and minimized when unavoidable.[17] The infant is an important part of the family system; the family will assume his/her care after discharge and mourn for him/her after death. Most of the studies have focused on mother-child interaction; the father and the rest of the family appear to be sadly neglected. Fathering, as well as mothering, is a learned behavior. The father is much more involved in and responsive toward his infant than our culture has acknowledged and "a critical issue is that the care of the infant be acknowledged as natural and appropriate male behavior."[21] Including the father in early contact with the infant is as important as including the mother; parenting takes time and patience. Parents of the sick infant are under a great deal of strain and support and encouragement are needed by both. The term "parental bonding" is much more relevant in our work with families, for as Doctor Parke concludes, "bringing the father back into the family from the start and demonstrating that he is a social as well as a biological necessity" should be a task for all nursery personnel.[21]

STRATEGIES FOR INTERVENTION

Parents of premature, sick or defective infants are faced with specific tasks during each stage of the crisis; the stages include: (1) labor and delivery, (2) hospitalization and (3) the end of hospitalization through discharge or death. Coping skills and new problem-solving strategies for a successful resolution of the crisis can be taught and developed; the family's capacity to deal with the crisis of the birth and hospitalization can be strengthened by a supportive staff. From observations in our unit, along with follow-up interviews with parents over a 2-year period, the following suggestions for effective intervention are recommended. (Also included is a stage-by-stage description with appropriate tasks.)

Stage 1. Delivery of a Premature, Sick or Defective Baby

TASK 1. — The parents must begin to grieve for the actual loss of the normal healthy child they expected and begin to anticipate the possible loss of their abnormal child.

Intervention. — As soon as possible after delivery, see both parents together; if the father is not present, see the mother alone or with a "significant other." Introduce yourself and give them the baby's picture that was taken on admission to the NICU. Find out what the parents know and what they want to know. Explain the baby's condition and point out that the baby will not be going home with the family when the mother goes home. Listen to what they are asking; answer one question at a time. Give reasons immediately for special care and admission to the NICU; stress the need to take things a day at a time. Combine the good news with the bad: "Your baby had to be taken to the NICU because . . . ; but you will be able to see him/her anytime; he/she is getting the best of care." Capitalize the positive while including the negative. Then, have the family repeat to you what you have said; emphasize that contact will be maintained and find out whether the father would like to come to the nursery alone while the mother still is in the delivery suite or if he will wait until she can be brought in a wheelchair. Before the mother is assigned a room, try to get her a room alone or with someone other than a mother of a new, healthy baby. Parents should also be given an information sheet that contains all necessary NICU information about visiting, general suggestions and names of the primary physician, nurse and social worker; phone numbers should be listed. If the mother is alone, give her the information sheet and give another to other family members. Reassure her that she will see her new baby as soon as possible. Many mothers note that they feel "very left out" initially, with information communicated to other family members first. All remembered being "very scared" the first few days. If the baby's death seems imminent, try to get the mother to the nursery immediately.

Rationale. — By seeing the parents as soon as possible, you are establishing a link between them and their new baby and beginning a trusting relationship with them. The initial contact is both supportive and informative, giving parents a realistic picture of the situation. The picture makes the baby real, and the immediate news that the baby will not be going home with them concretizes the uniqueness of the situation and the baby's condition. Immediate specific details of the baby's condition strengthen the parents' perception and include them in the baby's care. Every baby admitted to our NICU unit has his/her picture taken for the parents; the pictures belong to the parents and are cherished by them long after the baby goes home or, in some cases, dies. Too often, parents are the last ones to be included in the "bad news" and, therefore, are deprived of valuable grief time. Regardless of the baby's condition, each baby has his/her picture taken; for the parents, as one mother said, "The unknown is much more frightening than the known."

TASK 2. — The parents must begin to accept their sick and/or defective infant and develop new coping skills to deal with a disruption in their normal patterns.

Intervention. — Bring the parents to the NICU as soon as possible. On the way to the nursery, prepare them for what to expect in the unit: the sights and the sounds and how their baby will look. Give the new parents time with their baby and encourage them to have as much physical contact as possible; all the equipment should be explained to them and they should be encouraged to participate, in some way, in the infant's care. This initial visit is a critical time for parents; their subsequent involvement often is related to their first impressions: how welcome they feel, how much the staff encourages them to feel that this is their baby and how comfortable they feel with their new baby. Be sensitive to the parents' feelings of ambivalence, which are not often verbalized but usually present; help them to ventilate these feelings to alleviate guilt and to establish a therapeutic relationship with them. As one father said after he first saw his new premature son on a respirator, "I don't know whether to get ready for his death or hope that he will eventually come home. It's almost too hard to think about either way." Be where the family "is at"; do not start talking about blood gases when the family asks about the eye patches.

Rationale. — As indicated by attachment studies, early and consistent contact is to be encouraged. This is also the appropriate time to (1) begin establishing a relationship with the parents, (2) help parents adjust to the nursery and (3) identify potential areas of concern. Although high mourning was found to be related to the extent of contact, the completeness of the grief resolution appears also to relate to the parents' opportunity to be a parent; contact provides tangible evidence of the baby's existence. A relationship is made and not merely fantasized; from observations in our unit, it became apparent that families more easily reached a stage of acceptance of the loss and had less incidence of pathologic grief reaction when: (1) contact with their infant was made early and often, (2) communications with the staff were considered to be mutually satisfying and (3) parents felt included in decisions made about the care of their baby. Methods of medical management can facilitate coping; feelings of anger, guilt, sadness and joy should be explored in the hospital setting. Allow and encourage parents to ventilate their feelings within a supportive structure. Most parents are confused and distressed by their feelings of ambivalence about their new baby; help them deal with these feelings. Appropriate verbalization can help with tension discharge. Do not use a "can opener" approach but be sensitive to signals that parents are ready to share some of their discomforting feelings.

TASK 3. — The parents must begin to conserve their energies to cope with the ongoing stress of the sick infant; begin to help other family members deal with unique stress and mobilize other supports available to them.

Intervention. — Shortly after delivery, a brief interview should be scheduled with the parents. The information will provide a more complete assessment of the baby's family. Find out if the family has had other crises, their feelings about the pregnancy, available social supports, other children, parents' ages, occupation, marital and education history, previous mental health history. Make this assessment available to the nursery staff; tell the family the reasons for the interview. If possible, have a primary nurse continue with the family.

Reassure parents of the legitimacy of their feelings of confusion and bewilderment; help prepare them for the unpredictableness of the situation, for the events that most likely will occur and for the idiosyncrasies of your nursery. Prepare the parents for future physical responses: feelings of depression, restlessness, not being able to sleep or eat and exhaustion. Help the parents deal with other family members by including them in family meetings and by phone, if the parents request. Be available for questions about siblings, grandparents and friends. Have a comfortable room available to the parents near the nursery. Answer all questions; listen for repetition, which is helping parents come to terms with the knowledge that their baby is sick. Listen for early statements of self-blame, anger, diffused or focused inappropriately, and early dysfunctional communication among the family members.

Rationale. — In the first interview, and following contacts with the family, it is important to be able to identify factors that may interfere with a satisfactory relationship between the parents and the infant. The family history, prenatal history, flexibility of the family and history of previous crises provide initial diagnostic material about the family's ability to cope under stress and the potential for adaptive responses and the availability of resources.

Since one of the primary needs of a person in crisis is a reduction in confusion and bewilderment caused by the tension,[20] useful intervention at this point is a reassurance of the legitimacy of the parents' feelings. They also require ongoing information concerning the infant's medical status. Keep the channels of communication open; insist that the parents receive consistent, complete information. If the parents are helped to see their feelings as natural in coping with the stressful situation, it will be easier for them to deal with these feelings and process new information.

By involving other family members, you are helping the parents to seek needed support and making other family members feel more comfortable in this unusual situation. The parents will need help in explanations for their other children. Many parents delay telling the other children, using excuses that they "are too young to understand," "are not aware anyway" or may simply want to protect them. Children do absorb the feelings and reactions of their parents. They can acquire either an appropriate acceptance or an inappropriate reaction by incorporating or reacting to their parents.[11] Use of euphemisms such as "gone to sleep," "taken away" or "not feeling well" can confuse and upset a young child; if parents avoid any discussion of the illness or defect, the child will quickly perceive that his feelings should be hidden and denied. Lack of information and openness can only serve to compound the child's fears and fantasies about what may happen to him or his parents. Children must be appropriately included so that they, too, can feel a part of, and not excluded from, the family crisis. In this way, the staff can set an example of openness to the parents. Early feelings of resentment toward the new baby who appears to be taking up so much of their parents' time and energy should be explored with the children. Parents need to be reassured that sibling rivalry, even at this stage, is normal. The NICU must make some provision for siblings to visit, touch and relate with their new brother or sister.

During this time, well-meaning friends and relatives, often uncertain as to what to say, will avoid the new parents or offer unrealistic optimism. Parents need to be prepared for their friends' and family's often inappropriate, although well-meaning, attempts to comfort.

Early intervention and help with the parents' grief begins immediately. The NICU staff can help by responding to both the manner and content of the manifestations of the grief; the ease of passing through the emotional changes in the stages of grieving depends, to a large extent, on the attitudes of the staff. Our reactions directly affect the parents. A review of these stages (originally described by Kubler-Ross) will help in dealing with the grieving parents: (1) *denial* is "usually a temporary defense and will soon be replaced by partial acceptance";[16] look for continual repetition of questions, unrealistically optimistic statements and inability to hear what is being said, particularly the "bad news." Listen to the recurring questions that cover the underlying conflict; state facts without judgment; relate to the pain. Let denial stand; be ready to help the family with their other emotions as they appear; (2) *anger* is a difficult stage for both family and NICU staff. Initially, the anger may be unfocused, or diffused, and sometimes directed at the hospital, God, church or other family members — often toward the staff. Allow parents to express and focus their anger; help them find appropriate outlets and understand where it is coming from; often the intensity of their feelings, at this point, will drive others away; do not take the anger personally; (3) *bargaining* is an attempt to postpone or ward off threatening events by self-imposed promises; look for the parents' attempts "to make the baby better" by staying with him/her constantly, depriving themselves of any rest, hoping to prevent deterioration in the baby's condition; do not give false assurance; it is helpful to explore with the parents their fears and feelings of self-blame that are there; (4) *depression* is a phase most easily identified; the parents appear sad and tearful, sometimes with very little affect. Listen to the "If only I . . ." statements verbalized, the parents' feelings of guilt, usually unrealistic, that accompany this stage. Parents feel powerless to help their infant; be supportive, involve them in the baby's care and give them as many choices as possible related to that care; (5) *acceptance* usually does not take place while the baby still is in the hospital; look for signs of this and support it; parents will begin to ask about community resources for the developmentally delayed child; they will begin to discuss more comfortably the child's problems with others. Stress with the family that accepting the loss is not forgetting but rather integrating the reality into their lives; it includes the capacity to reinvest in other relationships, the relief from physical symptoms (lump in the throat, tearfulness, sighing) when discussing the loss, be it a death or a permanently handicapped child.

Stage 2. Hospitalization

TASK 1.—The parents must begin to adapt to a physical and mental state of ongoing stress.

Intervention. — Provide a comfortable room for the family to be with their baby. If it is not possible for the infant to be moved, try to make the parents' time with their baby as natural as possible under the circumstances. A comfortable rocking chair with a screen for some privacy is a good idea. Try to help the parents conserve their energy. Parents should be encouraged to call and visit the nursery anytime, but they are also given permission to take some time for themselves. Reassure them that their baby is in good hands. Continue to keep parents well informed about their baby, listening to their asked questions and anticipating unasked questions. Give verbal as well as nonverbal support; parents remember the staff person who stands by when they are distressed; they recall clearly the pat on the arm, the shoulder to lean on when they are feeling low.

Keep a family contact sheet (Fig. 12–1) and encourage all nursery staff to record on it. Look for those high-risk signals involved in the chronic stressful situation: consistently unrealistic expectations; denial of the situation; flat affect; inability to process information; infrequent visitation or, conversely, never leaving the NICU; neglecting their own needs; exhaustion; and overreacting to daily events. Relate to the parents' feelings underlying their questions; relate to their anguish but continue to deal with the reality. Share their joy if the baby continues to improve; reassure them that their baby's problem was not the result of something they did or did not do. Take one question at a time. Help parents to have sustained physical contact with their baby.

Rationale. — During this stage, the most exhausting and stressful aspect is the realization that the crisis may continue for days, weeks or months. It is crucial that the family conserve their energy; this is particularly essential if the baby has multiple defects such as meningomyelocele and will be a long-term management problem. The stress will not go away; to help the parents learn effective ways of dealing with their chronic grief is as important as the medical care provided for the infant. Help by keeping a focus on the crisis. Many times when the parents ask questions about medical information, an answer about their emotional concerns is what is needed. For example, when par-

FAMILY CONTACT SHEET

Patient _____

Phone: _____

Date:							
Type of Contact:							
Phone							
Visit							
Other							
Relative:							
Mother							
Father							
Grandmother							
Grandfather							
Other							
Impressions:							
Affectionate							
Cried							
Nervous							
Concerned							
Unconcerned							
Touched/held baby							
Would not touch/ hold baby							
Had questions							
No questions							
Confused							
Spoke to:							
Asked about? (Be specific)							
Other Impressions or Issues:							

Fig. 12–1.—An example of a family contact sheet.

ents ask about their baby's breathing or blood gases, help them identify their fears concerning his/her later development, his/her potential for normality. It is not necessary to respond in this way to every question, but be sensitive always to the unasked questions, which usually are of more intensity and therefore more difficult to verbalize. When possible, capitalize on the positive.

Reduction of the anxiety level will come through physical care of the baby; care of their baby is best learned in the nursery with helpful, skilled staff to encourage and teach. The family contact sheet describes the number and type of contacts made by the family. Because it is unrealistic in a busy NICU to have only one staff member communicate with the family, this kind of chart provides a record of contacts and the content of previous communication with the nursery. Much of the stress inherent in such a situation can be reduced by communication between the family and staff; one can refer to the sheet and quickly get an idea of the contact pattern. Klaus and Kennell[15] note that fewer than 3 phone calls in 2 weeks represent a "severe mother disorder"; the family's absence or reduced involvement may signal to the staff to examine the family situation and their reaction to the birth.

TASK 2. — The parents will be coming to terms with many feelings of ambivalence toward their new baby and dealing with simultaneous emotions of attachment and withdrawing.

Intervention. — At this point, it is very important for the staff to be available to parents for the verbalizations of joy, pain, anger and frustration. Answer questions as they come up; encourage the family to share their concerns. Be direct and truthful; this cannot be overemphasized. A trusting relationship with the staff is essential for therapeutic intervention, and when families sense a lack of completeness in a report, this will affect further communication. Well-meaning attempts to "protect" parents should be avoided. Do not take away all hope; do not build up false hopes. Include the families in the decisions about their baby — both large and small. (In follow-up interviews with the parents, the most resented responses were the staff's suggestions that there "was no hope" and well-meaning suggestions to "give up hope for the baby." Both were extremely upsetting to parents, as were reports that parents sensed were overly optimistic.)

Involve the parents in the baby's care; if the mother wants to breast feed, and it seems that the baby soon will be taking milk by mouth, have her begin to collect her milk and freeze it in small quantities in sealable plastic bags. For the very sick infants, parents can apply lotion to the infant's skin and lips; encourage physical contact. Whenever possible, have the parents hold, feed and touch their infant. Involve the parents in a program of infant stimulation; parents should be encouraged to bring in mobiles for him/her. Give the parents ongoing explanations of the equipment and what procedures are being performed and why.

Rationale. — During this stage, feelings of disappointment and anxiety will increase tremendously, for it is at this time that the parents begin to prepare for either the baby's homecoming or possible death. The shock has worn off and the pressures of continued hospitalization increase. The hospital should sustain support and ventilation of the feelings that have intensified. They need to have their feelings legitimized by the staff, who appreciate the strain involved in the baby's care and hospitalization. Self-blame is a common reaction in the parents of the sick and/or defective infant. The guilt may be irrational, unreasonable or inappropriate; it often is related to feelings of ambivalence toward the pregnancy or an eager need for the baby. A more complete understanding of the parents' situation will help in dealing with them.

This perhaps is the most difficult stage facing the parents. During this period, the shock has worn off; the parents are faced with an indefinite period of ups and downs, including anxiety about the baby, disturbances in their routines, often an exchange of their roles in which father stays home with the other children while mother stays with the new baby, communication problems if the infant is transferred to another hospital, physical exhaustion, worries over the mounting hospital bill and intense ambivalence about the child, particularly if there is a realistic fear that he/she will be permanently disabled. Keep in mind that adaptive coping behaviors reinforced at the time of the crisis are stronger later on.

TASK 3. — The parents will begin to come to terms with the uniqueness of their baby and prepare for the end of hospitalization, through either discharge or death.

Intervention. — Have the parents provide most of the care for their infant while visiting; set up several predischarge conferences to review the care, stressing both the special needs and the potential for normality. Have the parents spend increased periods of time in the nursery and encourage parent-child interaction by gradually relinquishing infant care to the family; staff can also serve as a therapeutic intermediary between the separated parents and child. Help the parents take the necessary precautions with the infant while enjoying the interaction. Have literature available for parents to read and begin to help them to connect with community agencies related to their special needs. Offer basic information regarding the child's development and care. Local community parent groups are especially helpful to the new parents of special-needs children. Self-help groups now are available in most communities.

For babies who will be long-term management problems, stress the positive and the helpfulness of outside resources while relating to the anxiety that the parents feel before discharge. Ask questions about their concerns about the hospital bill. Most parents will not bring this up but it is an area of major concern to them, often affecting them for several years after discharge. Know what your hospital's policy is concerning patient finances, particularly enormous NICU bills; be familiar with your state's regulations concerning insurance coverage for the newborn and the availability of SSI (Supplemental Security Income) for the permanently handicapped child. Be able to inform parents of benefits for which their infant may be eligible. Take responsibility for bringing up these issues; parents often will hesitate.

With the parents' permission, include others who will participate in the baby's care after discharge; parents will need much assistance at first, and your inclusion of friends or family who can help will provide much-needed relief to the parents in the weeks and months after discharge. Have siblings visit as often as possible and encourage them to participate in their new brother's/sister's care; they need to get to know him/her before discharge.

If it becomes apparent that the baby will not survive, begin to prepare the family for the events that most likely will occur. Be aware of how the loss will affect each of the family members; be aware of the differences but do not maximize them; mothers mention a real sense of failure, feelings that others will criticize or blame them for the loss, after their child dies. Often they have left a job for the birth of their first child. Their future plans are unsettled; there is a sense of uncertainty. Fathers report feelings of helplessness about the baby's deteriorating condition, an inability to comfort the mother and a sense of disorder in the family that affects everyone. Often the father needs more reassurance that his grief is normal; it is less socially acceptable for men to mourn openly. The Western concept, although it is changing, still does not encourage overt male expression of tender, empathetic feelings and dependency.[2]

Help the family to identify what they fear most; once they can recognize their own special feeling of loss, the grief is more easy to deal with. Continue to talk with the parents together, whenever possible; check out how and what information is exchanged within the family system. Be sensitive to one partner trying to protect the other; often the father will try to protect the baby's mother from the "bad news." In assuming this task, the father often is trying to protect himself from intense feelings that he perceives as too difficult to deal with. Do not allow him to take on this impossible task; help him to see that open communication will provide relief to both; explore this with both parents together.

Be willing to share yourself; it shows that you feel and are not made helpless by these feelings. Be in touch with your own feelings and, when appropriate, share these with the family. Give the family permission to cry and mourn openly; if the parents can prepare themselves slowly, if allowed to grieve and cry, they will be more able to separate themselves when their baby dies. Reassure them that you will be with them in the dying process, but not necessarily at the time of death. Stress the naturalness and normalcy of their emotions.

Rationale. — As soon as discharge is being considered, the parents can begin to actualize their hopes by participating in the baby's care and by gathering information concerning his/her needs after discharge. During this stage, healthy crisis resolution is encouraged by helping parents develop patterns of seeking and using help within the hospital, community and their own family. Specific assignments focusing on discharge will help to strengthen the nurturing relationship between the parents and child; tasks will also relieve some of the parents' anticipatory anxieties by forming new relationships and resources that will bring satisfaction to them after the baby is home. Having parents begin to make plans and prepare for discharge is also diagnostically significant. If the parents are unable or unwilling to begin to prepare for the discharge, this must be explored with them. Their reluctance to ask for or accept help from others may be the result of several factors: inability to accept the child, longstanding personality disorders; family isolation, current rivalry situation, such as between the mother and her mother, blaming, unresolved conflicts about the baby, hostility toward others for the situation or increased stress between the parents leading to dysfunctional communication, bickering, rejecting and being unsupportive of each other. Preventive intervention, perhaps with referral to an outside agency for supportive individual and family counseling, is indicated if the problem appears to be chronic.

If the baby's death seems inevitable, parents will need help with the intensity of their feelings. Pressures around the time of death can be high; the death itself is made less painful by a staff that continues to include the family in the baby's care and status. When hope for survival is gone, help the family sustain their "mini-hopes,"[26] that is, hope for short periods of time, in order to keep going.

Repeat to them that they are experiencing normal reactions to a significant loss; they will need help in dealing with the other children's reactions. Lack of information for both the parents and children increases fears and fantasies. It is helpful for the parents to realize that their children's reactions to death relate to their ages: for the child between the ages of 0 and 5, he/she senses withdrawal and fears a loss of love at the time of a death in the family; he/she responds and reacts to changes in his parents; for the child between the ages of 5 and 10, the fears relate to implications of death and he/she fears for himself/herself; between ages of 10 and 12, the child may experience some "survivor guilt," but it generally is supportive to others in the family.[18]

Stage 3. End of Hospitalization (Death or Discharge)

TASKS ON DISCHARGE. — The parents begin to work through feelings of high anxiety as they assume the role of primary caregiver to their infant; they will continue to integrate the positive and negative aspects of their feelings toward the new infant.

Intervention. — Offer encouragement to the parents concerning their own parenting abilities. Provide them with names and phone numbers of familiar nursery staff personnel who can be available to them after discharge. Schedule a follow-up appointment for the parents and new infant; give them date and time before they leave the hospital. Prepare the family for the anticipated stresses to them when the baby gets home. Support their own feelings of excitement that the baby finally is going home. Support their ability to be parents and give them permission to feel less than adequate at first. Make sure that they have been connected with the appropriate community agencies and, if indicated, mental health clinics for supportive follow-up counseling.

Rationale. — If the parents see the infant as continuing to pose a threat of death or delay, this can seriously hinder the parent-child relationship as well as the child's development. They need encouragement to see the child as normal as is possible. When the handicapped child is discharged, the parents must have a realistic picture of his/her present and future capabilities. Unrealistically high or low expectations will exacerbate an already stressful situation. Parents who have been made aware of the normal adjustment process to a handicapped child are much more likely to ask for help when it is needed. Give them permission not to know all the answers.

TASKS ON DEATH.—The parents will begin to accept the death of their infant; they must begin to grieve for their loss.

Intervention.—Be aware that although the infant's death is a tremendous loss for the family, it often brings relief with it. Tell the parents immediately, and, if the contact is made by phone, tell them of the death at that time. Many parents have reported later that having a few minutes at home alone with their grief helped tremendously. After the family arrives at the hospital, allow them the opportunity to touch, hold, view, dress and/or take pictures of the baby. (Before this, prepare them for the altered skin color, temperature and stiffness of the body.) Some families wish no physical contact; all should be given the opportunity; do not remove the body from the nursery until the family arrives, if at all possible.

Give verbal and nonverbal support; the events surrounding the infant's death usually are remembered with clarity. Do not use platitudes; allow the family to be sad. Take time to help the parents make the difficult decisions concerning the autopsy, disposal of the body and funeral. Help the family understand their options; find out about their fears and concerns about the autopsy. Find out if the family knows what is involved and what it means to them. (One family was surprised to hear that the baby's limbs and head were not cut off during the autopsy; they agreed to one after they realized that they still could have a funeral with an open casket.) The fact that an autopsy might give the family more information about their baby's illness and death is a significant factor in their decision. In our unit, an autopsy conference is scheduled for 6–8 weeks after the death; the family is told about this conference at the time of the death and given an appointment before they leave the hospital. (Even if the family does not give permission for an autopsy, a conference is scheduled.)

Prepare the family for future physical and psychologic responses related to the grief process: feelings of "going crazy," restlessness, loss of appetite, eating too much or too little, headaches, feelings of guilt, occasional aimlessness. Stress that grief has a purpose; do not rush it. It is both energy- and time-consuming; encourage the family to give in to it for a while. Do not encourage either parent to rush into activities "to forget." Give them permission to be angry, to share these feelings with each other. Include other family members, clergy and others who might give support in the grieving process. Parents of infants who die usually have relatively little support from the family or community. Encourage them to call if they feel a need to talk and reassure them that you will call them in 1 week. Prepare the family for the pain of "putting away the nursery" and encourage families to do this together.

For contact with the family after they leave the hospital, the following schedule is suggested: call the family twice before the death/autopsy conference, which, as stated, should take place within 6–8 weeks after the death. During the first few weeks, when the family is in the early stages of grieving, supportive contact is appropriate; the more technical discussion of the autopsy should be delayed until the family is more prepared to process the information. This usually occurs within 2 months after the death. Call the family again at suggested critical points of 6-month and 1-year anniversaries of the death.

Rationale.—The attachment process in the NICU, especially with the critically ill infant, often is tenuous. We have found that an acceptance of the finality of death is related to the staff's openness. That openness can be encouraged by example. Use of the words "death," "died," "autopsy" in a gentle, supportive manner serves to make the fact of the loss real; so, too, does the "death rite" with the body in the nursery. This may be the first time for some parents to have the opportunity to feel that this is really their baby by holding him/her. By avoiding euphemisms and keeping the body in the nursery for the parents, we are helping them to confront their loss with confidence and openness.

Being available with concrete information and suggestions shortly after the death is most important. Most parents are too distraught, no matter how expected the death, to accomplish problem solving alone. Help from others can relieve much of the strain at this point. Parents of dead and dying infants experience extreme isolation and usually are unprepared for the intensity of their reaction. This is related to hospital staff's reticence to discuss an infant's death because of their own frustration and sense of failure. What information is given rarely is heard the first time; it needs repeating. As one bereaved mother related, "The first few hours and days were a blur; I couldn't remember or concentrate on anything; but I felt that the staff cared and that got me through." Specific suggestions combined with a caring attitude are essential.

Survivors need to know what is normal in the grieving process; it is a great relief to know that their confusing combination of emotions is part of the normal healing process of grief. Our experience indicates that the acute symptoms abate within a period of 1–2 months (although acceptance may not be achieved for years) and that the parents deal much better with their loss when they are prepared for their feelings. Our observations indicate several significant reactions after the death of an infant: (1) the "phantom child syndrome," in which the child continues to be a part of the family, its image kept alive by the grieving parents, who have accepted the death but continue to "see" their deceased child grow up; (2) strong resentment toward other pregnant women, new mothers and babies, especially on the part of the mother; this usually lasts just a short while after the death but is a common reaction; (3) extreme reaction to stories of abused and neglected children; (4) "anniversary phenomenon," in which there is a resurgence of sadness on the date the baby was born, died, Mother's Day and during holidays; (5) a second, mini-death when the nursery is "put away"; this, for many parents, is a second funeral—painful, but an important task in the process of closure; (6) hollow feelings of incompleteness, described by one mother as a "feeling that I put something down and will never find it"; (7) intense feelings about getting pregnant again; for a short period after the death, the parents verbalize either "I'll never go through it again" or "We want another baby immediately"; this intensity usually disappears within a few weeks, at which time the parents become more realistic in their plans for the future.

By including others in the grieving process, the staff facilitates the communication process; verbalization aids in working through the grief. If the mother is a single parent, take responsibility to identify "significant others" and include him or her in the counseling. A word of caution: be careful to deal first and primarily with the parents. Often well-meaning relatives may interfere with the couple's communication. Be sensitive to this and focus on the couple.

The death/autopsy conference should include the family, physician, nurse and social worker; the conference offers an additional sense of closure to the family and helps actualize the loss through verbalization and memory recall of the events. At the conference, all technical questions are answered and the autopsy results are reviewed. Invariably, the parents will have additional questions about what they should or should not have done to prevent their child's death. Give reassurance that they were not responsible for what happened; differentiate between real and neurotic guilt and help parents deal with these feelings of guilt. Discuss future children with the parents and, if indicated, make a referral for genetic counseling. Sometimes this is best done at the same time as the autopsy/death conference. Talk about pleasant events, as well as the family's remaining feelings of anger and sadness. Help the parents recall positive, valuable aspects of the experience; provide a setting in which they feel comfortable verbalizing their search for a reason or meaning for their tragedy. Find out if the parents have resumed their normal activities, if they have begun to make future plans. Be sensitive to the symptoms of a pathologic grief response and let parents know that you will contact them again in about 3 months. Most parents report many mixed feelings in returning to the hospital where their baby died. They are happy to see the staff again and relive some of the poignant moments of their baby's life. They are also surprised at how intensely their memories affect them. There is an experience of "regriefing" for many parents in returning to the hospital; they encounter many of the original feelings. Prepare the family for this experience.

CARE OF THE STAFF

NICU work is exciting and satisfying; it is also physically and psychologically draining. There is intense involvement among staff, patients and families, with many demands continually placed on the staff. Because of this, it is crucial that the staff be provided with a structured setting that is mutually supportive. Our experience has been that regular group meetings within the unit can provide this needed support. Membership varies from week to week but usually includes nurses, residents, staff physicians and the unit social worker. The goals are: (1) information sharing, (2) ventilation of feelings and support, (3) release of tension in a protective setting and (4) exploration of feelings.

Topics vary from specific problems concerning an individual or family to general discussions of more global subjects such as ethical dilemmas in the NICU. Most often the staff members struggle with their own feelings, sometimes of frustration and failure, sometimes of joy and sense of accomplishment. There is sharing and confronting and we have found the group to be an invaluable aid in providing better service to our patients and their families.

REFERENCES
1. Ambuel, J., and Harris, B.: Failure to thrive: A study of failure to grow in height or weight, Ohio Med. J. 59:997, 1963.
2. Antel, K.: Psychologic involvement in pregnancy by expectant fathers, JOGN Nursing, July/August, p. 40, 1975.
3. Benfield, D. G., Leib, S., and Reuter, J.: Grief response of parents after referral of the critically ill newborn to a regional center, N. Engl. J. Med. 294:975, 1976.
4. Breslin, R.: Delivery of social work service in newborn special care unit. Presented at the First National Workshop on the Delivery of Hospital Social Work Services in Obstetrics/Gynecology and Services to the Newborn, Yale-New Haven Medical Center, 1974.

5. Caplan, G. Patterns of parental response to the crisis of premature birth, Psychiatry 23:365, 1970.
6. Corney, R. T., and Horton, F. T.: Pathological grief following spontaneous abortion, Am. J. Psychiatry 131:825, 1974.
7. Erikson, E. H.: *Childhood and Society* (New York: W. W. Norton & Company, 1950).
8. Fanaroff, A. A., Kennell, J. H., and Klaus, M. H.: Follow-up of low birth weight infants — the predictive value of maternal visiting patterns, Pediatrics 49:287, 1972.
9. Fischhoff, J., and O'Brien, N.: After a child dies, Pediatrics 88:140, 1976.
10. Golan, N.: Social work intervention in medical crises, Hosp. Community Psychiatry 23:41, 1972.
11. Hardgrove, C., and Warrick, L. H.: How shall we tell the children?, Am. J. Nursing 74:448, 1974.
12. Jackson, P. L.: Chronic grief, Am. J. Nursing 74:1289, 1974.
13. Kaplan, D. M., and Mason, E. A.: Maternal reactions to premature birth viewed as an acute emotional disorder, Am. J. Orthopsychiatry 3:539, 1960.
14. Kennell, J. H., Slyter, H., and Klaus, M. H.: The mourning response of parents to the death of a newborn infant, N. Engl. J. Med. 283:344, 1970.
15. Klaus, M. H., and Kennell, J.: Care of the Mother, in Klaus, M., and Fanaroff, A. (eds.), *Care of the High-risk Neonate* (Philadelphia: W. B. Saunders Company, 1973).
16. Kubler-Ross, E.: *On Death and Dying* (New York: Macmillan Publishing Co., Inc., 1969).
17. Leifer, A. D., Leiderman, P. H., Barnett, C. R., and Williams, J. A.: Effects of mother-infant separation and maternal attachment behavior, Child Dev. 43:1203, 1972.
18. I ewis, M.: *Clinical Aspects of Child Development* (Philadelphia: Lea & Febiger, 1971).
19. Lindemann, E.: Symptomatology and management of acute grief, Am. J. Psychiatry 101:141, 1944.
20 Parad, H. J. (ed.): *Crisis Intervention: Selected Readings* (New York: Family Service Association of America, 1965).
21. Parke, R. D. (ed.): Father-infant interaction, in Maternal Attachment and Mothering Disorders, A Round Table, Johnson & Johnson Baby Products Company, 1975, p. 61.
22. Parks, R. M.: Parental reactions to the birth of a handicapped child, Health Soc. Work 2:52, 1977.
23. Rapoport, L.: Crisis Intervention as a Mode of Brief Treatment, in Roberts, R. W., and Nee, R. H. (eds.), *Theories of Social Casework* (Chicago: University of Chicago Press, 1972).
24. Shaheen, E., Alexander, D., Truskowsky, M., and Barbero, G.: Failure to thrive — a retrospective profile, Clin. Pediatr. 7:255, 1968.
25. Solnit, A. J., and Stark, M. H.: Mourning and the Birth of a Defective Child, in Eissler, R. S., *et al.* (eds.), *Psychoanalytic Study of the Child* (New York: International University Press, 1961), Vol. 16.
26. Worden, J. W.: Excerpts from a paper delivered at the Mississippi Conference on Social Welfare, April, 1976.

Index